Fitness
and
Wellness

SEVENTH
EDITION

www.wadsworth.com

wadsworth.com is the
World Wide Web site for Wadsworth and is
your direct source to dozens of online
resources.

At *wadsworth.com* you can find out about supplements, demonstration software, and student resources.
You can also send e-mail to many of our
authors and preview new
publications and exciting new
technologies.

wadsworth.com
Changing the way the world learns®

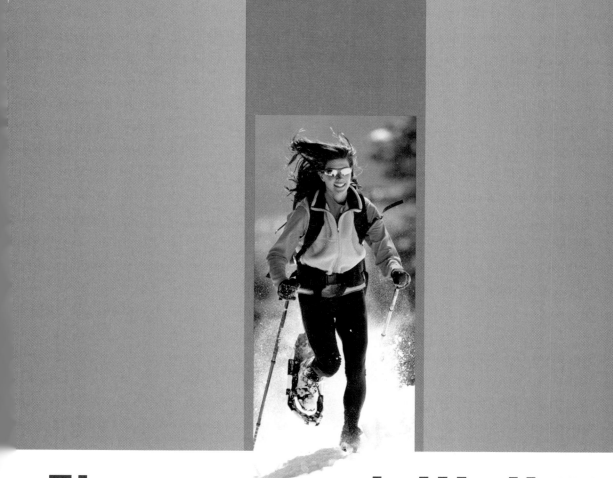

Fitness and Wellness

SEVENTH EDITION

WERNER W. K. HOEGER
Boise State University

SHARON A. HOEGER
Fitness and Wellness, Inc.

THOMSON
™
WADSWORTH

Australia • Brazil • Canada • Mexico • Singapore
Spain • United Kingdom • United States

THOMSON

WADSWORTH

Fitness and Wellness, Seventh Edition
Werner W. K. Hoeger, Sharon A. Hoeger

EXECUTIVE EDITOR: Nedah Rose
ASSISTANT EDITOR: Colin Blake
TECHNOLOGY PROJECT MANAGER: Donna Kelley
MARKETING MANAGER: Jennifer Somerville
MARKETING ASSISTANT: Michele Colella
MARKETING COMMUNICATIONS MANAGER: Jessica Perry
PROJECT MANAGER,
EDITORIAL PRODUCTION: Sandra Craig
CREATIVE DIRECTOR: Rob Hugel

ART DIRECTOR: Lee Friedman
PRINT BUYER: Karen Hunt
PERMISSIONS EDITOR: Joohee Lee
PRODUCTION, COMPOSITION, ILLUSTRATION: Ash Street Typecrafters, Inc.
TEXT AND COVER DESIGNER: Norman Baugher
COPY EDITOR: Carol Lombardi
COVER IMAGE: © Alan Becker/Getty Images
PRINTER: Quebecor World / Taunton

Library of Congress Control Number: 2005938696

ISBN 0-495-01256-4

**Thomson Higher Education
10 Davis Drive
Belmont, CA 94002-3098
USA**

For more information about our products, contact us at:
**Thomson Learning Academic Resource Center
1-800-423-0563**
For permission to use material from this text or product,
submit a request online at
http://www.thomsonrights.com.
Any additional questions about permissions can be
submitted by e-mail to thomsonrights@thomson.com.

CONTENTS

© Steve Lupton/CORBIS

CHAPTER 6
Weight Management   127

© Gulliver/zefa/CORBIS

CHAPTER 7
Stress Management   151

© Ariel Skelley/CORBIS

This book could help you live a longer, healthier life. It offers information that can start you on the path to fitness and wellness by helping you create and follow a healthy lifestyle.

The good news is that life-long health, fitness, and wellness are within the grasp of most people. Debilitating conditions can largely be prevented by living a healthy lifestyle.

The bad news is that too many people are unhealthy primarily because their lifestyles do not include sufficient physical activity or proper nutrition. The current epidemic of physical inactivity and obesity is so harmful to health that it increases the deterioration rate of the human body and leads to premature aging, illness, and death.

Because fitness and wellness needs vary significantly from one individual to another, all exercise and wellness prescriptions must be personalized to obtain best results. The information in the following chapters and the subsequent activities at the end of each chapter will enable all readers to develop a personal lifetime program that promotes fitness, preventive health care, and personal wellness. The activities have been prepared on tear-out sheets so they can be turned in to class instructors.

What the Book Covers

As you study this book and complete the end-of-chapter Activities, you will learn to

- Determine whether medical clearance is needed for your safe participation in exercise.
- Conduct nutrient analyses and follow the recommendations for adequate nutrition.
- Develop sound diet and weight-control programs.
- Assess the health-related components of your own fitness (cardiorespiratory endurance, muscular strength and endurance, muscular flexibility, and body composition).
- Write personalized exercise prescriptions for cardiorespiratory endurance, muscular strength and endurance, and muscular flexibility.

- Understand stress, lessen your vulnerability to stress, and implement a stress management program if necessary.
- Implement a cardiovascular disease risk-reduction program.
- Follow guidelines to reduce your personal risk of developing cancer.
- Implement a smoking cessation program, if applicable.
- Understand the health consequences of chemical dependency and irresponsible sexual behaviors and learn guidelines for preventing sexually transmitted infections.
- Distinguish between myths and facts of exercise and health-related concepts.
- Learn behavior modification techniques to help you adhere to a lifetime fitness and wellness program.

New and Enhanced Features of the Seventh Edition

The seventh edition of *Fitness & Wellness* has been updated to include a wealth of new information reported in the literature and at professional health, physical education, and sports medicine meetings. The following are the most significant updates in this seventh edition:

- Chapter 1 now includes information on the prevalence of physical activity in the United States, a discussion on the benefits of physical activity based on diverse public health recommendations (30, 60, or 60 to 90 minutes per day), and the concept of physiologic fitness. A new section on SMART goals will help students write goals and specific objectives to reach these goals.
- Chapter 2 has been revised to conform with the newly released *ACSM's Guidelines for Exercise Testing and Prescription* (2006). The concepts of responders, nonresponders, and the principle of individuality were also added to the chapter. The role of body mass index (BMI) as the most widely

used technique to determine overweight and obesity in the general population is discussed in greater detail. New emphasis is placed on the waist circumference measurement (WC) in combination with BMI to help identify individuals with increased risk for disease. Chapter Activities were also revised to conform with updated standards for BMI and WC, including the assessment of recommended body weight based on BMI.

- Chapter 3 includes an introduction to pedometer use to help students monitor daily physical activity. A new Activity to monitor daily physical activity, the concepts of responders and nonresponders, and the principle of individuality were also added. The guidelines for cardiorespiratory endurance, muscular fitness, and muscular flexibility prescription were reviewed to conform with the new 2006 American College of Sports Medicine guidelines for exercise testing and prescription. The relationship between flexibility and injury prevention, the best time to conduct stretching exercises, and revised recommendations for the prevention and treatment of back pain are also included.

- Chapter 4 presents a new figure summarizing the most popular physical activities in the United States. Updated information and evaluations of aerobic activity choices have been added so readers can make more informed choices about their fitness programs.

- Chapter 5 has been extensively revised to incorporate the new MyPyramid guidelines and the 2005 Dietary Guidelines for Americans from the U. S. Department of Agriculture. The topics of nutrient supplementation, antioxidants, and eating disorders have also been updated.

- Chapter 6 includes an update on the health consequences of being overweight or obese along with new information on low-carbohydrate/high protein diets; the binge-eating disorder; the benefits of dietary calcium on weight management; the relationship between strength training, diet, and muscle mass; and estimated energy requirement equations (EER) to determine daily caloric intake from the DRI committee of the Institute of Medicine of the National Academy of Sciences.

- Chapter 7 now includes the characteristics of good stress managers. The benefits of meditation and yoga on health and wellness were also updated.

- Chapter 8 provides statistical updates on the incidence and prevalence of cardiovascular disease and cancer. New information and updates on cardiovascular risk reduction, inflammation, homocysteine, LDL-cholesterol, dietary guidelines to decrease blood lipids, blood pressure guidelines, sodium and potassium recommendations to manage and prevent high blood pressure, and exercise recommendations for hypertensive individuals are included in this chapter. Cancer prevention guidelines are also updated here.

- Chapter 9's Q&A now contains several new questions about current fitness and wellness recommendations—in particular, the guidelines for exercise and pregnancy and the selection of personal trainers have been revised.

Ancillaries

The following ancillaries are available to qualified adopters of *Fitness & Wellness*, seventh edition. Please consult your local sales representative for details.

- **Instructor's Manual with Test Bank.** The Instructor's Manual includes detailed outlines of each chapter with specific transparency and PowerPoint references, classroom activities, learning objectives, lab descriptions, discussion questions, references, and a transparency acetate list. Each chapter contains a list and description of relevant Web sites for resources to aid instructors and offer health activities on the Web. The full test bank contains approximately 30 multiple choice, true-false, matching, fill-in-the-blank and essay questions per chapter.

- **ExamView Computerized Testing.** Create, deliver, and customize tests and study guides (both print and online) in minutes with this easy-to-use assessment and tutorial system. ExamView offers both a Quick Test Wizard and an Online Test Wizard that guide you step-by-step through the process of creating tests, while the unique "WYSIWYG" capability allows you to see the test you are creating on the screen exactly as it will print or display online. You can build tests of up to 250 questions using up to 12 question types. Using ExamView's complete word processing capabilities, you can enter an unlimited number of new questions or edit existing questions.

- **Transparency Acetates.** Approximately 80 full-color transparencies correlated to the text to enhance your lectures. The transparencies include figures, tables, and illustrations from the text, as well as a number of enrichments from other sources.

- **Multimedia Manager for Fitness and Wellness.** This link tool includes a wide array of lecture specific PowerPoint slides, images from the Hoeger texts, digitized ABC video clips, an electronic instructor's manual and an electronic test bank.

- **Web Tutor Toolbox for Web CT and Blackboard.** With WebTutor's text-specific, pre-formatted content and total flexibility, you can easily create and manage your own personal Web site! WebTutor's course management tool gives you the ability to provide virtual office hours, post syllabi, set up threaded discussions, track student progress with the quizzing material, and much more. For students, WebTutor offers real-time access to a full array of study tools, including chapter outlines, summaries, learning objectives, practice quizzes, and Web links. WebTutor also provides robust communication tools, such as a course calendar, asynchronous discussion, real time chat, a whiteboard, and an integrated e-mail system.

- **Profile Plus 2007 for** *Lifetime Physical Fitness & Wellness*, **9th Edition and** *Fitness & Wellness*, **7th Edition.** The most comprehensive software package available! Profile Plus allows students to generate personalized fitness and wellness profiles, conduct self-assessments, analyze their diets, tailor exercise prescriptions to their individual needs, keep an exercise log, and much more!

- **Diet Analysis+ 8.0 Online and Win/Mac CD-ROM.** This market-leading diet assessment program allows students to create their own personal profiles based on height, weight, age, sex, and activity level. Its dynamic interface makes it easy for students to track the types and serving sizes of the foods they consume, from one day to 365 days! Now including even more exciting features, the updated 8.0 version includes an 18,000+ food database, a 500+ activity database, ten reports for analysis (including MyPyramid), the ability to print single- and multiple-day reports, a food recipe feature, the latest Dietary References, and goals and actual percentages of essential nutrients, vitamins, and minerals. Students can use this information to adjust their diet and gain a better understanding of how nutrition relates to their personal health goals.

- **Personal Daily Log.** This log contains an exercise pyramid, tips for achieving test success, a body composition record form, body mass index chart, cardiorespiratory exercise record form, strength training record form, and much more.

- **Wellness Worksheets.** Forty detachable self-assessments and a complete wellness inventory are included.

- **Integrative Medicine: The Mind-Body Prescription.** This supplementary text explains the relationship between Western medical practice and more traditional therapies. The topics include the evolution of integrative medicine, a detailed list of Internet sources, a comprehensive list of herbs and their interactions, and more.

- **Careers in Health, Physical Education and Sport.** This comprehensive guide to finding and establishing a career in the field of Health, Physical Education, and Sport encourages students to establish personal goals, develop action plans, and research fields of study ranging from entry-level to post-graduate positions.

- **Trigger Video Series.** Designed to promote or "trigger" classroom discussion on a variety of important topics. This 60-minute video focuses on changing concepts of fitness. Contains five 8–10 minute clips, followed by questions for answer or discussion, and material appropriate to the chapters concerning fitness in our books.

- **Relaxation Video.** Exclusive to Thomson Wadsworth, this outstanding video covers the causes, symptoms, and effects of stress and helps students develop life-long strategies for stress management. The video demonstrates such relaxation techniques as progressive muscle relaxation and guided meditation. It also shows students how to use exercise and visualization as preventative measures against stress. This video includes visualizations that help students start and adhere to an exercise program, as well as visualizations that can enhance sports performance.

- **ABC Videos for Health and Wellness.** These videos allow you to integrate the news-gathering and programming power of the ABC News networks into the classroom to show students the relevance of course topics to their everyday lives. The videos include news clips correlated directly with the text and can help you launch a lecture, spark a discussion, or demonstrate an application. Students can see firsthand how the principles they learn in the course apply to the stories they hear in the news.

- **Wadsworth Video Library for Health, Fitness and Wellness.** A comprehensive library of videos is available to adopters of this textbook. Topics include weight control, fitness, AIDS, sexual communication, peer pressure, compulsive and addictive behaviors and the relationship between alcohol and violence. Contact your local sales representative for a detailed list of video options.

- **Health, Fitness and Wellness Internet Explorer 3.0.** A handy full-color trifold brochure containing dozens of useful health and wellness Internet links.

- **The Wadsworth Health, Fitness and Wellness Resource Center Web Site.** http://www.thomsonedu.com/health

When you adopt this text, you and your students will have access to a rich array of teaching and learning resources you won't find anywhere else. This outstanding site features both student and instructor resources for this text, including self-quizzes, Web links, and suggested online readings for students—as well as downloadable supplementary resources, PowerPoint® presentations, and more for instructors.

Acknowledgments

We would like to thank the following reviewers for their valuable comments and contributions to the Seventh Edition:

Cheryl J. Cohen, Western Illinois University

Peggy J. Foss, University of Michigan - Dearborn

Janet S. Hamilton, Clayton College and State University

Carlyn L. Martin, St. Cloud State University

Patricia A. Ochoa, Chattanooga State Technical Community College

Ben Reuter, Florida Southern College

Judy Stewart, Motlow State Community College

William Kelley, Green Mountain College

Shawnee Bonnett, Del Mar College

Robert Dvorak, Houston Baptist University

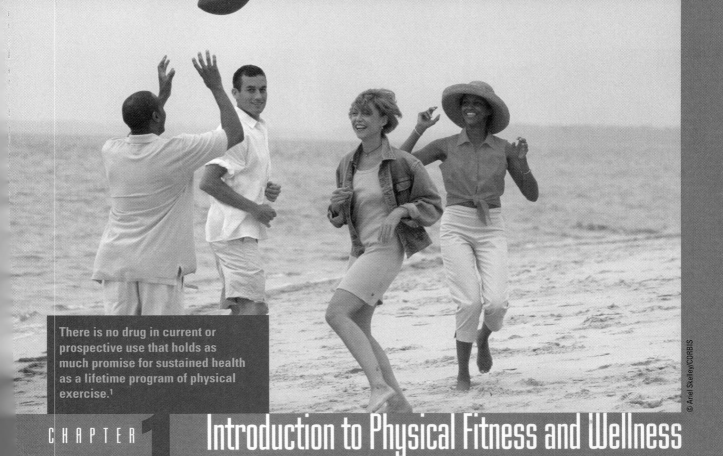

There is no drug in current or prospective use that holds as much promise for sustained health as a lifetime program of physical exercise.[1]

CHAPTER 1 Introduction to Physical Fitness and Wellness

OBJECTIVES

- Understand the importance of sound physical fitness and wellness.
- Define physical fitness and list components of health-related and skill-related fitness.
- Learn the benefits of a comprehensive fitness and wellness program.
- Learn motivational and behavior modification techniques to enhance compliance with a healthy lifestyle program.
- Determine whether medical clearance is required for safe participation in exercise.

Prepare for a healthy change in lifestyle by completing the Behavior Change Plan on your CD-ROM.

Most people believe school will teach them how to make a better living. A fitness and wellness course will teach you how to live better—how to truly live your life to its fullest potential. Real success is about more than money: Making a good living will not help you unless you live a wellness lifestyle that will allow you to enjoy what you have. Your lifestyle is the most important factor affecting your personal well-being, but most people don't know how to make the right choices to live their best life.

During the last three decades, the benefits of physical activity have been substantiated by scientific evidence linking increased physical activity and positive lifestyle habits to better health and improved quality of life. Even though some people live long because of favorable genetic factors, the quality of life during middle age and the "golden years" is more often related to wise choices initiated during youth and continued throughout life.

Based on the abundance of scientific research on physical activity and exercise, a clear distinction has been established between physical activity and exercise. **Physical activity** is defined as bodily movement produced by skeletal muscles that requires the expenditure of energy and produces progressive health benefits. Examples of physical activity are walking to and from work and the store, taking the stairs instead of elevators and escalators, gardening, doing household chores, dancing, and washing the car by hand. Physical inactivity, by contrast, implies a level of activity that is lower than that required to maintain good health.

Photos © Fitness & Wellness, Inc.

Physical activity and exercise lead to less disease, a longer life, and enhanced quality of life.

Exercise is considered a type of physical activity that requires planned, structured, and repetitive bodily movement to improve or maintain one or more components of physical fitness. A regular weekly program of walking, jogging, cycling, aerobics, swimming, strength training, and stretching exercises are all examples of exercise.

Unfortunately, the current way of life in North America does not provide the human body with sufficient physical exercise to maintain adequate health. Furthermore, many lifestyle patterns are such a serious threat to health that they actually speed up deterioration of the human body. In a few short years, lack of wellness leads to loss of vitality and gusto for life, as well as premature morbidity and mortality.

The typical North American is not a good role model in terms of physical fitness. According to the Centers for Disease Control and Prevention, the majority of U.S. adults are not sufficiently physically active to promote good health. The data indicate that only 46 percent of adults meet the minimal recommendation of 30 minutes of moderate physical activity at least 5 days per week, 25 percent report no leisure physical activity at all, and 16 percent are completely inactive (that is, spending less than 10 minutes per week in moderate- or vigorous-intensity physical activity). The prevalence of physical activity by state in the United States is displayed in Figure 1.1.

Even though most people in the United States believe a positive lifestyle has a great impact on health and longevity, most do not know how to implement a fitness and wellness program that will yield the desired results. Patty Neavill is an example of someone who frequently tried to change her life but was unable to do so because she did not know how to implement a sound exercise and weight control program. At age 24, Patty, a college sophomore, was discouraged with her weight, level of fitness, self-image, and quality of life in general.

She had struggled with weight most of her life. Like thousands of other people, she had made many unsuccessful attempts to lose weight. Patty put aside her fears and decided to enroll in a fitness course. As part of the course requirement, she took a battery of fitness tests at the beginning of the semester. Patty's cardiorespiratory fitness and strength ratings were poor, her flexibility classification was average, she weighed more than 200 pounds, and she was 41 percent body fat.

Following the initial fitness assessment, Patty met with her course instructor, who prescribed an exercise and nutrition program such as the one presented in this book. Patty fully committed to carry out the prescription. She walked or jogged five times a week, worked out with weights twice a week, and played volleyball or basketball two to four times each week. Her daily caloric intake was set in the range of 1,500 to 1,700 calories. She took care to meet the minimum required amounts from the basic food groups each day, which contributed about 1,200 calories to her diet. The remainder of the calories came primarily from complex carbohydrates. At the end of the 16-week semester, Patty's cardiorespiratory fitness, strength, and flexibility ratings had all improved to the "good" category, she had lost 50 pounds, and her percent body fat had dropped to 22.5!

A thank-you note from Patty to the course instructor at the end of the semester read:

Thank you for making me a new person. I truly appreciate the time you spent with me. Without

F I G U R E **1.1** U. S. Prevalence of Recommended Physical Activity, 2003.*

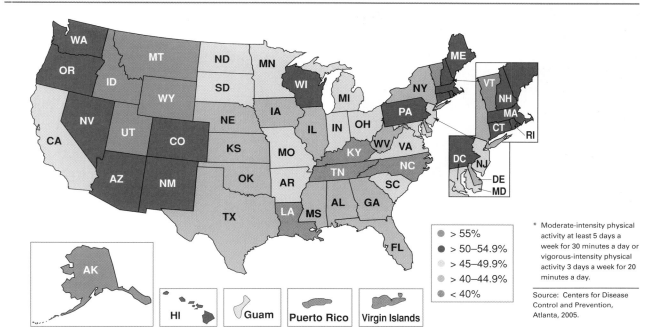

* Moderate-intensity physical activity at least 5 days a week for 30 minutes a day or vigorous-intensity physical activity 3 days a week for 20 minutes a day.

- \> 55%
- \> 50–54.9%
- \> 45–49.9%
- \> 40–44.9%
- < 40%

Source: Centers for Disease Control and Prevention, Atlanta, 2005.

your kindness and motivation, I would have never made it. It's great to be fit and trim. I've never had this feeling before and I wish everyone could feel like this once in their life.

Thank you, Your trim Patty!

Patty never had been taught the principles governing a sound weight loss program. She needed this knowledge and, like most Americans who never have experienced the process of becoming physically fit, she needed to be in a structured exercise setting to truly feel the joy of fitness.

Of even greater significance, Patty maintained her aerobic and strength-training programs. A year after ending her calorie-restricted diet, her weight actually increased by 10 pounds—but her body fat decreased from 22.5 percent to 21.2 percent. As discussed in Chapter 6, the weight increase is related mostly to changes in lean tissue lost during the weight-reduction phase. Despite only a slight drop in weight during the second year following the calorie-restricted diet, Patty's 2-year follow-up revealed a further decrease in body fat, to 19.5 percent. Patty understands the new quality of life reaped through a sound fitness program.

Lifestyle, Health, and Quality of Life

Research findings have shown that physical inactivity and negative lifestyle habits pose a serious threat to health. Movement and physical activity are basic functions for which the human organism was created. Advances in modern technology, however, have all but eliminated the need for physical activity in daily life. Physical activity no longer is a natural part of our existence. This epidemic of physical inactivity is the second greatest threat to U. S. public health and has been termed **Sedentary Death Syndrome**, or **SeDS**. (The number-one threat is tobacco use—the largest cause of preventable deaths.)

Today we live in an automated society. Most of the activities that used to require strenuous physical exertion can be accomplished by machines with the simple pull of a handle or push of a button. If people go to a store that is only a couple of blocks away, most drive their automobiles and then spend a couple of minutes driving around the parking lot to find a spot 10 yards

K E Y   T E R M S

Physical activity Bodily movement produced by skeletal muscles that requires energy expenditure and produces progressive health benefits.

Exercise A type of physical activity that requires planned, structured, and repetitive bodily movement done to improve or maintain one or more components of physical fitness.

Sedentary Death Syndrome (SeDS) Deaths that are attributed to a lack of regular physical activity.

The epitome of physical inactivity is to drive around a parking lot for several minutes in search of a parking spot 10 to 20 yards closer to the store's entrance.

FIGURE **1.2** Leading causes of death in the United States: 2003.

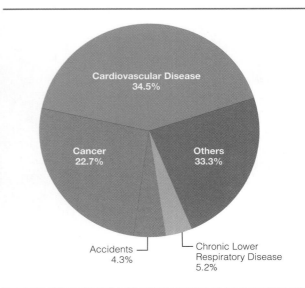

Source: U.S. Department of Health and Human Services, Centers for Disease Control and Prevention, *National Vital Statistics Report; Deaths: Preliminary Data for 2003*, 53:15 (February 28, 2005).

closer to the store's entrance. The groceries do not even have to be carried out any more. A store employee willingly takes them out in a cart and places them in the vehicle. During a visit to a multi-level shopping mall, nearly everyone chooses to ride the escalators instead of taking the stairs.

Automobiles, elevators, escalators, telephones, intercoms, remote controls, electric garage door openers —all are modern-day commodities that minimize the amount of movement and effort required of the human body.

One of the most significant detrimental effects of modern-day technology has been an increase in **chronic diseases** related to a lack of physical activity. These include hypertension (high blood pressure), heart disease, chronic low-back pain, and obesity, among others. They sometimes are referred to as **hypokinetic diseases**. ("Hypo" means low or little, and "kinetic" implies motion.) Lack of adequate physical activity is a fact of modern life that most people can avoid no longer. If we want to enjoy contemporary commodities and still expect to live life to its fullest, a personalized lifetime exercise program must become a part of our daily lives.

With the developments in technology, three additional factors have changed our lives significantly and have had a negative effect on human health: nutrition, stress, and environment. Fatty foods, sweets, alcohol, tobacco, excessive stress, and environmental hazards (such as wastes, noise, and air pollution) have detrimental effects on peoples' health.

The leading causes of death in the United States today (see Figure 1.2) are lifestyle-related. More than 57 percent of all deaths in the United States are caused by cardiovascular disease and cancer.[2] Almost 80 percent of these deaths could be prevented by adhering to a healthy lifestyle. The third leading cause of death— chronic lower respiratory (lung) disease—is related largely to tobacco use. Accidents are the fourth leading cause of death. Even though not all accidents are preventable, many are. Fatal accidents often are related to abusing drugs and not wearing seat belts.

According to Dr. David Satcher, former U. S. Surgeon General, more than 50 percent of the people who die in the United States each year die because of what they do. Estimates indicate that more than half of disease is lifestyle-related, a fifth is attributed to environmental factors, and a tenth is influenced by the health care the individual receives. Only 16 percent is related to genetic factors. Thus, the individual controls as much as 84 percent of disease and quality of life. The data also indicate that 83 percent of deaths that occur before age 65 are preventable. In essence, most people in the United States are threatened by the very lives they lead today.[3]

Presently, the average **life expectancy** in the United States is 77.6 years (about 75 for men and 80 for women). Unlike previous life expectancy calculations, the World Health Organization (WHO) has calculated **healthy life expectancy (HLE)** estimates for 191 nations. The United States ranks 24th in this report with an HLE of 70 years. Japan is first with an HLE of 74.5 years (see Figure 1.3).

FIGURE **1.3** Year 2000 life expectancy (right values) and healthy life expectancy (left values) for selected countries.

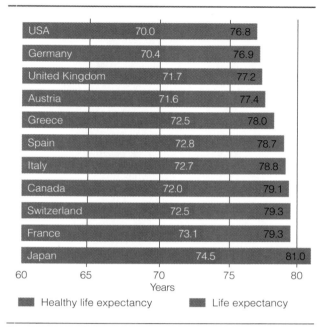

Country	Healthy life expectancy	Life expectancy
USA	70.0	76.8
Germany	70.4	76.9
United Kingdom	71.7	77.2
Austria	71.6	77.4
Greece	72.5	78.0
Spain	72.8	78.7
Italy	72.7	78.8
Canada	72.0	79.1
Switzerland	72.5	79.3
France	73.1	79.3
Japan	74.5	81.0

Years

■ Healthy life expectancy   ■ Life expectancy

Source: World Health Organization, http://www.who.int/inf-pr-2000/en/pr2000-life.html. Retrieved June 4, 2000.

The ranking for the United States is a major surprise for a developed country with one of the best medical care systems in the world. The rating indicates that Americans die earlier and spend more time disabled than people in most other advanced countries. The WHO points to several factors that may account for this unexpected finding:

1. The extremely poor health of some groups, such as Native Americans, rural African Americans, and the inner-city poor. Their health status is more characteristic of poor, developing nations than a rich industrialized country.
2. The HIV epidemic, which causes more deaths and disability than in other developed nations.
3. The high use of tobacco products.
4. A high incidence of coronary heart disease.
5. Fairly high levels of violence, notably homicides, compared with other developed countries.

Surgeon General's Report on Physical Activity and Health

A landmark report on the influence of regular physical activity on health was released in July of 1996 by the U.S. Surgeon General.[4] The significance of this historic document cannot be underestimated. Until 1996 the Surgeon General had released only two prior reports: one on smoking and health in 1964 and one on nutrition and health in 1988. The 1996 document on physical activity and health is a summary of more than 1,000 scientific studies from the fields of epidemiology, exercise physiology, medicine, and the behavioral sciences.

The report states that regular, moderate physical activity provides substantial benefits in health and well-being for the vast majority of Americans who are not physically active. Among these benefits are a significant reduction in the risk of developing or dying from heart disease, diabetes, colon cancer, and high blood pressure.

Regular physical activity also is important for healthy muscles, bones, and joints; and it seems to reduce symptoms of depression and anxiety, improve mood, and enhance the ability to perform daily tasks throughout life. If individuals already are moderately active, greater health benefits can be achieved by increasing the amount of physical activity.

According to the Surgeon General, improving health through physical activity is a serious public health problem that we must meet head-on. Almost half of all adults do not achieve the daily recommended amount of physical activity, and about 50 percent of young individuals between the ages of 13 and 21 are not vigorously active on a regular basis. The report also stated that physical inactivity is more prevalent in women than men, African Americans and Hispanics than Caucasians, older than younger adults, lower income than more affluent people, and less educated than more educated adults.

This report became a call to nationwide action. Regular, moderate physical activity can prevent premature death, unnecessary illness, and disability. It also can help to control health-care costs and maintain a high quality of life into old age. In the report, moderate physical activity was defined as physical activity that uses 150 calories of energy per day, or 1,000 calories per week. For health benefits, people should strive to achieve

KEY TERMS

Chronic diseases Illnesses that develop and last over a long time.

Hypokinetic diseases Diseases related to a lack of physical activity.

Life expectancy Number of years a person is expected to live based on the person's birth year.

Healthy life expectancy (HLE) Number of years a person is expected to live in good health; this number is obtained by subtracting ill-health years from overall life expectancy.

at least 30 minutes of physical activity per day most days of the week.

Examples of moderate physical activity are walking, cycling, playing basketball or volleyball, swimming, water aerobics, dancing fast, pushing a stroller, raking leaves, shoveling snow, washing or waxing a car, washing windows or floors, and even gardening.

Because of the growing epidemic of obesity in the United States, a 2002 guideline by American and Canadian scientists from the Institute of Medicine of the National Academy of Sciences increased the recommendation to 60 minutes of moderate-intensity physical activity every day.[5] This recommendation was based on evidence indicating that people who maintain healthy weight typically accumulate 1 hour of physical activity each day.

Subsequently, the 2005 Dietary Guidelines for Americans released by the USDA recommended that up to 60 minutes of moderate- to vigorous-intensity physical activity per day may be necessary to prevent weight gain, and between 60 and 90 minutes of daily moderate-intensity physical activity is recommended to sustain weight loss for previously overweight people.[6] Although health benefits are derived with 30 minutes per day, people with a tendency to gain weight need to be physically active daily for an hour to an hour and a half to prevent weight gain. Further, 60 to 90 minutes of activity per day provides additional health benefits, including a lower risk of cardiovascular disease and diabetes.

Critical Thinking

Do you consciously incorporate physical activity into your daily lifestyle? Can you provide examples? Do you think you get sufficient daily physical activity to maintain good health?

Wellness

After the initial fitness boom swept across the United States in the 1970s, it became clear that improving physical fitness alone was not always enough to lower the risk for disease and ensure better health. For example, individuals who run 3 miles a day, lift weights regularly, participate in stretching exercises, and watch their body weight can be classified as having good or excellent fitness. If these same people, however, have high blood pressure, smoke, are under constant stress, consume too much alcohol, and eat too many fatty foods, they are exposing themselves to **risk factors** for disease of which they may not be aware.

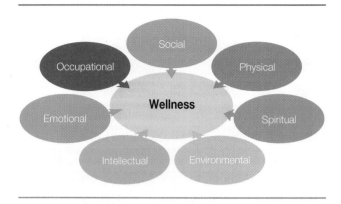

FIGURE **1.4** Dimensions of wellness.

Good health no longer is viewed as simply the absence of disease. The notion of good health has evolved notably in the last few years and continues to change as scientists learn more about lifestyle factors that bring on illness and affect wellness. Once the idea took hold that fitness by itself would not necessarily decrease the risk for disease and ensure better health, the wellness concept developed in the 1980s.

Wellness is an all-inclusive umbrella covering a variety of health-related factors. A wellness lifestyle requires the implementation of positive programs to change behavior and thereby improve health and quality of life, prolong life, and achieve total well-being. To enjoy a wellness lifestyle, a person has to practice behaviors that will lead to positive outcomes in seven dimensions of wellness: physical, emotional, intellectual, social, environmental, spiritual, and occupational (Figure 1.4). These dimensions are interrelated; one frequently affects the others. For example, a person who is "emotionally down" often has no desire to exercise, study, go to work, socialize with friends, or attend church.

The concept behind the seven dimensions of wellness shows that high-level wellness clearly goes beyond optimum fitness and the absence of disease. Wellness incorporates fitness, proper nutrition, stress management, disease prevention, social support, self-worth, nurturance (a sense of being needed), spirituality, personal safety, substance control and not smoking, regular physical examinations, health education, and environmental support.

For a wellness way of life, individuals must be physically fit and manifest no signs of disease, and they also must avoid all risk factors for disease (such as physical inactivity, hypertension, abnormal cholesterol levels, cigarette smoking, excessive stress, faulty nutrition, or careless sex). Even though an individual tested in a fitness center might demonstrate adequate or even excellent fitness, indulgence in unhealthy lifestyle behaviors will increase the risk for chronic diseases and decrease the person's well-being. Additional information on wellness and how to implement a wellness program is given in Chapter 8.

Unhealthy behaviors contribute to the staggering U. S. health-care costs. Risk factors for disease carry a heavy price tag. About 13 percent of the gross national product (GNP), or $1.7 trillion, was spent in health-care costs in 2003. Expenditures are projected to reach about 16 percent of the GNP by the year 2010. According to estimates, 1 percent of Americans account for 30 percent of these costs. Half of the people use up about 97 percent of the health-care dollars.

In terms of yearly health care costs per person, the United States spends more per person than any other industrialized nation. In 2003, U. S. health care costs per capita were about $5,800 and are expected to reach almost $9,000 in 2010. Yet, overall, the health-care system ranks only 37th in the world. One of the reasons for the low overall ranking is the overemphasis on state-of-the art cures instead of prevention programs. The United States is the best place in the world to treat people once they are sick, but the system does a poor job of keeping people healthy in the first place. The United States also fails to provide good health care for all; 44 million residents do not have health insurance.

Physical Fitness

Individuals are physically fit when they can meet both the ordinary and the unusual demands of daily life safely and effectively without being overly fatigued and still have energy left for leisure and recreational activities. **Physical fitness** can be classified into health-related, skill-related, and physiologic fitness.

Health-Related Fitness

Health-related fitness has four components: cardiorespiratory endurance, muscular strength and endurance, muscular flexibility, and body composition (see Figure 1.5):

1. *Cardiorespiratory endurance*: the ability of the heart, lungs, and blood vessels to supply oxygen to the cells to meet the demands of prolonged physical activity (also referred to as aerobic exercise).
2. *Muscular strength and endurance*: the ability of the muscles to generate force.
3. *Muscular flexibility*: the achievable range of motion at a joint or group of joints without causing injury.

FIGURE **1.5** Health-related components of physical fitness.

4. *Body composition:* the amount of lean body mass and adipose tissue (fat mass) in the human body.

Skill-Related Fitness

Fitness in motor skills is essential in activities such as basketball, racquetball, golf, hiking, soccer, and water skiing. Good skill-related fitness also enhances overall quality of life by helping people cope more effectively in emergency situations (see Chapter 4). The components of **skill-related fitness** are agility, balance, coordination, power, reaction time, and speed (see Figure 1.6):

1. *Agility*: the ability to change body position and direction quickly and efficiently. Agility is important in sports such as basketball, soccer, and racquetball, in which the participant must change direction rapidly and at the same time maintain proper body control.
2. *Balance:* the ability to maintain the body in equilibrium. Balance is vital in activities such as gymnastics, diving, ice skating, skiing, and even football and wrestling, in which the athlete attempts to upset the opponent's equilibrium.

KEY TERMS

Risk factors Characteristics that predict the chances for developing a certain disease.

Wellness The constant and deliberate effort to stay healthy and achieve the highest potential for well-being.

Physical fitness The general capacity to adapt and respond favorably to physical effort.

Health-related fitness A physical state encompassing cardiorespiratory endurance, muscular strength and endurance, muscular flexibility, and body composition.

Skill-related fitness Components of fitness important for successful motor performance in athletic events and in lifetime sports and activities.

FIGURE **1.6** Motor skill-related components of physical fitness.

Good skill-related fitness enhances success in sports performance.

© Fitness & Wellness, Inc.

3. *Coordination*: integration of the nervous system and the muscular system to produce correct, graceful, and harmonious body movements. This component is important in a wide variety of motor activities such as golf, baseball, karate, soccer, and racquetball, in which hand–eye or foot–eye movements, or both, must be integrated.

4. *Power*: the ability to produce maximum force in the shortest time. The two components of power are muscle speed and force (strength). An effective combination of these two components allows a person to produce explosive movements such as required in jumping; putting the shot; and spiking, throwing, and hitting a ball.

5. *Reaction time*: the time required to initiate a response to a given stimulus. Good reaction time is important for starts in track and swimming; for quick reactions when playing tennis at the net; and in sports such as ping-pong, boxing, and karate.

6. *Speed*: the ability to propel the body or a part of the body rapidly from one point to another. Examples of activities that require good speed for success are soccer, basketball, stealing a base in baseball, and sprints in track.

Physiologic Fitness

Physiologic fitness is a new term used primarily in the field of medicine in reference to biological systems that are affected by physical activity and the role the latter plays in the prevention of illness, including cardiovascular disease, diabetes, obesity, and osteoporosis.

In terms of preventive medicine, the main emphasis of fitness programs should be on the health-related components. As these components improve, so does physiologic fitness. Skill-related fitness is crucial for success in sports and athletics, and it also contributes to wellness. Improving skill-related fitness affords an individual more enjoyment and success in lifetime sports, and regular participation in skill-related fitness activities also helps develop health-related fitness. Further, total fitness is achieved by taking part in specific programs to improve health-related and skill-related components alike.

Benefits of Fitness and Wellness

The benefits to be enjoyed from participating in a regular fitness and wellness program are many. In addition to a longer life (see Figures 1.7, 1.8, and 1.9 on pages 9–10), the greatest benefit of all is that physically fit people who lead a positive lifestyle have a healthier and better quality of life. These people live life to its fullest and have fewer health problems than inactive individuals who also indulge in negative lifestyle habits.

Compiling an all-inclusive list of the benefits to be reaped through participation in a fitness and wellness program is a challenge, but the following list summarizes many of these benefits:

- Improves and strengthens the cardiorespiratory system.
- Promotes better muscle tone, muscular strength, and endurance.
- Improves muscular flexibility.
- Enhances athletic performance.
- Helps maintain recommended body weight.
- Helps preserve lean body mass.
- Increases resting metabolic rate.
- Improves the body's ability to use fat during physical activity.
- Improves posture and physical appearance.
- Improves functioning of the immune system.
- Lowers the risk for chronic diseases and illness (such as cardiovascular diseases and cancer).
- Decreases the mortality rate from chronic diseases.

- Thins the blood so it doesn't clot as readily (thereby decreasing the risk for coronary heart disease and strokes).
- Helps the body manage cholesterol more effectively.
- Prevents or delays the development of high blood pressure and lowers blood pressure in people with hypertension.
- Helps prevent and control diabetes.
- Helps achieve peak bone mass in young adults and maintain bone mass later in life, thereby decreasing the risk for osteoporosis.
- Helps people sleep better.
- Helps prevent chronic back pain.
- Relieves tension and helps in coping with life stresses.
- Raises levels of energy and job productivity.
- Extends longevity and slows the aging process.
- Promotes psychological well-being through better morale, self-image, and self-esteem.
- Reduces feelings of depression and anxiety.
- Motivates a person toward positive lifestyle changes (improving nutrition, quitting smoking, controlling alcohol and drug use).
- Speeds recovery time following physical exertion.
- Speeds recovery following injury or disease.
- Regulates and improves overall body functions.
- Helps maintain independent living, especially in older adults.
- Enhances quality of life: People feel better and live a healthier and happier life.

In addition to the benefits listed, **epidemiological** research studies linking physical activity habits and mortality rates have shown lower premature mortality rates in physically active people. Pioneer work in this area demonstrated that, as the amount of weekly physical activity increased, the risk of cardiovascular deaths decreased.[7] In this study, conducted among 16,936 Harvard alumni, the greatest decrease in cardiovascular deaths was observed in alumni who burned more than 2,000 calories per week through physical activity (see Figure 1.7).

Another major study subsequently upheld the findings of the Harvard alumni study.[8] Based on data from 13,344 individuals who were followed over an average of 8 years, the results confirmed that the level of cardiorespiratory fitness is related to mortality from all causes. These findings showed a graded and consistent inverse relationship between physical fitness and mortality, regardless of age and other risk factors.

In essence, the higher the level of cardiorespiratory fitness, the longer the life (see Figure 1.8). The death rate from all causes for the low-fit men was 3.4 times higher than for the high-fit men. For the low-fit women, the death rate was 4.6 times higher than for the high-fit

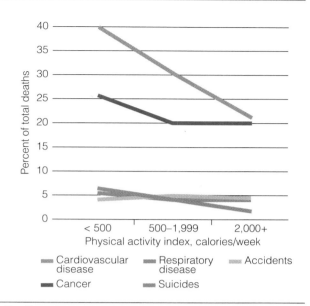

FIGURE **1.7** Death rates by physical activity index.

Note: The graph represents cause-specific death rates per 10,000 person-years of observation among 16,936 Harvard alumni, 1962–1978, by physical activity index; adjusted for differences in age, cigarette smoking, and hypertension.

Source: "A Natural History of Athleticism and Cardiovascular Health" by R. S. Paffenbarger, R. T. Hyde, A. L. Wing, and C. H. Steinmetz. *Journal of the American Medical Association* 252 (1989): 491–495. Used by permission.

women. The study also reported a greatly reduced rate of premature deaths, even at moderate fitness levels, which most adults can achieve easily. People gain further protection when they combine higher fitness levels with reduction in other risk factors such as hypertension, elevated cholesterol, cigarette smoking, and excessive body fat.

Additional research that looked at changes in fitness and mortality found a substantial (44 percent) reduction in mortality risk when the study participants abandoned a sedentary lifestyle and became moderately fit.[9] The lowest death rate was found in people who were fit and remained fit, and the highest rate was found in men who remained unfit (see Figure 1.9).

Further research in this area substantiated the previous findings and also indicated that primarily vigorous activities are associated with greater longevity.[10] Vigorous activity was defined as activity that requires a MET

KEY TERMS

Physiologic fitness Biological systems that are affected by physical activity; also the role of activity in disease prevention.

Epidemiological The study of epidemic diseases.

FIGURE **1.8** Death rates by physical fitness levels.

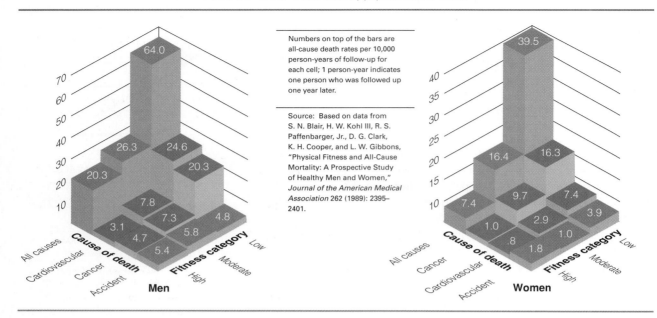

Numbers on top of the bars are all-cause death rates per 10,000 person-years of follow-up for each cell; 1 person-year indicates one person who was followed up one year later.

Source: Based on data from S. N. Blair, H. W. Kohl III, R. S. Paffenbarger, Jr., D. G. Clark, K. H. Cooper, and L. W. Gibbons, "Physical Fitness and All-Cause Mortality: A Prospective Study of Healthy Men and Women," *Journal of the American Medical Association* 262 (1989): 2395–2401.

FIGURE **1.9** Effects of fitness changes on mortality rates.

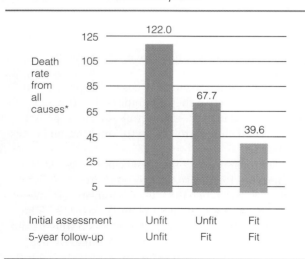

	Initial assessment	5-year follow-up
	Unfit	Unfit
	Unfit	Fit
	Fit	Fit

* Death rate per 10,000 man-years observation. Based on data from "Changes in Physical Fitness and All-Cause Mortality: A Prospective Study of Healthy Men," *Journal of the American Medical Association* 273 (1995): 1193–1198.

Source: S. N. Blair, H. W. Kohl III, C. E. Barlow, R. S. Paffenbarger, Jr., L. W. Gibbons, and C. A. Macera, "Changes in Physical Fitness and All-Cause Mortality: A Prospective Study of Healthy and Unhealthy Men," *Journal of the American Medical Association* 273 (1995): 1193–1198.

level equal to or greater than 6 METs (see Chapter 4, Table 4.1, page 98). This level represents exercising at an energy level of 6 times the resting energy requirement. Examples of vigorous activities used in the previous study include brisk walking, jogging, swimming laps, squash, racquetball, tennis, and shoveling snow. Results also indicated that vigorous exercise is as important as maintaining recommended weight and not smoking.

The results of these studies indicate clearly that fitness improves wellness, quality of life, and longevity. If people are able, vigorous exercise is preferable because it is associated most closely with longer life.

National Health Objectives for the Year 2010

Every 10 years, the U. S. Department of Health and Human Services releases a list of objectives for preventing disease and promoting health. From its onset in 1980, this 10-year plan has helped instill a new sense of purpose and focus for public health and preventive medicine. These national health objectives are intended as realistic goals to improve the health of all Americans as we start the first decade of the new millennium. Two unique goals of the new 2010 objectives are that they emphasize increased quality and years of healthy life, and they seek to eliminate health disparities among all

FIGURE **1.10** Selected national health objectives for the year 2010.

1. Increase quality and years of healthy life.
2. Eliminate health disparities.
3. Improve the health, fitness, and quality of life of all Americans through the adoption and maintenance of regular, daily physical activity.
4. Promote health and reduce chronic disease risk, disease progression, debilitation, and premature death associated with dietary factors and nutritional status among all people in the United States.
5. Reduce disease, disability, and death related to tobacco use and exposure to secondhand smoke.
6. Increase the quality, availability, and effectiveness of educational and community-based programs designed to prevent disease and improve the health and quality of life of the American people.
7. Promote health for all people through a healthy environment.
8. Reduce the incidence and severity of injuries from unintentional causes, as well as violence and abuse.
9. Promote worker health and safety through prevention.
10. Improve access to comprehensive, high quality health care.
11. Ensure that every pregnancy in the United States is intended.
12. Improve maternal and pregnancy outcomes and reduce rates of disability in infants.
13. Improve the quality of health-related decisions through effective communication.
14. Decrease the incidence of functional limitations due to arthritis, osteoporosis, and chronic back conditions.
15. Decrease cancer incidence, morbidity, and mortality.
16. Promote health and prevent secondary conditions among persons with disabilities.
17. Enhance the cardiovascular health and quality of life of all Americans through prevention and control of risk factors, and promotion of healthy lifestyle behaviors.
18. Prevent HIV transmission and associated morbidity and mortality.
19. Improve the mental health of all Americans.
20. Raise the public's awareness of the signs and symptoms of lung disease.
21. Increase awareness of healthy sexual relationships and prevent all forms of sexually transmitted diseases.
22. Reduce the incidence of substance abuse by all people, especially children.

Source: U.S. Department of Health and Human Services.

groups of people. The objectives address three important points:[11]

1. Personal responsibility. Individuals need to become ever more health-conscious. Responsible and informed behaviors are the key to good health.
2. Health benefits for all people. Lower socioeconomic conditions and poor health often are interrelated. Extending the benefits of good health to all people is crucial to the health of the nation.
3. Health promotion and disease prevention. A shift from treatment to preventive techniques will drastically cut health-care costs and help all Americans achieve a better quality of life.

Development of these health objectives involves more than 10,000 people representing 300 national organizations, including the Institute of Medicine of the National Academy of Sciences, all state health departments, and the federal Office of Disease Prevention and Health Promotion. A summary of key 2010 objectives is provided in Figure 1.10. Living according to the fitness and wellness principles provided in this book will enhance the quality of your life and also will allow you to

be an active participant in achieving the Healthy People 2010 Objectives.

The Path to Fitness and Wellness

Current scientific data and the fitness movement that began more than three decades ago in the United States have led many people to see the advantages of participating in fitness programs that will improve and maintain health. Because fitness and wellness needs vary from one person to another, exercise and wellness prescriptions must be personalized for best results. This book provides the necessary guidelines for developing a lifetime program to improve fitness and promote preventive health care and personal wellness. As you study the book and complete the assignments in each chapter, you will learn to

- Determine whether medical clearance is required for you to participate safely in exercise.
- Assess your overall level of physical fitness, including cardiorespiratory endurance, muscular strength and endurance, muscular flexibility, and body composition.

- Prescribe personal programs for total fitness development.
- Learn behavior modification techniques that will allow you to change unhealthy lifestyle patterns.
- Develop sound diet and weight-control programs.
- Implement a healthy lifestyle program that includes prevention of cardiovascular diseases and cancer, stress management, and smoking cessation, if applicable.
- Discern myths from facts pertaining to exercise and health-related concepts.

Behavior Modification

Scientific evidence of the benefits derived from living a healthy lifestyle continues to mount each day. Although the data are impressive, most people still don't adhere to a healthy lifestyle. To understand why this is so, one has to examine what motivates people and what actions are required to make permanent changes in behavior, called **behavior modification.**

Let's look at an all-too-common occurrence on college campuses. Most students understand that they should be exercising. They contemplate enrolling in a fitness course. The motivating factor might be enhanced physical appearance, health benefits, or simply fulfillment of a college requirement. They sign up for the course, participate for a few months, finish the course—and stop exercising! A wide array of excuses are offered: too busy, no one to exercise with, already have the grade, inconvenient open-gym hours, or job conflicts. A few months later, they realize once again that exercise is vital and repeat the cycle (see Figure 1.11).

The information in this book will be of little value to you if you are unable to abandon negative habits and adopt and maintain new, healthy behaviors. Before looking at the physical fitness and wellness guidelines, you will need to take a critical look at your behaviors and lifestyle—and most likely make some permanent changes to promote your overall health and wellness.

Changing Behavior

The very first step in addressing behavioral change is to recognize that indeed a problem exists. Five general categories of behaviors are addressed in the process of willful change:

1. Stopping a negative behavior
2. Preventing relapse of a negative behavior
3. Developing a positive behavior
4. Strengthening a positive behavior
5. Maintaining a positive behavior

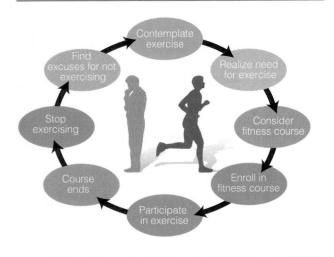

FIGURE **1.11** Exercise–exercise dropout cycle.

Changing chronic, unhealthy behaviors to stable, healthy behaviors is often challenging. Change usually does not happen all at once but, rather, is a lengthy process with several stages.

The simplest model of change is the two-stage model of unhealthy behavior and healthy behavior. This model states that either you do it or you don't. Most people who use this model attempt self-change but end up asking themselves why they're unsuccessful: They just can't do it (start and adhere to exercise or quit smoking, for example). Their intention to change may be good, but to accomplish it, they need knowledge about how to achieve change. The following discussion may help.

To aid in this process, psychologists James Prochaska, John Norcross, and Carlo DiClemente developed a behavioral change model.[12] The model's five stages are important to understanding the process of willful change. The stages of change describe underlying processes that people go through to change most problem behaviors and adopt healthy behaviors. Most frequently, the model is used to change health-related behaviors such as physical inactivity, smoking, nutrition, weight control, stress, and alcohol abuse.

The five stages of change are precontemplation, contemplation, preparation, action, and maintenance. A sixth stage of change, termination/adoption, was subsequently added to this model.

After years of study, researchers found that applying specific behavior-change techniques during each stage of the model increases the rate of success for change. Understanding each stage of this model will help you determine where you are in relation to your personal healthy-lifestyle behaviors. It also will help you identify techniques to make successful changes.

Precontemplation

People in the **precontemplation stage** are not considering or do not want to change a specific behavior. They typically deny having a problem and presently do not intend to change. These people are usually unaware or underaware of the problem. Other people around them, including family, friends, health-care practitioners, and coworkers, however, identify the problem quite clearly.

Precontemplators do not care about the problem behavior and might even avoid information and materials that address the issue. They avoid free screenings and workshops that could help identify and change the problem, even if they receive financial incentives for attending. Frequently these people actively resist change and seem resigned to accept the unhealthy behavior as their "fate."

Precontemplators are the most difficult people to reach for behavioral change. They often think that change isn't even a possibility. Educating them about the problem behavior is critical to helping them start contemplating the process of change. It is said that knowledge is power, and the challenge is to find ways to help them realize that they will be ultimately responsible for the consequences of their behavior. Sometimes they initiate change only when under pressure from others.

Contemplation

In the **contemplation stage,** people acknowledge that they have a problem and begin to think seriously about overcoming it. Although they are not quite ready for change yet, they are weighing the pros and cons. People may remain in this stage for years, but in their mind they are planning to take some action within the next 6 months or so. Education and peer support are valuable during this stage.

Preparation

In the **preparation stage,** people are seriously considering and planning to change a behavior within the next month. They are taking initial steps for change and may even try it for a short while, such as stopping smoking for a day or exercising a few times during this month. In this stage, people define a general goal for behavior change (say, to quit smoking by the last day of the month) and write specific objectives to accomplish this goal (see the discussion on SMART Goals, pages 17–18). Continued peer and environmental support are recommended during the preparation phase.

Action

The **action stage** requires the most commitment of time and energy by the individual. Here people are actively doing things to change or modify the problem behavior or to adopt a new health behavior. The action stage requires that the person follow the specific guidelines set forth for that specific behavior. For example, a person has actually stopped smoking completely, is exercising aerobically three times per week according to exercise prescription guidelines (see Chapter 3), or is maintaining a healthy diet.

Relapse, in which the individual regresses to a previous stage, is common during this stage. Once people maintain the action stage for 6 consecutive months, they move into the maintenance stage.

Maintenance

During the **maintenance stage,** the person continues to adhere to the behavior change for up to 5 years. The maintenance phase requires continually adhering to the specific guidelines that govern the target behavior (for example, complete smoking cessation, aerobic exercise three times per week, or proper stress management techniques). At this time, a person works to reinforce the gains made through the various stages of change and strives to prevent lapses and relapses.

Termination/Adoption

Once a person has maintained a behavior more than 5 years, he or she enters the **termination/adoption stage** without fear of relapse. In the case of negative behaviors

K E Y   T E R M S

Behavior modification The process used to permanently change negative behaviors in favor of positive behaviors that will lead to better health and well-being.

Precontemplation stage Stage of change in which people are unwilling to change their behavior.

Contemplation stage Stage of change in which people are considering changing behavior in the next 6 months.

Preparation stage Stage of change in which people are getting ready to make a change within the coming month.

Action stage Stage of change in which people are actively changing a negative behavior or adopting a new, healthy behavior.

Relapse Slipping or falling back into unhealthy behavior(s) or failing to maintain healthy behaviors.

Maintenance stage Stage of change in which people maintain behavioral change for up to 5 years.

Termination/adoption stage Stage of change in which people have eliminated an undesirable behavior or maintained a positive behavior for more than 5 years.

that have been terminated, this stage of change is referred to as termination. If the person has adopted a positive behavior for more than 5 years, this stage is designated the adoption stage. Many experts believe that after this period of time, any former addictions, problems, or lack of compliance with healthy behaviors no longer present an obstacle in the quest for wellness. The change has become a part of one's lifestyle. This phase is the ultimate goal for everyone who seeks a healthier lifestyle.

Use the form provided in Figure 1.12 to determine where you stand in respect to behaviors that you want to change or new ones that you wish to adopt. As you fill out this form, you will realize that you are at different stages for different behaviors. For instance, you may be in the termination stage for aerobic exercise and smoking, in the action stage for strength training, but only in the contemplation stage for a healthy diet. Realizing where you are at with respect to different behaviors will help you design a better action plan for a healthy lifestyle.

Using the form provided in Activity 1.1, pages 21–22, select two or three behaviors that you have targeted for the next 3 months. Developing new behavioral patterns takes time, and trying to work on too many components at once most likely will lower your chances for success. Start with components in which you think you will have a high chance for success.

Critical Thinking

What factors do you think keep you from participating in a regular exercise program? How about factors that keep you from managing your daily caloric intake?

Motivation and Locus of Control

Motivation often explains why some people succeed and others do not. Although motivation comes from within, external factors are what trigger the inner desire to accomplish a given task. These external factors, then, control behavior.

Understanding **locus of control** is helpful to the study of motivation. People who believe they have control over events in their lives are said to have an internal locus of control. People with an external locus of control, by contrast, believe that what happens to them is a result of chance or environmental factors and is unrelated to their behavior. The latter group often has difficulty getting out of the precontemplation or contemplation stages.

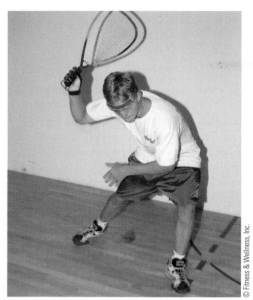

Many people refrain from physical activity because they lack the necessary skills to enjoy and reap the benefits of regular participation.

People with an internal locus of control are apt to be healthier and have an easier time initiating and adhering to a wellness program than those who perceive that they have little control and think of themselves as powerless and vulnerable. The latter people also are at greater risk for illness. When illness does strike, restoring a sense of control is vital to regaining health.

Few people have either a completely external or a completely internal locus of control. They fall somewhere along a continuum. The more external, the greater is the challenge in changing and adhering to exercise and other healthy lifestyle behaviors. Fortunately, a person can develop a more internal locus of control. Understanding that most events in life are not determined genetically or environmentally helps people pursue goals and gain control over their lives. Three impediments, however, can keep people from entering the preparation or action stages: problems of competence, confidence, and motivation.

1. *Problems of competence.* Lacking the skills to get a given task done leads to less competence. If your friends play basketball regularly but you don't know how to play, you might not be inclined to participate. The solution to this problem of competence is to master the skills you need for participation. Most people are not born with all-inclusive natural abilities, including playing sports.

A college professor continuously watched a group of students play an entertaining game of basketball

FIGURE **1.12** Identifying your current stage of change.

Please indicate which response most accurately describes your current _____
behavior (in the blank space identify the behavior: smoking, physical activity, stress, nutrition, weight control, etc.).
Next, select the statement below (select only one) that best represents your current behavior pattern. To select the
most appropriate statement, fill in the blank for one of the first three statements if your current behavior is a problem behavior. (For example, you might say, "I currently smoke and I do *not* intend to change in the foreseeable
future," or "I currently *do not* exercise but I am contemplating changing in the next 6 months.") If you have already
started to make changes, fill in the blank in one of the last three statements. (In this case, you might say: "I currently
eat a low-fat diet but I have done so only within the last 6 months," or "I currently *practice adequate stress management techniques* and I have done so for more than 6 months.") As you can see, you may use this form to identify
your stage of change for any type of health-related behavior.

1. I currently _____ and I do not intend to change in the foreseeable future.

2. I currently _____ but I am contemplating changing in the next 6 months.

3. I currently _____ regularly but intend to change in the next month.

4. I currently _____ but I have done so only within the last 6 months.

5. I currently _____ and I have done so for more than 6 months.

6. I currently _____ and I have done so for more than 5 years.

STAGES OF CHANGE

1 =	Precontemplation	4 =	Action
2 =	Contemplation	5 =	Maintenance
3 =	Preparation	6 =	Termination/Adoption

every Friday at noon. Having no basketball skills, he
was reluctant to play (contemplation stage). Eventually,
however, the desire to join in the fun was strong enough
that he enrolled in a beginning course at the college so
he would learn to play the game (preparation stage). To
his surprise, most of the students were impressed that
he was willing to do this. Now, with greater competence,
he is able to join in on Friday's "pick-up games" (action
phase).

Another alternative is to select an activity in which
you are skilled. It may not be basketball, but it well
could be aerobics. And don't be afraid to try new activities. Similarly, if your body weight is a problem, you
could learn to cook low-fat meals. Try different recipes
until you find foods you like.

Patty's story at the beginning of this chapter exem-
plifies a lack of competence. Patty was motivated and
knew she could do it, but she lacked the skills to reach
her goal. All along, Patty was fluctuating between the
contemplation and action stages. Once she mastered
the skills, she was able to achieve and maintain her goal.

2. *Problems of confidence.* Problems with confidence arise when you have the skills but you don't

believe you can get it done. Fear and feelings of inade-
quacy often interfere with the ability to perform the task.

Don't talk yourself out of something until you have
given it a fair try. If the skills are there, the sky is the
limit. Initially, try to visualize yourself doing the task
and getting it done. Repeat this several times, then
actually give it a try. You will surprise yourself.

Sometimes, lack of confidence sets in when the
task seems to be insurmountable. In these situations,
dividing a goal into smaller, realistic objectives helps
to accomplish the task. You may know how to swim,
but the goal of swimming a continuous mile could take
you several weeks to accomplish. Set up your training
program so you swim a little farther each day until you
are able to swim the entire mile. If you don't meet your
objective on a given day, try it again, reevaluate, cut back
a little, and, most important, don't give up.

KEY TERMS

Motivation The desire and will to do something.

Locus of control The extent to which a person believes he or
she can influence the external environment.

3. *Problems of motivation*. With problems of motivation, both the competence and the confidence are there but individuals are unwilling to change because the reasons for change are not important to them. For example, a person begins contemplating a smoking cessation program when the reasons for quitting outweigh the reasons for smoking.

The lack of knowledge and lack of goals are the primary causes of unwillingness to change (precontemplators). Knowledge often determines goals, and goals determine motivation. How badly you want something dictates how hard you'll work at it. Many people are unaware of the magnitude of the benefits of a wellness program. When it comes to a healthy lifestyle, however, there may not be a second chance. A stroke, a heart attack, or cancer can have irreparable or fatal consequences. Greater understanding of what leads to disease may be all that is needed to initiate change.

Also, feeling physically fit is difficult to explain unless you have experienced it yourself. What Patty expressed to her instructor—fitness, self-esteem, confidence, health, and quality of life—cannot be conveyed to someone who is constrained by sedentary living. In a way, wellness is like reaching the top of a mountain. The quiet, the clean air, the lush vegetation, the flowing water in the river, the wildlife, and the majestic valley below are difficult to explain to someone who has spent a lifetime within city limits.

Behavior Modification Principles

Over the course of many years, we all develop habits that we would like to change at some point. The adage "old habits die hard" comes to mind. Acquiring positive behaviors that will lead to better health and well-being requires continual effort. When wellness is concerned, the sooner we implement a healthy lifestyle program, the greater are the health benefits and quality of life that lie ahead. Adopting the following behavior modification principles can help change behavior.

Self-Analysis

The first step in modifying behavior is a decisive desire to do so. If you have no interest in changing a behavior, you won't do it (precontemplator). A person who has no intention of quitting smoking will not quit, regardless of what anyone says or how strong the evidence is against it. As part of your self-analysis, you may want to prepare a list of reasons for continuing or discontinuing the behavior. When the reasons for changing outweigh the reasons for not changing, you are ready for the next step (contemplation stage).

Behavior Analysis

Now you have to determine the frequency, circumstances, and consequences of the behavior to be altered or implemented. If the desired outcome is to consume less fat, you first must find out what foods in your diet are high in fat, when you eat them, and when you don't eat them (preparation stage). Knowing when you don't eat fatty foods points to circumstances under which you exert control of your diet and will help as you set goals.

Goal Setting

A **goal** motivates change in behavior. The stronger the goal, or desire, the more motivated you will be either to change unwanted behaviors or to implement new healthy behaviors. The final topic of this chapter, SMART Goals, will help you write goals and prepare an action plan to achieve those goals. This will aid with behavior modification.

Social Support

Surrounding yourself with people who will work toward a common goal with you or will encourage you along the way will be helpful. Attempting to quit smoking, for instance, is easier when the person is around others who are trying to quit as well. The person also may get help from friends who have quit already. Peer support is a strong incentive for behavior change. During this process, people who will not be supportive should be avoided. Friends who have no desire to quit smoking may tempt the person to smoke and encourage relapse. People who achieved the same goal earlier might not be supportive either. For instance, someone might say, "I can do six consecutive miles." The response should be, "I'm proud that I can jog three consecutive miles."

Monitoring

During the action and maintenance stages, continuous behavior monitoring increases awareness of the desired outcome. Sometimes this principle in itself is sufficient to cause change. For example, keeping track of daily food intake reveals sources of fat in the diet. This can help a person cut down gradually or completely eliminate some high-fat foods before consuming them. If the goal is to increase daily intake of fruit and vegetables, keeping track of the number of servings eaten each day raises awareness and may help increase their intake.

A Positive Outlook

Having a positive outlook means taking an optimistic approach from the beginning and believing in yourself.

Social support enhances regular participation and the process of behavior modification.

Following the guidelines in this chapter will help you pace yourself so you can work toward change. Also, you may become motivated by looking at the outcomes—how much healthier you will be, how much better you will look, or how much farther you can jog.

Reinforcement

People tend to repeat behaviors that are rewarded and disregard those that are not rewarded or are punished. If you have successfully cut down your fat intake during the week, reward yourself by going to a show or buying a new pair of shoes. Do not reinforce yourself with destructive behaviors such as eating a high-fat dinner. If you fail to change a desired behavior (or to implement a new one), you may want to put off buying those new shoes. When a positive behavior becomes habitual, give yourself an even better reward. Treat yourself to a weekend away from home, buy a new bike, or get that tennis racket you always wanted.

SMART Goals

Only a well-conceived action plan will help you attain goals. Determining what you want to accomplish is the starting point, but to reach your goal you need to write

SMART goals. The SMART acronym means that goals are *S*pecific, *M*easurable, *A*cceptable, *R*ealistic, and *T*ime-specific.

1. *Specific.* When writing goals, state exactly and in a positive manner what you would like to accomplish. For example, if you are overweight at 150 pounds and at 27 percent body fat, simply stating "I will lose weight" is not a specific goal. Instead, re-write your goal to state "I will reduce my body fat to 20 percent body fat (137 pounds) in 12 weeks."

Be sure to write down your goals. An unwritten goal is simply a wish. A written goal, in essence, becomes a contract with yourself. Show this goal to a friend or an instructor and have him or her witness the contract you made with yourself by signing alongside your signature.

Once you have identified and written down a specific goal, write the specific **objectives** that will help you reach that goal. These objectives are the necessary steps required to reach your goal. For example, a goal might be to achieve recommended body weight. Several specific objectives could be to

(a) lose an average of 1 pound (or 1 fat percentage point) per week
(b) monitor body weight before breakfast every morning
(c) assess body composition every 3 weeks
(d) limit fat intake to less than 25 percent of total daily caloric intake
(e) eliminate all pastries from the diet during this time, and
(f) walk/jog in the proper target zone for 60 minutes, six times per week.

2. *Measurable.* Whenever possible, goals and objectives should be measurable. For example, "I will lose weight" is not measurable, but "I will reduce body fat to 20 percent" is measurable. Also note that all of the sample specific objectives (a) through (f) in Item 1 above are measurable. For instance, you can figure out easily whether you are losing a pound or a percentage point per week; you can conduct a nutrient analysis to assess your average fat intake; or you can monitor your weekly exercise sessions to make sure you are meeting this specific objective.

3. *Acceptable.* Goals that you set for yourself are more motivational than goals that someone else sets for

KEY TERMS

Goal The ultimate aim toward which effort is directed.

SMART An acronym for Specific, Measurable, Attainable, Realistic, and Time-specific goals.

Objectives Steps required to reach a goal.

you. These goals will motivate and challenge you and should be consistent with other goals that you have. As you set an acceptable goal, ask yourself: Do I have the time, commitment, and necessary skills to accomplish this goal? If not, you need to restate your goal so that it is acceptable to you.

In instances where successful completion of a goal involves others, such as an athletic team or an organization, an acceptable goal must be compatible with those of the other people involved. If a team's practice schedule is set Monday through Friday from 4:00 to 6:00 P.M., it is unacceptable for you to train only three times per week or at a different time of the day.

Acceptable goals are also embraced with positive thoughts. Visualize and believe in your success. As difficult as some tasks may seem, where there's a will, there's a way. A plan of action, prepared according to the guidelines in this chapter, will help you achieve your goals.

4. *Realistic.* Goals should be within reach. If you currently weigh 190 pounds and your target weight (at 20 percent body fat) is 140 pounds, setting a goal to lose 50 pounds in a month would be unsound, if not impossible. Such a goal does not allow for the implementation of adequate behavior modification techniques or ensure weight maintenance at the target weight. Unattainable goals only set you up for failure, discouragement, and loss of interest.

On the other hand, do not write goals that are too easy to achieve and do not challenge you. If a goal is too easy, you may lose interest and stop working toward it.

At times, problems arise even with realistic goals. Try to anticipate potential difficulties as much as possible, and plan for ways to deal with them. If your goal is to jog for 30 minutes on six consecutive days, what are the alternatives if the weather turns bad? Possible solutions are to jog in the rain, find an indoor track, jog at a different time of day when the weather is better, or participate in a different aerobic activity such as stationary cycling, swimming, or step aerobics.

Monitoring your progress as you move toward a goal also reinforces behavior. Keeping an exercise log or doing a body composition assessment periodically enables you to determine your progress at any given time.

5. *Time-specific.* A goal always should have a specific date set for completion. The above example to reach 20 percent body fat in 12 weeks is time-specific. The chosen date should be realistic but not too distant in the future. Allow yourself enough time to achieve

the goal, but not too much time, as this could affect your performance. With a deadline, a task is much easier to work toward.

Goal Evaluation

In addition to the SMART guidelines provided above, you should conduct periodic evaluations of your goals. Reevaluations are vital for success. You may find that after you have fully committed and put all your effort into a goal, that goal may be unreachable. If so, reassess the goal.

Recognize that you will face obstacles and that you will not always meet your goals. Use your setbacks and learn from them. Rewrite your goal and create a plan that will help you get around self-defeating behaviors in the future. Once you achieve a goal, set a new one to improve upon or maintain what you have achieved. Goals keep you motivated.

In addition to previously discussed guidelines, throughout this book you will find information on behavioral change. For example, Chapter 3 includes the Exercise Readiness Questionnaire, tips to start and adhere to an exercise program, and how to set your fitness goals; Chapter 4 offers tips to enhance your aerobic workout; Chapter 6 gives suggestions on how to adhere to a lifetime weight management program; Chapter 7 sets forth stress management techniques; and Chapter 8 outlines a six-step smoking cessation plan.

A Word of Caution Before You Start Exercise

Even though exercise testing and participation is relatively safe for most apparently healthy men and women under age 45 and 55 respectively, a small but real risk exists for exercise-induced abnormalities in people with a history of cardiovascular problems and those who are at higher risk for disease.[13] These people should be screened before initiating or increasing the intensity of an exercise program.

Before you start an exercise program or participate in any exercise testing, you should fill out the health history questionnaire provided in Activity 1.2. A "yes" answer to any of these questions may signal the need for a physician's approval before you participate. If you don't have any "yes" responses, you may proceed to Chapter 2 to assess your current level of fitness.

LifeScan will help you learn more about the health risks you might be taking each day. Take the health questionnaire to determine your personal lifestyle risks. Your results provide a score for general results, nutrition results, and height/weight results. Your ranking among the top ten causes of death is provided, as well as suggestions on how to improve.
http://wellness.uwsp.edu/other/lifescan/lifescan.htm

ASSESS YOUR KNOWLEDGE

Evaluate how well you understand the concepts presented in this chapter using the Assess Your Knowledge and Practice Quizzes options on your Profile Plus CD-ROM.

1. Bodily movement produced by skeletal muscles is called
   a. physical activity.
   b. kinesiology.
   c. exercise.
   d. aerobic exercise.
   e. muscle strength.
2. Most people in the United States
   a. get adequate physical activity on a regular basis.
   b. meet health-related fitness standards.
   c. regularly participate in skill-related activities.
   d. Choices a, b, and c are correct.
   e. None of the above choices is correct.
3. The leading cause of death in the United States is
   a. cancer.
   b. accidents.
   c. chronic lower respiratory disease.
   d. diseases of the cardiovascular system.
   e. drug-related illness.
4. The constant and deliberate effort to stay healthy and achieve the highest potential for well-being is defined as
   a. health.
   b. physical fitness.
   c. wellness.
   d. health-related fitness.
   e. metabolic fitness.
5. Which of the following is *not* a component of health-related fitness?
   a. cardiorespiratory endurance
   b. body composition
   c. agility
   d. muscular strength and endurance
   e. muscular flexibility
6. Research on the effects of fitness on mortality indicates that the largest drop in premature mortality is seen between
   a. the average and excellent fitness groups.
   b. the least fit and moderately fit groups.

   c. the good and high fitness groups.
   d. the moderately fit and good fitness groups.
   e. The drop is similar between all fitness groups.
7. What is the greatest benefit of being physically fit?
   a. absence of disease
   b. a higher quality of life
   c. improved sports performance
   d. better personal appearance
   e. maintenance of ideal body weight
8. Which of the following is a stage in the behavioral modification model?
   a. recognition
   b. motivation
   c. relapse
   d. preparation
   e. goal setting
9. A precontemplator is a person who
   a. has no desire to change a behavior.
   b. is looking to make a change in the next six months.
   c. is preparing for change in the next 30 days.
   d. willingly adopts healthy behaviors.
   e. is talking to a therapist to overcome a problem behavior.
10. A SMART goal is effective when it is
    a. realistic.
    b. measurable.
    c. specific.
    d. acceptable.
    e. All are correct choices.

Correct answers can be found on page 261.

Behavior Modification: Stages of Change

Name _____   Date _____

Course _____   Section _____

Instructions

Please indicate which response most accurately describes your stage of change for three different behaviors (in the blank space identify the behavior: smoking, physical activity, stress, nutrition, weight control, etc.). Next, select the statement (select only one) that best represents your current behavior pattern. To select the most appropriate statement, fill in the blank for one of the first three statements if your current behavior is a problem behavior. (For example, you might say, "I currently smoke and I do *not* intend to change in the foreseeable future," or "I currently *do not* exercise but I am contemplating changing in the next 6 months.")

If you have already started to make changes, fill in the blank in one of the last three statements. (In this case, you might say: "I currently *eat a low-fat diet* but I have done so only within the last 6 months," or "I currently *practice adequate stress management techniques* and I have done so for more than 6 months.") You may use this technique to identify your stage of change for any type of health-related behavior.

Now write a specific goal (see pages 17–18) and identify three behavior modification principles (pages 16–17) that will aid you with the process of change.

Behavior 1: _____

1. I currently _____ and I do not intend to change in the foreseeable future.

2. I currently _____ but I am contemplating changing in the next 6 months.

3. I currently_____ regularly but intend to change in the next month.

4. I currently_____ but I have done so only within the last 6 months.

5. I currently _____ and I have done so for more than 6 months.

6. I currently _____ and I have done so for more than 5 years.

Stage of change: (see Figure 1.12, page 15). _____

Specific goal and date to be accomplished: _____

Principles of behavior modification to be used: _____

Behavior 2: _____

1. I currently _____ and I do not intend to change in the foreseeable future.

2. I currently _____ but I am contemplating changing in the next 6 months.

3. I currently_____ regularly but intend to change in the next month.

4. I currently_____ but I have done so only within the last 6 months.

5. I currently _____ and I have done so for more than 6 months.

6. I currently _____ and I have done so for more than 5 years.

Stage of change: (see Figure 1.12, page 15). _____

Specific goal and date to be accomplished: _____

Principles of behavior modification to be used: _____

Behavior 3: _____

1. I currently _____ and I do not intend to change in the foreseeable future.

2. I currently _____ but I am contemplating changing in the next 6 months.

3. I currently _____ regularly but intend to change in the next month.

4. I currently _____ but I have done so only within the last 6 months.

5. I currently _____ and I have done so for more than 6 months.

6. I currently _____ and I have done so for more than 5 years.

Stage of change: (see Figure 1.12, page 15). _____

Specific goal and date to be accomplished: _____

Principles of behavior modification to be used: _____

Stages of Change

1 = Precontemplation   4 = Action
2 = Contemplation   5 = Maintenance
3 = Preparation   6 = Termination/Adoption

Self-Reflection

In your own words, indicate barriers (what may keep you from changing) that you may encounter during the process of change and how can you best prepare to overcome these barriers.

_____

_____

_____

_____

_____

_____

_____

_____

_____

Clearance for Exercise Participation

Name _____   Date _____

Course _____   Section _____

I. Health History

Even though participation in exercise is relatively safe for most apparently healthy individuals, the reaction of the cardiovascular system to increased levels of physical activity cannot always be totally predicted. Consequently, there is a small but real risk of certain changes occurring during exercise participation. These changes include abnormal blood pressure, irregular heart rhythm, fainting, and in rare instances a heart attack or cardiac arrest. Therefore, you must provide honest answers to this questionnaire.

Have you ever had or do you now have any of the following conditions?

☐ Yes ☐ No   1. Cardiovascular disease (any type of heart or blood vessel disease, including strokes)

☐ Yes ☐ No   2. Elevated blood lipids (cholesterol and triglycerides)

☐ Yes ☐ No   3. Chest pain at rest or during exertion

☐ Yes ☐ No   4. Shortness of breath or other respiratory problems

☐ Yes ☐ No   5. Uneven, irregular, or skipped heartbeats (including a racing or fluttering heart)

☐ Yes ☐ No   6. Elevated blood pressure

☐ Yes ☐ No   7. Often feel faint or have spells of severe dizziness

☐ Yes ☐ No   8. Obesity (BMI of 30 or above)

☐ Yes ☐ No   9. Diabetes

☐ Yes ☐ No   10. Any joint, bone, or muscle problems (e.g., arthritis, low-back pain, rheumatism)

☐ Yes ☐ No   11. An eating disorder (anorexia nervosa, bulimia, binge-eating)

☐ Yes ☐ No   12. Any other concern regarding your ability to participate safely in an exercise program? If so, explain:

Indicate if any of the following two conditions apply:

☐ Yes ☐ No   13. Do you smoke cigarettes?

☐ Yes ☐ No   14. Men—Are you age 45 or older?

☐ Yes ☐ No   15. Women—Are you age 55 or older?

Exercise may not be recommended under some of the conditions listed above; others may simply indicate special consideration. If any of the conditions apply, you should consult your physician before participating in an exercise program. You also should promptly report to your instructor any exercise-related abnormalities you experienced during the course of the semester.

Student's Signature: _____   Date: _____

II. Do you feel that it is safe for you to proceed with an exercise program? Explain any concerns or limitations that you may have regarding your safe participation in a comprehensive exercise program to improve cardiorespiratory endurance, muscular strength and endurance, and muscular flexibility.

_____

_____

_____

_____

_____

_____

_____

_____

III. In a few words, describe your previous experiences with sports participation, whether you have taken part in a structured exercise program, and express your own feelings about exercise participation.

_____

_____

_____

_____

_____

_____

_____

_____

_____

© Paul Barton/CORBIS

CHAPTER 2

Assessment of Physical Fitness

OBJECTIVES

- Identify the health-related components of physical fitness.
- Be able to assess cardiorespiratory fitness.
- Understand the difference between muscular strength and muscular endurance.
- Learn to assess muscular strength fitness.
- Be able to assess muscular flexibility.
- Understand the components of body composition.
- Be able to assess body composition.
- Learn to determine recommended body weight.
- Learn to assess disease risk based on Body Mass Index (BMI) and waist circumference.

This chapter covers the health-related components of physical fitness—cardiorespiratory endurance, muscular strength and endurance, muscular flexibility, and body composition, along with basic techniques frequently used to assess these components. This information will help you determine your level of physical fitness regularly as you engage in an exercise program. Fitness testing in a comprehensive program is important to

1. Educate yourself regarding the various fitness components.
2. Assess your fitness level for each health-related fitness component and compare the results to health fitness and physical fitness standards.
3. Identify areas of weakness for training emphasis.
4. Motivate you to participate in exercise.
5. Use as a starting point for your personalized exercise prescriptions.
6. Evaluate the progress and effectiveness of your program.
7. Make adjustments in your exercise prescription, if necessary.
8. Reward yourself for complying with your exercise program (although a change to a higher fitness level is a reward in and of itself).

You are encouraged to conduct at least pre- and post-exercise program fitness tests. A personal fitness profile is provided in Activity 2.1, page 49, for you to record the results of each fitness test in this chapter (pre-test). At the end of the term, you can use the back of Activity

Test your cardiorespiratory endurance by participating in the activities on your CD-ROM.

An exercise tolerance test with 12-lead electrocardiographic monitoring (stress ECG) may be required of some individuals prior to participation in exercise.

2.1, page 50, to record the results of your post-test. You also may choose to use the computer software available with this textbook.

In Chapter 3 you will write personal fitness goals for this course (see Activity 3.4, pages 83–86). You should base these goals on the actual results of your initial fitness assessments. As you proceed with your exercise program, you should allow a minimum of 8 weeks before doing your post-fitness assessments.

As discussed in Chapter 1, exercise testing or exercise participation is not advised for individuals with certain medical or physical conditions. Therefore, before starting an exercise program or participating in any exercise testing, you should fill out the Clearance for Exercise Participation questionnaire given in Chapter 1, Activity 1.2, page 23. A "yes" answer to any of the questions suggests that you consult a physician before initiating, continuing, or increasing your level of physical activity.

Responders Versus Nonresponders

Individuals who follow similar training programs show a wide variation in physiological responses. Heredity plays a crucial role in how each person responds to and improves after beginning an exercise program. Several studies have documented that following exercise training, most individuals, called **responders**, readily show improvements, but a few, **nonresponders**, exhibit small or no improvements at all. This concept is referred to as the **principle of individuality**.

After several months of aerobic training, VO_{2max} increases are between 15 and 20 percent on the average, although individual responses can range from 0 percent (in a few selected cases) to more than 50 percent improvement, even when all participants follow exactly the same training program. Non-fitness and low-fitness participants, however, should not label themselves nonresponders based the previous discussion. Nonresponders constitute less than 5 percent of exercise participants. Although additional research is necessary, lack of improvement in cardiorespiratory endurance among nonresponders might be related to low levels of leg strength. A lower body strength-training program has been shown to help these individuals improve VO_{2max} through aerobic exercise.[1]

Following assessment of cardiorespiratory fitness, if your fitness level is less than adequate, do not let that discourage you, but make it a priority to be physically active every day. In addition to regular exercise; lifestyle behaviors such as walking, taking stairs, cycling to work, parking farther from the office, doing household tasks, gardening, and doing yardwork provide substantial benefits. In this regard, monitoring daily physical activity and exercise habits should be used in conjunction with fitness testing to evaluate compliance among nonresponders. After all, it is through increased daily activity that we reap the health benefits that improve quality of life.

Fitness Assessment Battery

No single test can provide a complete measure of physical fitness. Because health-related fitness has four components, a battery of tests is necessary to determine an individual's overall level of fitness. In the next few pages are descriptions of several tests used to assess the health-related fitness components. When interpreting the results of fitness tests, you can apply either of two standards: health fitness and physical fitness.

Health Fitness Standard

As illustrated in Figure 2.1, although fitness (defined as VO_{2max}—see discussion of cardiorespiratory endurance on page 28) improvements with a moderate aerobic activity program are not as notable, significant health benefits are reaped with such a program. These health improvements are quite striking, and only slightly greater benefits are obtained through a more intense exercise program. Health benefits include a reduction in blood lipids, lower blood pressure, weight loss, stress release, and lower risk for diabetes, other diseases, and premature mortality.

FIGURE **2.1** Health and fitness benefits based on type of lifestyle and physical activity program.

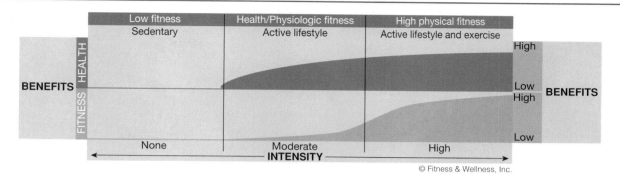

© Fitness & Wellness, Inc.

More specifically, improvements in the **metabolic profile** (better insulin sensitivity and glucose tolerance and improved cholesterol levels) can be notable in spite of little or no improvement in aerobic capacity or weight loss. These improvements in the metabolic profile through an active lifestyle and moderate physical activity are referred to as **metabolic fitness**.

The health fitness or criterion-referenced standards used in this book are based on epidemiological data linking minimum fitness values to disease prevention and better health. Attaining the **health fitness standards** requires only moderate amounts of physical activity. For example, a 2-mile walk in less than 30 minutes, five to six times per week, seems to be sufficient to achieve the health fitness standard for cardiorespiratory endurance.

Physical Fitness Standard

The **physical fitness standard** is set higher than the health fitness standard and requires a more vigorous exercise program. Physically fit people of all ages have the freedom to enjoy most of life's daily and recreational activities to their fullest potential. Current health fitness standards may not be enough to achieve these objectives.

Sound physical fitness gives the individual a level of independence throughout life that many people no longer enjoy. Most older people should be able to carry out activities similar to those they conducted in their youth, though not with the same intensity. Although a person does not have to be an elite athlete, activities such as changing a tire, chopping wood, climbing several flights of stairs, playing a game of basketball, mountain biking, playing soccer with grandchildren, walking several miles around a lake, and hiking through a national park require more than the "average fitness" level of the American people.

If the main objective of the fitness program is to lower the risk for disease, attaining the health fitness standards may be enough to ensure better health. But if the individual wants to participate in moderate to vigorous fitness activities, achieving a high physical fitness standard is recommended. For the purposes of this book, both health fitness and physical fitness standards are given for each fitness test. You will have to decide your personal objectives for the fitness program.

Cardiorespiratory Endurance

As a person breathes, part of the oxygen in the air is taken up in the lungs and transported in the blood to the heart. The heart then pumps the oxygenated blood through the circulatory system to all organs and tissues of the body. At the cellular level, oxygen is used to

KEY TERMS

Responders Individuals who exhibit improvements in fitness as a result of exercise training.

Nonresponders Individuals who exhibit small or no improvements in fitness compared with others who undergo the same training program.

Principle of individuality Training concept that genetics plays a major role in individual responses to exercise training and these differences should be considered when designing exercise programs for different people.

Metabolic profile Result of the assessment of diabetes and cardiovascular disease risk through plasma insulin, glucose, lipid, and lipoprotein levels.

Metabolic fitness Improvements in the metabolic profile through a moderate-intensity exercise program in spite of little or no improvement in health-related fitness components.

Health fitness standard The lowest fitness requirements for maintaining good health, decreasing the risk for chronic diseases, and lowering the incidence of muscular-skeletal injuries.

Physical fitness standard Required criteria to achieve a high level of physical fitness; ability to do moderate to vigorous physical activity without undue fatigue.

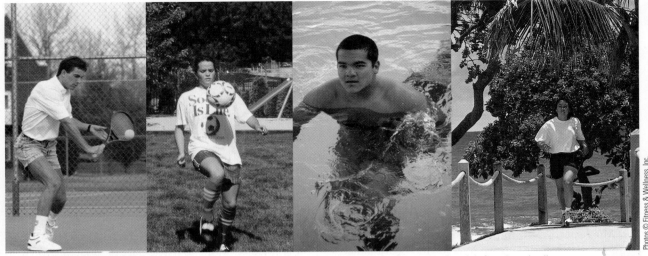

Aerobic activities promote cardiorespiratory development and help decrease the risk for chronic diseases.

Photos © Fitness & Wellness, Inc.

convert food substrates, primarily carbohydrates and fats, into the energy necessary to conduct body functions, maintain a constant internal equilibrium, and perform physical tasks.

Some examples of activities that promote **cardiorespiratory endurance**, or aerobic fitness, are walking, jogging, cycling, rowing, swimming, cross-country skiing, aerobic dance, soccer, basketball, and racquetball. Guidelines to develop a lifetime cardiorespiratory endurance exercise program are given in Chapter 3, and an introduction and description of benefits of leading aerobic activities are given in Chapter 4.

A sound cardiorespiratory endurance program contributes greatly to good health. The typical American is not exactly a good role model in terms of cardiorespiratory fitness. A poorly conditioned heart that has to pump more often just to keep a person alive is subject to more wear-and-tear than is a well-conditioned heart. In situations that place strenuous demands on the heart, such as doing yardwork, lifting heavy objects or weights, or running to catch a bus, the unconditioned heart may not be able to sustain the strain.

Everyone who initiates a cardiorespiratory exercise program can expect a number of benefits from training. Among these are lower resting heart rate, blood pressure, blood lipids (cholesterol and triglycerides), recovery time following exercise, and risk for hypokinetic diseases (those associated with physical inactivity and sedentary living). Simultaneously, cardiac muscle strength and oxygen-carrying capacity increase.

Cardiorespiratory endurance is determined by the **maximal oxygen uptake** or VO_{2max}, the maximum amount of oxygen the human body is able to utilize per minute of physical activity. This value can be expressed in liters per minute (l/min) or milliliters per kilogram (2.2 pounds) of body weight per minute (ml/kg/min). The relative value in ml/kg/min is used most often because it considers total body mass (weight) in kilograms. When comparing two individuals with the same absolute value, the one with the lesser body mass will have a higher relative value, indicating that more oxygen is available to each kilogram (2.2 pounds) of body weight. Because all tissues and organs of the body need oxygen to function, higher oxygen consumption indicates a more efficient cardiorespiratory system.

CT   Critical Thinking

Your relative maximal oxygen uptake can be improved without engaging in an aerobic exercise program. How can you accomplish this, and would you benefit from doing so?

Physical exertion requires more energy to perform the activity. As a result, the heart, lungs, and blood vessels have to deliver more oxygen to the cells to supply the required energy. During prolonged exercise, an individual with a high level of cardiorespiratory endurance is able to deliver the required amount of oxygen to the tissues with relative ease. The cardiorespiratory system of a person with a low level of endurance has to work much harder, because the heart has to pump more often to supply the same amount of oxygen to the tissues, and consequently fatigues faster. Hence, a higher capacity to deliver and utilize oxygen (oxygen uptake) indicates a more efficient cardiorespiratory system.

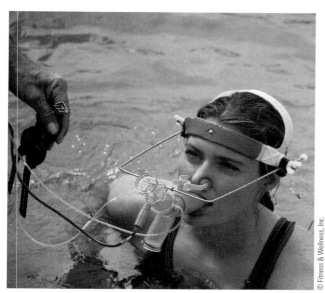

Maximal oxygen uptake (VO₂max) can be determined through direct gas analysis as shown during a water aerobics exercise test.

Absolute oxygen uptake, expressed in l/min, is valuable in determining the caloric expenditure of physical activity. The human body burns about 5 calories for each liter of oxygen consumed and oxygen uptake ranges from about .3 to .5 l/min during resting conditions to over 5 l/min during maximal exercise. During aerobic exercise, the average person trains at between 50 and 75 percent of maximal oxygen uptake.

A person with a maximal absolute oxygen uptake of 3.5 l/min who trains at 60 percent of maximum uses 2.1 (3.5 × .60) liters of oxygen per minute of physical activity. At 5 calories per liter, this indicates that 10.5 calories are burned during each minute of exercise (2.1 × 5). If the activity is carried out for 30 minutes, 315 calories (10.5 × .30) have been burned. Because a pound of body fat represents 3,500 calories, the previous example indicates that this individual would have to exercise for a total of 333 minutes (3,500 ÷ 10.5) to burn the equivalent of a pound of body fat. At 30 minutes per exercise session, approximately 11 sessions would be required to expend the 3,500 calories.

Assessing Cardiorespiratory Endurance

Even though most cardiorespiratory endurance tests probably are safe to administer to apparently healthy individuals (those with no major coronary risk factors or symptoms), the American College of Sports Medicine recommends that a physician be present for all maximal exercise tests on apparently healthy men over age 45 and women over age 55.[2]

A maximal test is any test that requires the participant's all-out or nearly all-out effort, such as the 1.5-Mile Run Test or a maximal exercise treadmill test (stress electrocardiogram). For submaximal exercise tests (such as a walking test), a physician should be present when testing higher-risk and symptomatic individuals and people with medical conditions, regardless of age.

1.5-Mile Run Test

The test used most often to determine cardiorespiratory endurance is the 1.5-Mile Run Test. The fitness category is determined according to the time a person takes to run or walk a 1.5-mile course. The only equipment necessary to conduct this test is a stopwatch and a track or a premeasured 1.5-mile course.

Although the 1.5-Mile Run Test is quite simple to administer, a note of caution is in order: Given that the objective is to cover the distance in the shortest time, it is considered a maximal exercise test. The 1.5-Mile Run Test should be limited to conditioned individuals who have been cleared for exercise. It is not recommended for unconditioned beginners, symptomatic individuals, those with known cardiovascular disease or risk factors for heart disease, men over age 45, or women over age 55. Unconditioned beginners are encouraged to have at least 6 weeks of aerobic training before they take the test.

Prior to taking the 1.5-Mile Run Test, you should do a few warm-up exercises—mild stretching exercises, some walking, and slow jogging. Next, time yourself during the 1.5-Mile Run to see how fast you cover the distance. If you notice any unusual symptoms during the test, do not continue. Stop immediately and see your physician or retake the test after another 6 weeks of aerobic training. At the end of the test, cool down by walking or jogging slowly for another 3 to 5 minutes. Use your performance time to look up your estimated VO₂max in Table 2.1 and the corresponding fitness category in Table 2.2.

For example, a 20-year-old male runs the 1.5-mile course in 10 minutes and 20 seconds. Table 2.1 shows a VO₂max of 49.5 ml/kg/min for a time of 10:20. According to Table 2.2, this VO₂max places him in the good cardiorespiratory fitness category.

KEY TERMS

Cardiorespiratory endurance Ability of the lungs, heart, and blood vessels to deliver adequate amounts of oxygen to the cells to meet the demands of prolonged physical activity.

Maximal oxygen uptake (VO₂max) Maximum amount of oxygen the human body is able to utilize per minute of physical activity.

© Fitness & Wellness, Inc.

TABLE 2.1 Estimated Maximal Oxygen Uptake (in ml/kg/min) for 1.5-Mile Run Test

TIME	VO_{2max}	TIME	VO_{2max}	TIME	VO_{2max}
6:10	80.0	10:30	48.6	14:50	34.0
6:20	79.0	10:40	48.0	15:00	33.6
6:30	77.9	10:50	47.4	15:10	33.1
6:40	76.7	11:00	46.6	15:20	32.7
6:50	75.5	11:10	45.8	15:30	32.2
7:00	74.0	11:20	45.1	15:40	31.8
7:10	72.6	11:30	44.4	15:50	31.4
7:20	71.3	11:40	43.7	16:00	30.9
7:30	69.9	11:50	43.2	16:10	30.5
7:40	68.3	12:00	42.0	16:20	30.2
7:50	66.8	12:10	41.7	16:30	29.8
8:00	65.2	12:20	41.0	16:40	29.5
8:10	63.9	12:30	40.4	16:50	29.1
8:20	62.5	12:40	39.8	17:00	28.9
8:30	61.2	12:50	39.2	17:10	28.5
8:40	60.2	13:00	38.6	17:20	28.3
8:50	59.1	13:10	38.1	17:30	28.0
9:00	58.1	13:20	37.8	17:40	27.7
9:10	56.9	13:30	37.2	17:50	27.4
9:20	55.9	13:40	36.8	18:00	27.1
9:30	54.7	13:50	36.3	18:10	26.8
9:40	53.5	14:00	35.9	18:20	26.6
9:50	52.3	14:10	35.5	18:30	26.3
10:00	51.1	14:20	35.1	18:40	26.0
10:10	50.4	14:30	34.7	18:50	25.7
10:20	49.5	14:40	34.3	19:00	25.4

Adapted from "A Means of Assessing Maximal Oxygen Intake," by K. H. Cooper, *Journal of the American Medical Association*, 203 (1968), 201–204; *Health and Fitness Through Physical Activity*, by M. L. Pollock (New York: John Wiley and Sons, 1978); and *Training for Sport Activity*, by J. H. Wilmore (Boston: Allyn & Bacon, 1982).

1.0-Mile Walk Test*

The 1.0-Mile Walk Test calls for a 440-yard track (four laps to a mile) or a premeasured 1.0-mile course. Body weight in pounds must be determined prior to the walk. A stopwatch is required to measure total walking time and exercise heart rate.

You can proceed to walk the 1-mile course at a brisk pace so your exercise heart rate at the end of the test is above 120 beats per minute. At the end of the 1.0-mile walk, check your walking time and immediately count your pulse for 10 seconds. You can take your pulse on the wrist by placing two fingers over the radial artery (inside of the wrist on the side of the thumb) or over the carotid artery in the neck just below the jaw next to the voice box, as shown above.

Next, multiply the 10-second pulse count by 6 to obtain the exercise heart rate in beats per minute. Now convert the walking time from minutes and seconds to decimal-based minute units. Each minute has 60 seconds, so the seconds are divided by 60 to obtain the decimal fraction of a minute. For instance, a walking time of 12 minutes and 15 seconds equals $12 + (15 \div 60)$, or 12.25 minutes. To obtain the estimated VO_{2max} in ml/kg/min for the 1.0-Mile Walk Test, plug your values into the following equation:

$$VO_{2max} = 88.768 - (0.0957 \times W) + (8.892 \times G) - (1.4537 \times T) - (0.1194 \times HR)$$

---

* Source: "Validation of the Rockport Fitness Walking Test in College Males and Females," by F. A. Dolgener, L. D. Hensley, J. J. Marsh, and J. K. Fjelstul, *Research Quarterly for Exercise and Sport*, 65 (1994), 152–158.

TABLE 2.2 Cardiorespiratory Fitness Category According to Maximal Oxygen Uptake (in ml/kg/min)

GENDER	AGE	FITNESS CATEGORY				
		POOR	FAIR	AVERAGE	GOOD	EXCELLENT
MEN	≤29	≤24.9	25–33.9	34–43.9	44–52.9	≥53
	30–39	≤22.9	23–30.9	31–41.9	42–49.9	≥50
	40–49	≤19.9	20–26.9	27–38.9	39–44.9	≥45
	50–59	≤17.9	18–24.9	25–37.9	38–42.9	≥43
	60–69	≤15.9	16–22.9	23–35.9	36–40.9	≥41
WOMEN	≤29	≤23.9	24–30.9	31–38.9	39–48.9	≥49
	30–39	≤19.9	20–27.9	28–36.9	37–44.9	≥45
	40–49	≤16.9	17–24.9	25–34.9	35–41.9	≥42
	50–59	≤14.9	15–21.9	22–33.9	34–39.9	≥40
	60–69	≤12.9	13–20.9	21–32.9	33–36.9	≥37

▨ Health fitness or criterion-referenced standard
▨ High physical fitness standard

Taking the pulse at the radial artery.

Taking the pulse at the carotid artery.

where:

W = weight in pounds
G = gender (use 0 for women and 1 for men)
T = total time for the mile walk in minutes
HR = exercise heart rate in beats per minute at the end of the mile walk

For example, a woman who weighs 140 pounds completed the mile walk in 14 minutes and 39 seconds with an exercise heart rate of 148 beats per minute. The estimated VO_{2max} is:

W = 140 lbs
G = 0 (female gender = 0)
T = 14:39 = 14 + (39 ÷ 60) = 14.65 min
HR = 148 bpm
VO_{2max} = 88.768 − (0.0957 × 140) + (8.892 × 0)
     − (1.4537 × 14.65) − (0.1194 × 148)
VO_{2max} = 36.4 ml/kg/min

As with the 1.5-Mile Run Test, the fitness categories based on VO_{2max} are found in Table 2.2. Record your cardiorespiratory fitness test results on your fitness profile in Activity 2.1, Pre-Test, page 49.

Muscular Strength and Endurance

Many people are under the impression that muscular strength and endurance are necessary only for athletes and those whose jobs require heavy muscular work. Actually, strength and endurance are important components of total physical fitness and have been shown to be essential to everyone.

Adequate levels of strength enhance a person's health and well-being throughout life. Strength is crucial for top performance in daily activities such as sitting, walking, running, lifting and carrying objects, doing housework, and even enjoying recreational activities. Strength is also valuable in improving personal appearance and self-image, developing sports skills, and meeting

certain emergencies in life in which strength is necessary to cope effectively.

Muscular strength also seems to be the most important health-related component of physical fitness in the older adult population. Whereas proper cardiorespiratory endurance helps maintain a healthy heart, good strength levels do more to promote independent living than any other fitness component. More than anything else, older adults want to enjoy good health and function independently. Many, however, are confined to nursing homes because they lack sufficient strength to move about. They usually cannot walk very far, and some have to be helped in and out of beds, chairs, and tubs.

A strength-training program can have a tremendous impact on quality of life. Research has shown leg strength improvements as high as 200 percent in previously inactive adults over age 90.[3] As strength improves, so does the ability to move about, the capacity for independent living, and life enjoyment during the "golden years." More specifically, good strength enhances quality of life in the following ways:

- It increases lean (muscle) tissue.
- It helps increase and maintain **resting metabolism**.
- It improves balance and restores mobility.
- It makes lifting and reaching easier.
- It decreases the risk for injuries and falls.
- It stresses the bones, thus preserving bone density, and decreasing the risk for osteoporosis.

Muscular Strength and Muscular Endurance

Although **muscular strength** and **muscular endurance** are interrelated, the two have a basic difference. Muscular strength is the ability to exert maximum force against resistance. Muscular endurance (also called localized muscular endurance) is the ability of the muscle to exert submaximal force repeatedly over a period of time. Muscular endurance depends to a large extent on muscular strength and to a lesser extent on cardiorespiratory endurance. Weak muscles cannot repeat an action several times or sustain it for long. Keeping these concepts in mind, strength tests and training

KEY TERMS

Resting metabolism The energy required to maintain the body's vital processes in the resting state.

Muscular strength Ability to exert maximum force against resistance.

Muscular endurance Ability of a muscle to exert submaximal force repeatedly over a period of time.

programs have been designed to measure and develop absolute muscular strength, muscular endurance, or a combination of the two.

Determining Strength

Muscular strength usually is determined using the **one repetition maximum (1 RM)** technique. Although this assessment gives a good measure of absolute strength, it does require a considerable amount of time to administer. Muscular endurance commonly is established by the number of repetitions an individual can perform against a submaximal resistance or by the length of time a person can sustain a given contraction.

Muscular Endurance Test

We live in a world in which muscular strength and endurance are both required, and muscular endurance depends to a large extent on muscular strength. Accordingly, a muscular endurance test that uses three exercises to assess the upper body, lower body, and mid-body muscle groups have been selected to determine your level of strength. To perform the test, you will need a stopwatch, a metronome, a bench or gymnasium bleacher 16¼" high, and a partner.

The exercises conducted for this test are the Bench Jump, Modified Dip (men) or Modified Push-Up (women), and Bent-Leg Curl-Up. Individuals who are susceptible to low-back injury may do the Abdominal Crunch instead of the Bent-Leg Curl-Up test (see discussion on page 33). All tests should be conducted with the aid of a partner. The correct procedures for performing these exercises follow.

Bench Jump

For the Bench Jump, use a bench or gymnasium bleacher 16¼" high, and attempt to jump up onto and down off of the bench as many times as you can in 1 minute. If you cannot jump the full minute, step up and down. A repetition is counted each time both feet return to the floor.

Modified Dip

The Modified Dip is an upper-body exercise that is done by men only. Using a bench or gymnasium bleacher, place your hands on the bench with the fingers pointing forward. Have a partner hold your feet in front of you. Bend your hips at approximately 90 degrees (you also may use three sturdy chairs; put your hands on two chairs placed by the sides of your body and your feet on the third chair in front of you).

Bench jump.

Modified-Dip.

Next, lower your body by flexing your elbows until you reach a 90 degree angle at this joint, and then return to the starting position. The repetition does not count if you fail to reach 90 degrees. Perform the repetitions to a two-step cadence (down–up), regulated with a metronome set at 56 beats per minute. Perform as many continuous repetitions as possible. If you fail to follow the metronome cadence, you no longer can count the repetitions.

Modified Push-Up

Women perform the Modified Push-Up instead of the Modified Dip. Lie down on the floor (face down), bend your knees (feet up in the air), and place your hands on the floor by your shoulders with the fingers pointing forward. Your lower body will be supported at the knees (rather than the feet) throughout the test. Your chest must touch the floor on each repetition.

Perform the repetitions to a two-step cadence (up–down) regulated with a metronome set at 56 beats per minute. Do as many continuous repetitions as possible. If you fail to follow the metronome cadence, you cannot count any more repetitions.

Modified push-up.

© Fitness & Wellness, Inc.

Bent-Leg Curl-Up

For the Bent-Leg Curl-Up, lie down on the floor, face up, and bend both legs at the knees at approximately 100 degrees. Your feet should be on the floor, and you must hold them in place yourself throughout the test. Cross your arms in front of your chest, each hand on the opposite shoulder.

Now raise your head off the floor, placing your chin against your chest. This is the starting and finishing position for each curl-up. The back of the head may not come in contact with the floor; the hands cannot be removed from the shoulders; and neither the feet nor the hips can be raised off the floor at any time during the test. The test is terminated if any of these four conditions occur. When you curl up, your upper body must come to an upright position before going back down. The repetitions are performed to a two-step cadence (up–down) regulated with the metronome set at 40 beats per minute.

For this exercise you should allow a brief practice period of 5 to 10 seconds to familiarize yourself with the cadence (the up movement is initiated with the first beat, then you must wait for the next beat to initiate the down movement; one repetition is accomplished every two beats of the metronome). Count as many repetitions as you are able to perform following the proper cadence. The test is terminated if you fail to maintain the appropriate cadence or if you accomplish 100 repetitions. Have your partner check the angle at the knees throughout the test to make sure that you maintain the 100 degree angle as closely as possible.

Abdominal Crunch

The Abdominal Crunch is recommended only for individuals who are unable to perform the Bent-Leg Curl-Up because of susceptibility to low-back injury. Exercise form must be monitored carefully during the test.

Several authors and researchers[4] have indicated that participants have difficulty maintaining proper form during this test. They often slide their bodies, bend their

Bent-leg Curl-up.

Photos © Fitness & Wellness, Inc.

elbows, or shrug their shoulders during the test. These actions make the test easier and misrepresent performance. Biomechanical factors also limit the ability to perform this test.[5] Further, lack of spinal flexibility does not allow some individuals to move the required (3½") range of motion.[6] Others are unable to keep their heels on the floor during the test. Some research has questioned the validity of this test as an effective measure of abdominal strength or abdominal endurance.[7] With these caveats in mind, the procedure is as follows.

Tape a 3½" × 30" strip of cardboard onto the floor. Lie on the floor in a supine position (face up) with your knees bent at approximately 100 degrees and your legs slightly apart. Your feet should be on the floor, and you must hold them in place yourself throughout the test. Straighten your arms, and place them on the floor alongside your trunk with your palms down and fingers fully extended. The fingertips of both hands should barely touch the closest edge of the cardboard.

Bring your head off the floor until your chin is 1" to 2" away from your chest. Keep your head in this position during the entire test. (Do not move your head by flexing or extending the neck.) You now are ready to begin the test.

Perform the repetitions to a two-step cadence (up–down) regulated with a metronome set at 60 beats per

KEY TERMS

One repetition maximum (1 RM) The maximal amount of resistance a person is able to lift in a single effort.

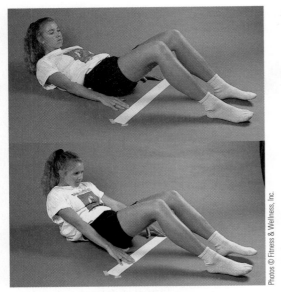

Photos © Fitness & Wellness, Inc.

Abdominal Crunch.

Photos © Fitness & Wellness, Inc.

Abdominal Crunch test using a
Crunch-Ster Curl-Up Tester.

minute. As you curl up, slide your fingers over the cardboard until your fingertips reach the far end (3½") of the board, then return to the starting position.

Allow a brief practice period of 5 to 10 seconds to familiarize yourself with the cadence. Initiate the up movement with the first beat and the down movement with the next beat. Accomplish one repetition every two beats of the metronome. Count as many repetitions as you are able to perform while following the proper cadence. You may not count a repetition if your fingertips fail to reach the distant end of the cardboard.

Terminate the test if you: (a) fail to maintain the appropriate cadence, (b) bend your elbows, (c) shrug your shoulders, (d) slide your body, (e) fail to keep your heels on the floor, (f) do not keep your chin close to your chest, (g) accomplish 100 repetitions, or (h) can no longer perform the test. Have your partner check the angle at the knees throughout the test to make sure you maintain the 100-degree angle as closely as possible. For this test, you also may use a Crunch-Ster Curl-Up Tester, available from Novel Products.*

Interpreting the Strength Test

According to the number of repetitions you performed on each test item, look up the percentile rank for each exercise in the far left column of Table 2.3. Based on your percentile ranks, you can determine your muscular endurance fitness category for each exercise using the guidelines provided in Table 2.4. Look up the number

*Novel Products, Inc., Figure Finder Collection, PO Box 408, Rockton, IL 61072-0408; 1-800-323-5143.

TABLE 2.3 Muscular Endurance Scoring Table

| | MEN | | | |
PERCENTILE RANK	BENCH JUMPS	MODIFIED DIPS	BENT-LEG CURL-UPS	ABDOMINAL CRUNCHES
99	66	54	100	100
95	63	50	81	100
90	62	38	65	100
80	58	32	51	66
70	57	30	44	45
60	56	27	31	38
50	54	26	28	33
40	51	23	25	29
30	48	20	22	26
20	47	17	17	22
10	40	11	10	18
5	34	7	3	16

| | WOMEN | | | |
PERCENTILE RANK	BENCH JUMPS	MODIFIED PUSH-UPS	BENT-LEG CURL-UPS	ABDOMINAL CRUNCHES
99	58	95	100	100
95	54	70	100	100
90	52	50	97	69
80	48	41	77	49
70	44	38	57	37
60	42	33	45	34
50	39	30	37	31
40	38	28	28	27
30	36	25	22	24
20	32	21	17	21
10	28	18	9	15
5	26	15	4	0

▮ High physical fitness standard   ▮ Health fitness standard

TABLE **2.4** Fitness Categories Based on Percentile Ranks

PERCENTILE RANK	FITNESS CATEGORY	POINTS
≥90	Excellent	5
70–80	Good	4
50–60	Average	3
30–40	Fair	2
≤20	Poor	1

TABLE **2.5** Muscular Strength/Endurance Fitness Categories by Total Points

TOTAL POINTS	STRENGTH ENDURANCE CATEGORY
≥13	Excellent
10–12	Good
7–9	Average
4–6	Fair
≤3	Poor

of points assigned for each fitness category in Table 2.4. Now total the points and determine your overall strength endurance fitness category according to the ratings provided in Table 2.5.

Record the results of your strength tests in Activity 2.1, Pre-Test, page 49.

Muscular Flexibility

Flexibility refers to the achievable range of motion at a joint or group of joints without causing injury. Most people who exercise don't take the time to stretch. And many of those who do stretch don't stretch properly. When joints are not regularly moved through their normal range of motion, muscles and ligaments shorten in time, and flexibility decreases.

Developing and maintaining some level of flexibility are important factors in all health enhancement programs—and even more so as we age. Good flexibility promotes healthy muscles and joints. Sportsmedicine specialists say that many muscular/skeletal problems and injuries, especially in adults, are related to a lack of flexibility. At times in daily life, we have to make rapid or strenuous movements we are not accustomed to making. Abruptly forcing a tight muscle beyond its normal range of motion often leads to injuries.

Improving elasticity of muscles and connective tissue around joints enables greater freedom of movement and increases the individual's ability to participate in many types of sports and recreational activities. Adequate flexibility also makes activities of daily living, such as turning, lifting, and bending much easier to perform. A person must take care, however, not to overstretch joints. Too much flexibility leads to unstable and loose joints, which may actually increase injury rate.

A decline in flexibility can cause poor posture and subsequent aches and pains that lead to limited movement of joints. Inordinate tightness is uncomfortable and debilitating. Approximately 80 percent of all low-back problems in the United States stem from improper alignment of the vertebral column and pelvic girdle, a direct result of inflexible and weak muscles. This backache syndrome costs U. S. industry billions of dollars each year in health services, lost productivity, and worker compensation.

Muscular flexibility is highly specific and varies from one joint to the other (hip, trunk, shoulder), as well as from one individual to the next. Muscular flexibility relates primarily to genetic factors and the index of physical activity. Beyond that, factors such as joint structure, ligaments, tendons, muscles, skin, tissue injury, adipose (fat) tissue, body temperature, age, and gender influence the range of motion about a joint.

On the average, women are more flexible than men and seem to retain this advantage throughout life. Aging decreases the extensibility of soft tissue, decreasing flexibility in both genders. The most significant contributors to loss of flexibility, however, are sedentary living and lack of physical activity.

Most experts agree that participating in a regular flexibility program has the following benefits:

- It helps to maintain good joint mobility.
- It increases resistance to muscle injury and soreness.
- It prevents low-back and other spinal column problems.
- It improves and maintains good postural alignment.
- It enhances proper and graceful body movement.
- It improves personal appearance and self-image.
- It facilitates the development of motor skills throughout life.

Flexibility exercises also have been prescribed successfully to treat **dysmenorrhea**[8] (painful menstruation) and general neuromuscular tension (stress). Regular **stretching** helps decrease the aches and pains caused

KEY TERMS

Flexibility The achievable range of motion at a joint or group of joints without causing injury.

Dysmenorrhea Painful menstruation.

Stretching Moving the joints beyond the accustomed range of motion.

by psychological stress and contributes to a decrease in anxiety, blood pressure, and breathing rate.[9]

Further, mild stretching exercises, in conjunction with calisthenics, are helpful in warm-up routines to prepare the body for more vigorous aerobic or strength-training exercises, and as cool-down routines following exercise to help the person return to a normal resting state. Fatigued muscles tend to contract to a shorter-than-average resting length, and stretching exercises help fatigued muscles reestablish their normal resting length.

Similar to muscular strength, good range of motion is critical in older life. Because of decreased flexibility, older adults lose mobility and are unable to perform simple daily tasks such as bending forward and turning. Many older adults do not turn their head or rotate their trunk to look over their shoulder but, rather, step around 90 degrees to 180 degrees to see behind them.

Physical activity and exercise also can be hampered severely by restricted range of motion. Because of the pain involved during activity, older people who have tight hip flexors (muscles) cannot jog or walk very far. A vicious circle ensues, because the condition usually worsens with further inactivity. A simple stretching program can alleviate or prevent this problem and help people return to an exercise program.

Assessing Flexibility

Two flexibility tests are used to produce a flexibility profile: the Modified Sit-and-Reach Test and the Total Body Rotation Test.

Modified Sit-and-Reach Test

To perform the Modified Sit-and-Reach Test, you will need the Acuflex I* sit-and-reach flexibility tester, or you may simply place a yardstick on top of a box approximately 12" high. To administer this test:

1. Warm up properly before the first trial.
2. Remove your shoes for the test. Sit on the floor with your hips, back, and head against a wall, legs fully extended, and the bottom of your feet against the Acuflex I or the sit-and-reach box.
3. Place your hands one on top of the other, and reach forward as far as possible without letting your hips, back, or head come off the wall.
4. Another person then should slide the reach indicator on the Acuflex I (or yardstick) along the top of the box until the end of the indicator touches the tips

Starting position for Modified Sit-and-Reach Test.

Modified Sit-and-Reach Test.

of your fingers. The indicator then must be held firmly in place throughout the rest of the test.

5. Your head and back now can come off the wall, and you may reach forward gradually three times, the third time stretching forward as far as possible on the indicator (or yardstick) and holding the final position at least 2 seconds. Be sure to keep the back of your knees against the floor throughout the test.
6. Record to the nearest half-inch the final number of inches you reached.
7. You are allowed two trials, and an average of the two scores is used as the final test score.

The percentile ranks and fitness categories for this test are given in Tables 2.6 and 2.4, respectively.

Total Body Rotation Test

An Acuflex II total body rotation flexibility tester or a measuring scale with a sliding panel is needed to administer the Total Body Rotation Test. The Acuflex II or scale is placed on the wall at shoulder height and should

*The Acuflex I and II flexibility testers for the Modified Sit-and-Reach and the Total Body Rotation tests can be obtained from Novel Products, Inc., Figure Finder Collection, PO Box 408, Rockton, IL 61072-0408; 1-800-323-5143.

TABLE 2.6 Modified Sit-and-Reach Scoring Table

MEN						WOMEN					
PERCENTILE RANK	AGE CATEGORY				FITNESS CATEGORY	PERCENTILE RANK	AGE CATEGORY				FITNESS CATEGORY
	<18	19–35	36–49	>50			<18	19–35	36–49	>50	
99	20.8	20.1	18.9	16.2		99	22.6	21.0	19.8	17.2	
95	19.6	18.9	18.2	15.8	Excellent	95	19.5	19.3	19.2	15.7	Excellent
90	18.2	17.2	16.1	15.0		90	18.7	17.9	17.4	15.0	
80	17.8	17.0	14.6	13.3	Good	80	17.8	16.7	16.2	14.2	Good
70	16.0	15.8	13.9	12.3		70	16.5	16.2	15.2	13.6	
60	15.2	15.0	13.4	11.5	Average	60	16.0	15.8	14.5	12.3	Average
50	14.5	14.4	12.6	10.2		50	15.2	14.8	13.5	11.1	
40	14.0	13.5	11.6	9.7	Fair	40	14.5	14.5	12.8	10.1	Fair
30	13.4	13.0	10.8	9.3		30	13.7	13.7	12.2	9.2	
20	11.8	11.6	9.9	8.8		20	12.6	12.6	11.0	8.3	
10	9.5	9.2	8.3	7.8	Poor	10	11.4	10.1	9.7	7.5	Poor
5	8.4	7.9	7.0	7.2		5	9.4	8.1	8.5	3.7	
1	7.2	7.0	5.1	4.0		1	6.5	2.6	2.0	1.5	

▓ High physical fitness standard

▓ Health fitness or criterion referenced standard

From *Lifetime Physical Fitness & Wellness: A Personalized Program*, by W. W. K. Hoeger (Belmont, CA: Wadsworth/Thomson Learning, 2007).

be adjustable to accommodate individual differences in height. If an Acuflex II is not available, you can build your own scale. Glue or tape one measuring tape above the sliding panel and another below it, both centered at the 15" mark. Each tape should be at least 30" long. Draw a line on the floor, centered at the 15" mark. Use the following procedure:

1. Warm up properly before beginning this test.
2. To start, stand sideways, an arm's length away from the wall, with your feet straight ahead, slightly separated, and your toes right up to the corresponding line drawn on the floor. Hold out the arm opposite the wall horizontally from the body and make a fist. The Acuflex II, measuring scale, or tapes should be shoulder height at this time.
3. Now rotate the body, the extended arm going backward (always maintaining a horizontal plane) and making contact with the panel, gradually sliding it forward as far as possible. If no panel is available, slide your fist alongside the tapes as far as possible. Hold the final position at least 2 seconds.
4. Position the hand with the little finger-side forward during the entire sliding movement. Proper hand position is crucial. Some people attempt to open the hand or push with extended fingers or slide the panel with the knuckles—none of which is acceptable. During the test you can bend your knees slightly, but you cannot move your feet; they always must point straight forward. You must keep your body as straight (vertical) as possible.

Acuflex II measuring device for Total Body Rotation Test.

Homemade measuring device for Total Body Rotation Test.

Use of measuring tapes for Total Body Rotation Test.

5. Conduct the test on either the right or the left side of the body. Two trials are allowed on the selected side. The farthest point reached, measured to the nearest half inch and held for at least 2 seconds, is recorded. The average of the two trials is the final test score.

TABLE 2.7 Total Body Rotation Scoring Table

	PERCENTILE RANK	LEFT ROTATION				RIGHT ROTATION				FITNESS CATEGORY
		AGE CATEGORY				AGE CATEGORY				
		<18	19–35	36–49	>50	<18	19–35	36–49	>50	
MEN	99	29.1	28.0	26.6	21.0	28.2	27.8	25.2	22.2	Excellent
	95	26.6	24.8	24.5	20.0	25.5	25.6	23.8	20.7	Excellent
	90	25.0	23.6	23.0	17.7	24.3	24.1	22.5	19.3	
	80	22.0	22.0	21.2	15.5	22.7	22.3	21.0	16.3	Good
	70	20.9	20.3	20.4	14.7	21.3	20.7	18.7	15.7	Good
	60	19.9	19.3	18.7	13.9	19.8	19.0	17.3	14.7	Average
	50	18.6	18.0	16.7	12.7	19.0	17.2	16.3	12.3	Average
	40	17.0	16.8	15.3	11.7	17.3	16.3	14.7	11.5	Fair
	30	14.9	15.0	14.8	10.3	15.1	15.0	13.3	10.7	Fair
	20	13.8	13.3	13.7	9.5	12.9	13.3	11.2	8.7	
	10	10.8	10.5	10.8	4.3	10.8	11.3	8.0	2.7	Poor
	05	8.5	8.9	8.8	0.3	8.1	8.3	5.5	0.3	Poor
	01	3.4	1.7	5.1	0.0	6.6	2.9	2.0	0.0	
WOMEN	99	29.3	28.6	27.1	23.0	29.6	29.4	27.1	21.7	Excellent
	95	26.8	24.8	25.3	21.4	27.6	25.3	25.9	19.7	Excellent
	90	25.5	23.0	23.4	20.5	25.8	23.0	21.3	19.0	
	80	23.8	21.5	20.2	19.1	23.7	20.8	19.6	17.9	Good
	70	21.8	20.5	18.6	17.3	22.0	19.3	17.3	16.8	Good
	60	20.5	19.3	17.7	16.0	20.8	18.0	16.5	15.6	Average
	50	19.5	18.0	16.4	14.8	19.5	17.3	14.6	14.0	Average
	40	18.5	17.2	14.8	13.7	18.3	16.0	13.1	12.8	Fair
	30	17.1	15.7	13.6	10.0	16.3	15.2	11.7	8.5	Fair
	20	16.0	15.2	11.6	6.3	14.5	14.0	9.8	3.9	
	10	12.8	13.6	8.5	3.0	12.4	11.1	6.1	2.2	Poor
	5	11.1	7.3	6.8	0.7	10.2	8.8	4.0	1.1	Poor
	1	8.9	5.3	4.3	0.0	8.9	3.2	2.8	0.0	

▓ High physical fitness standard

▓ Health fitness or criterion referenced standard

From *Lifetime Physical Fitness & Wellness: A Personalized Program*, by W. W. K. Hoeger (Belmont, CA: Wadsworth/Thomson Learning, 2007).

© Fitness & Wellness, Inc.

Total Body Rotation Test.

Proper hand position for Total Body Rotation Test.

© Fitness & Wellness, Inc.

6. Refer to Tables 2.7 and 2.4 to determine the respective percentile rank and fitness category for this test.

Interpreting Flexibility Tests

The fitness category for each flexibility test is obtained based on your percentile rank for each test, using the guidelines provided in Table 2.4. You also should look up

TABLE 2.8 Muscular Flexibility Fitness Categories by Total Points

TOTAL POINTS	FLEXIBILITY CATEGORY
≥9	Excellent
7–8	Good
5–6	Average
3–4	Fair
≤2	Poor

Good flexibility enhances the development of sports-related skills.

FIGURE 2.2 Typical body composition changes for adults in the United States.

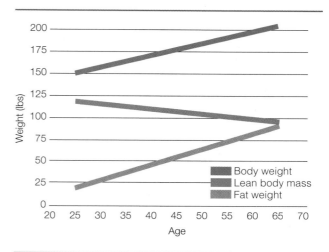

the number of points assigned for each fitness category in this table. Your overall flexibility fitness category is obtained by totaling these points and using the ratings provided in Table 2.8. Record your flexibility test results in Activity 2.1, Pre-Test, page 49.

Body Composition

Currently, starting at age 25, the average man and woman in the United States gains 1 to 2 pounds of weight per year. Thus, by age 65, the average American will have gained in excess of 40 pounds of weight. Because of the typical reduction in physical activity in our society, however, each year the average person also loses a half pound of lean tissue. Therefore, this span of 40 years has resulted in an actual fat gain of at least 60 pounds accompanied by a 20-pound loss of lean body mass[10] (see Figure 2.2). These changes cannot be detected unless body composition is assessed periodically.

Body composition refers to the fat and nonfat components of the human body. The fat component of the body usually is called fat mass or **percent body fat**. The nonfat component of the body is termed **lean body mass**.

Total fat in the human body is classified into two types: essential fat and storage fat. **Essential fat** is the body fat needed for normal physiological functions. Essential fat constitutes about 3 percent of the total weight in men and 12 percent in women (see Figure 2.3). The percentage is higher in women because it includes gender-specific fat, such as that found in the breast tissue, the uterus, and other gender-related fat deposits. Without it, human health deteriorates. **Storage fat**, the body fat stored in adipose tissue, is found mostly beneath the skin (subcutaneous fat) and around major organs in the body.

Obesity is a health hazard of epidemic proportions in the United States (Figure 2.4) and in most developed countries around the world. Obesity by itself has been associated with several serious health problems and accounts for 15 percent to 20 percent of the annual mortality rate in the United States. It is one of the six major risk factors for coronary heart disease. It also is a risk factor for other diseases of the cardiovascular system, including hypertension, congestive heart failure, elevated

KEY TERMS

Body composition The fat and nonfat components of the human body.

Percent body fat (fat mass) Fat component of the body.

Lean body mass Nonfat component of the body.

Essential fat Body fat needed for normal physiological functions.

Storage fat Body fat stored in adipose tissue.

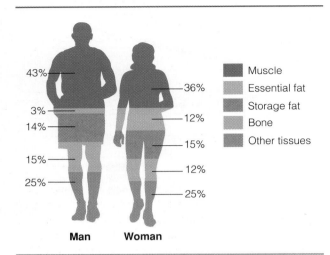

Man   **Woman**

Muscle
Essential fat
Storage fat
Bone
Other tissues

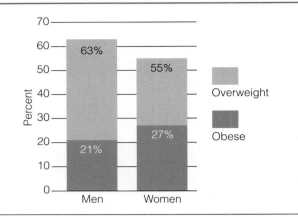

Source: "The Disease Burden Associated with Overweight and Obesity," by A. Must et al., *Journal of the American Medical Association*, 282 (1999), 1523–1529.

blood lipids, atherosclerosis, strokes, thromboembolitic disease, varicose veins, and intermittent claudication.

Underweight people, too, have health problems and a higher mortality rate. Although the social pressure to be thin has waned slightly in recent years, pressure to attain model-like thinness is still with us and contributes to the gradual increase in incidence of eating disorders (anorexia nervosa and bulimia nervosa, discussed in Chapter 5). Extreme weight loss can spawn medical conditions such as heart damage, gastrointestinal problems, shrinkage of internal organs, immune system abnormalities, disorders of the reproductive system, loss of muscle tissue, damage to the nervous system, and even death.

For many years, people relied on height/weight charts to determine **recommended body weight**, but we now know that these tables are highly inaccurate for many people. The standard height/weight tables, first published in 1912, were based on average weights (including shoes and clothing) for men and women who obtained life insurance policies between 1888 and 1905. The recommended weight on height/weight tables is obtained according to gender, height, and frame size. Because no scientific guidelines are given to determine frame size, most people choose their frame size based on the column where the weight comes closest to their own!

The proper way to determine recommended weight is to find out what percent of total body weight is fat and what amount is lean tissue (body composition). Once the fat percentage is known, recommended weight can be calculated from recommended body fat.

Obesity is related to an excess of body fat. If body weight is the only criterion, an individual can easily

be considered overweight according to height/weight charts, yet not be genuinely obese. Typical examples are football players, body builders, weight lifters, and other athletes with large muscle size. Some athletes who appear to be 20 or 30 pounds overweight really have little body fat.

At the other end of the spectrum, some people who weigh very little and are viewed by many as "skinny" or underweight actually can be classified as obese because of their high body fat content. People who weigh as little as 120 pounds but are more than 30 percent fat (about a third of their total body weight) are not rare. These people often are sedentary or are dieting constantly. Physical inactivity and constant negative caloric balance both lead to a loss in lean body mass (see Chapter 6). Body weight alone clearly does not always tell the true story.

Assessing Body Composition

Body composition can be assessed through several procedures. The most common techniques are skinfold thickness, girth measurements, bioelectrical impedance, hydrostatic or underwater weighing, and air displacement. These procedures all yield estimates of body fat; thus, each technique may yield slightly different values. Therefore, when assessing body composition, you should use the same technique for pre- and post-test comparisons.

Hydrostatic weighing and air displacement are most frequently used in the laboratory and research setting. Bioelectrical impedance is much simpler to administer, but its accuracy is questionable. In this technique,

Hydrostatic weighing (top) and air displacement (bottom) techniques used for assessing body composition.

Skinfold thickness technique used for assessing body composition.

facilities. In addition to measuring lean tissue and body fat, some of these methods provide information on total body water and bone mass. Among these techniques are dual energy X-ray absorptiometry (DEXA), magnetic resonance imaging (MRI), computed tomography (CT), and total body electrical conductivity (TOBEC). The technique discussed here is skinfold thickness, which does not require expensive equipment. Two additional techniques that assess excessive body weight, Body Mass Index and waist circumference are also discussed in this section.

Skinfold Thickness

Assessment of body composition is done most frequently using skinfold thickness. This technique is based on the principle that approximately half of the body's fatty tissue is directly beneath the skin. Valid and reliable measurements of this tissue give a good indication of percent body fat.

The skinfold thickness test is performed with the aid of pressure calipers. To reflect the total percentage of fat, three sites are measured:

For women: triceps, suprailium, and thigh
For men: chest, abdomen, and thigh

All measurements are taken on the right side of the body with the person standing. The correct anatomical landmarks for skinfolds are as follows and are also shown in Figure 2.5.

Chest: a diagonal fold halfway between the shoulder crease and the nipple
Abdomen: a vertical fold about ½ to 1 inch to the right of the umbilicus

sensors are applied to the skin and a weak (totally painless) electrical current is run through the body to estimate body fat, lean body mass, and body water. The technique is based on the principle that fat tissue is a less efficient conductor of electrical current than lean tissue is. The easier the conductance, the leaner the individual. Body weight scales with sensors on the surface are also available to perform this procedure, but again, the accuracy is questionable.

More sophisticated techniques to assess body composition are available, but the equipment is costly and not readily accessible to the general population. These procedures are used primarily in research and medical

K E Y   T E R M S

Recommended body weight The weight at which there appears to be no harm to human health.

FIGURE **2.5** Anatomical landmarks for skinfold measurements.

SKINFOLD MEASUREMENT

1. Select the proper anatomical sites. For men, use chest, abdomen, and thigh skinfolds. For women, use triceps, suprailium, and thigh skinfolds. Take all measurements on the right side of the body with the person standing.

2. Measure each site by grasping a double thickness of skin firmly with the thumb and forefinger, pulling the fold slightly away from the muscular tissue. Hold caliper perpendicular to the fold, and take the measurement one-half inch below the finger hold. Measure each site three times and read the values to the nearest .1 to .5 mm. Record the average of the two closest readings as the final value. Take the readings without delay to avoid excessive compression of the skinfold. Release and refold the skinfold between readings.

3. When doing pre- and post-assessments, conduct the measurement at the same time of day. The best time is early in the morning to avoid water hydration changes resulting from activity or exercise.

4. Obtain percent fat by adding the three skinfold measurements and looking up the respective values.

For example, if the skinfold measurements for an 18-year-old female are: (a) triceps = 16, (b) suprailium = 4, and (c) thigh = 30 (total = 50), the percent body fat is 20.6%.

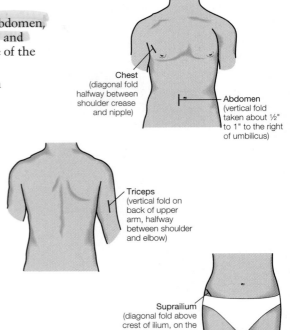

Chest
(diagonal fold halfway between shoulder crease and nipple)

Abdomen
(vertical fold taken about ½" to 1" to the right of umbilicus)

Triceps
(vertical fold on back of upper arm, halfway between shoulder and elbow)

Suprailium
(diagonal fold above crest of ilium, on the side of the hip)

Thigh
(vertical fold on front of thigh, midway between knee and hip)

Triceps: a vertical fold on the back of the upper arm, halfway between the shoulder and the arm

Thigh: a vertical fold on the front of the thigh, midway between the knee and the hip

Suprailium: a diagonal fold above the crest of the ilium (on the side of the hip)

Each site is measured by grasping a double thickness of skin firmly with the thumb and forefinger, pulling the fold slightly away from the muscle tissue. Hold the calipers perpendicular to the fold, and take the measurements ½" below the finger hold. Measure each site three times, and read the values to the nearest .1 to .5 mm. Record the average of the two closest readings as the final value. Take the readings without delay to avoid excessive compression of the skinfold. Releasing and refolding the skinfold is required between readings. Be sure to wear shorts or a loose-fitting t-shirt (no leotards) and do not use lotion on your skin the day when skinfolds are to be taken.

After determining the average value for each site, percent fat can be obtained by adding together all three skinfold measurements and looking up the respective values in Table 2.9 for women, Table 2.10 for men under age 40, and Table 2.11 for men over 40. You can record your results in Activity 2.1, Pre-Test, page 49. Then use the computation form in Activity 2.2, page 51, and the percent ranges in Table 2.12 to compute your recommended body weight.

The recommended percent body fat values given in Table 2.12 include essential fat and storage fat, discussed previously. For example, the recommended body fat range for women under age 30 is 17 to 25 percent. This indicates that only 5 to 13 percent of the total recommended fat is storage fat, and the other 12 percent is essential fat. The recommended range has been selected based on research indicating that some storage fat is required for optimal health and greater longevity.

The recommended body fat range selected in this book incorporates the recommendations of most health and fitness experts throughout the United States. If you desire to have just one target weight, you may select your body weight according to your personal preference, as long as it falls within the recommended range. The

TABLE 2.9 Percent Fat Estimates for Women, Calculated from Triceps, Suprailium, and Thigh Skinfold Thickness

SUM OF 3 SKINFOLDS	UNDER 22	23 TO 27	28 TO 32	33 TO 37	38 TO 42	43 TO 47	48 TO 52	53 TO 57	OVER 58
23– 25	9.7	9.9	10.2	10.4	10.7	10.9	11.2	11.4	11.7
26– 28	11.0	11.2	11.5	11.7	12.0	12.3	12.5	12.7	13.0
29– 31	12.3	12.5	12.8	13.0	13.3	13.5	13.8	14.0	14.3
32– 34	13.6	13.8	14.0	14.3	14.5	14.8	15.0	15.3	15.5
35– 37	14.8	15.0	15.3	15.5	15.8	16.0	16.3	16.5	16.8
38– 40	16.0	16.3	16.5	16.7	17.0	17.2	17.5	17.7	18.0
41– 43	17.2	17.4	17.7	17.9	18.2	18.4	18.7	18.9	19.2
44– 46	18.3	18.6	18.8	19.1	19.3	19.6	19.8	20.1	20.3
47– 49	19.5	19.7	20.0	20.2	20.5	20.7	21.0	21.2	21.5
50– 52	20.6	20.8	21.1	21.3	21.6	21.8	22.1	22.3	22.6
53– 55	21.7	21.9	22.1	22.4	22.6	22.9	23.1	23.4	23.6
56– 58	22.7	23.0	23.2	23.4	23.7	23.9	24.2	24.4	24.7
59– 61	23.7	24.0	24.2	24.5	24.7	25.0	25.2	25.5	25.7
62– 64	24.7	25.0	25.2	25.5	25.7	26.0	26.2	26.4	26.7
65– 67	25.7	25.9	26.2	26.4	26.7	26.9	27.2	27.4	27.7
68– 70	26.6	26.9	27.1	27.4	27.6	27.9	28.1	28.4	28.6
71– 73	27.5	27.8	28.0	28.3	28.5	28.8	29.0	29.3	29.5
74– 76	28.4	28.7	28.9	29.2	29.4	29.7	29.9	30.2	30.4
77– 79	29.3	29.5	29.8	30.0	30.3	30.5	30.8	31.0	31.3
80– 82	30.1	30.4	30.6	30.9	31.1	31.4	31.6	31.9	32.1
83– 85	30.9	31.2	31.4	31.7	31.9	32.2	32.4	32.7	32.9
86– 88	31.7	32.0	32.2	32.5	32.7	32.9	33.2	33.4	33.7
89– 91	32.5	32.7	33.0	33.2	33.5	33.7	33.9	34.2	34.4
92– 94	33.2	33.4	33.7	33.9	34.2	34.4	34.7	34.9	35.2
95– 97	33.9	34.1	34.4	34.6	34.9	35.1	35.4	35.6	35.9
98–100	34.6	34.8	35.1	35.3	35.5	35.8	36.0	36.3	36.5
101–103	35.2	35.4	35.7	35.9	36.2	36.4	36.7	36.9	37.2
104–106	35.8	36.1	36.3	36.6	36.8	37.1	37.3	37.5	37.8
107–109	36.4	36.7	36.9	37.1	37.4	37.6	37.9	38.1	38.4
110–112	37.0	37.2	37.5	37.7	38.0	38.2	38.5	38.7	38.9
113–115	37.5	37.8	38.0	38.2	38.5	38.7	39.0	39.2	39.5
116–118	38.0	38.3	38.5	38.8	39.0	39.3	39.5	39.7	40.0
119–121	38.5	38.7	39.0	39.2	39.5	39.7	40.0	40.2	40.5
122–124	39.0	39.2	39.4	39.7	39.9	40.2	40.4	40.7	40.9
125–127	39.4	39.6	39.9	40.1	40.4	40.6	40.9	41.1	41.4
128–130	39.8	40.0	40.3	40.5	40.8	41.0	41.3	41.5	41.8

Body density is calculated based on the generalized equation for predicting body density of women developed by A. S. Jackson, M. L. Pollock, and A. Ward, reported in *Medicine and Science in Sports and Exercise*, 12 (1980), 175–182. Percent body fat is determined from the calculated body density using the Siri formula.

TABLE 2.10 Percent Fat Estimates for Men Under Age 40 Calculated from Chest, Abdomen, and Thigh Skinfold Thickness

SUM OF 3 SKINFOLDS	UNDER 19	20 TO 22	23 TO 25	26 TO 28	29 TO 31	32 TO 34	35 TO 37	38 TO 40
8– 10	.9	1.3	1.6	2.0	2.3	2.7	3.0	3.3
11– 13	1.9	2.3	2.6	3.0	3.3	3.7	4.0	4.3
14– 16	2.9	3.3	3.6	3.9	4.3	4.6	5.0	5.3
17– 19	3.9	4.2	4.6	4.9	5.3	5.6	6.0	6.3
20– 22	4.8	5.2	5.5	5.9	6.2	6.6	6.9	7.3
23– 25	5.8	6.2	6.5	6.8	7.2	7.5	7.9	8.2
26– 28	6.8	7.1	7.5	7.8	8.1	8.5	8.8	9.2
29– 31	7.7	8.0	8.4	8.7	9.1	9.4	9.8	10.1
32– 34	8.6	9.0	9.3	9.7	10.0	10.4	10.7	11.1
35– 37	9.5	9.9	10.2	10.6	10.9	11.3	11.6	12.0
38– 40	10.5	10.8	11.2	11.5	11.8	12.2	12.5	12.9
41– 43	11.4	11.7	12.1	12.4	12.7	13.1	13.4	13.8
44– 46	12.2	12.6	12.9	13.3	13.6	14.0	14.3	14.7
47– 49	13.1	13.5	13.8	14.2	14.5	14.9	15.2	15.5
50– 52	14.0	14.3	14.7	15.0	15.4	15.7	16.1	16.4
53– 55	14.8	15.2	15.5	15.9	16.2	16.6	16.9	17.3
56– 58	15.7	16.0	16.4	16.7	17.1	17.4	17.8	18.1
59– 61	16.5	16.9	17.2	17.6	17.9	18.3	18.6	19.0
62– 64	17.4	17.7	18.1	18.4	18.8	19.1	19.4	19.8
65– 67	18.2	18.5	18.9	19.2	19.6	19.9	20.3	20.6
68– 70	19.0	19.3	19.7	20.0	20.4	20.7	21.1	21.4
71– 73	19.8	20.1	20.5	20.8	21.2	21.5	21.9	22.2
74– 76	20.6	20.9	21.3	21.6	22.0	22.2	22.7	23.0
77– 79	21.4	21.7	22.1	22.4	22.8	23.1	23.4	23.8
80– 82	22.1	22.5	22.8	23.2	23.5	23.9	24.2	24.6
83– 85	22.9	23.2	23.6	23.9	24.3	24.6	25.0	25.3
86– 88	23.6	24.0	24.3	24.7	25.0	25.4	25.7	26.1
89– 91	24.4	24.7	25.1	25.4	25.8	26.1	26.5	26.8
92– 94	25.1	25.5	25.8	26.2	26.5	26.9	27.2	27.5
95– 97	25.8	26.2	26.5	26.9	27.2	27.6	27.9	28.3
98–100	26.6	26.9	27.3	27.6	27.9	28.3	28.6	29.0
101–103	27.3	27.6	28.0	28.3	28.6	29.0	29.3	29.7
104–106	27.9	28.3	28.6	29.0	29.3	29.7	30.0	30.4
107–109	28.6	29.0	29.3	29.7	30.0	30.4	30.7	31.1
110–112	29.3	29.6	30.0	30.3	30.7	31.0	31.4	31.7
113–115	30.0	30.3	30.7	31.0	31.3	31.7	32.0	32.4
116–118	30.6	31.0	31.3	31.6	32.0	32.3	32.7	33.0
119–121	31.3	31.6	32.0	32.3	32.6	33.0	33.3	33.7
122–124	31.9	32.2	32.6	32.9	33.3	33.6	34.0	34.3
125–127	32.5	32.9	33.2	33.5	33.9	34.2	34.6	34.9
128–130	33.1	33.5	33.8	34.2	34.5	34.9	35.2	35.5

Body density is calculated based on the generalized equation for predicting body density of men developed by A. S. Jackson and M. L. Pollock, *British Journal of Nutrition*, 40 (1978), 497–504. Percent body fat is determined from the calculated body density using the Siri formula.

TABLE 2.11 Percent Fat Estimates for Men Over Age 40 Calculated from Chest, Abdomen, and Thigh Skinfold Thickness

SUM OF 3 SKINFOLDS	AGE							
	41 TO 43	44 TO 46	47 TO 49	50 TO 52	53 TO 55	56 TO 58	59 TO 61	OVER 62
8– 10	3.7	4.0	4.4	4.7	5.1	5.4	5.8	6.1
11– 13	4.7	5.0	5.4	5.7	6.1	6.4	6.8	7.1
14– 16	5.7	6.0	6.4	6.7	7.1	7.4	7.8	8.1
17– 19	6.7	7.0	7.4	7.7	8.1	8.4	8.7	9.1
20– 22	7.6	8.0	8.3	8.7	9.0	9.4	9.7	10.1
23– 25	8.6	8.9	9.3	9.6	10.0	10.3	10.7	11.0
26– 28	9.5	9.9	10.2	10.6	10.9	11.3	11.6	12.0
29– 31	10.5	10.8	11.2	11.5	11.9	12.2	12.6	12.9
32– 34	11.4	11.8	12.1	12.4	12.8	13.1	13.5	13.8
35– 37	12.3	12.7	13.0	13.4	13.7	14.1	14.4	14.8
38– 40	13.2	13.6	13.9	14.3	14.6	15.0	15.3	15.7
41– 43	14.1	14.5	14.8	15.2	15.5	15.9	16.2	16.6
44– 46	15.0	15.4	15.7	16.1	16.4	16.8	17.1	17.5
47– 49	15.9	16.2	16.6	16.9	17.3	17.6	18.0	18.3
50– 52	16.8	17.1	17.5	17.8	18.2	18.5	18.8	19.2
53– 55	17.6	18.0	18.3	18.7	19.0	19.4	19.7	20.1
56– 58	18.5	18.8	19.2	19.5	19.9	20.2	20.6	20.9
59– 61	19.3	19.7	20.0	20.4	20.7	21.0	21.4	21.7
62– 64	20.1	20.5	20.8	21.2	21.5	21.9	22.2	22.6
65– 67	21.0	21.3	21.7	22.0	22.4	22.7	23.0	23.4
68– 70	21.8	22.1	22.5	22.8	23.2	23.5	23.9	24.2
71– 73	22.6	22.9	23.3	23.6	24.0	24.3	24.7	25.0
74– 76	23.4	23.7	24.1	24.4	24.8	25.1	25.4	25.8
77– 79	24.1	24.5	24.8	25.2	25.5	25.9	26.2	26.6
80– 82	24.9	25.3	25.6	26.0	26.3	26.6	27.0	27.3
83– 85	25.7	26.0	26.4	26.7	27.1	27.4	27.8	28.1
86– 88	26.4	26.8	27.1	27.5	27.8	28.2	28.5	28.9
89– 91	27.2	27.5	27.9	28.2	28.6	28.9	29.2	29.6
92– 94	27.9	28.2	28.6	28.9	29.3	29.6	30.0	30.3
95– 97	28.6	29.0	29.3	29.7	30.0	30.4	30.7	31.1
98–100	29.3	29.7	30.0	30.4	30.7	31.1	31.4	31.8
101–103	30.0	30.4	30.7	31.1	31.4	31.8	32.1	32.5
104–106	30.7	31.1	31.4	31.8	32.1	32.5	32.8	33.2
107–109	31.4	31.8	32.1	32.4	32.8	33.1	33.5	33.8
110–112	32.1	32.4	32.8	33.1	33.5	33.8	34.2	34.5
113–115	32.7	33.1	33.4	33.8	34.1	34.5	34.8	35.2
116–118	33.4	33.7	34.1	34.4	34.8	35.1	35.5	35.8
119–121	34.0	34.4	34.7	35.1	35.4	35.8	36.1	36.5
122–124	34.7	35.0	35.4	35.7	36.1	36.4	36.7	37.1
125–127	35.3	35.6	36.0	36.3	36.7	37.0	37.4	37.7
128–130	35.9	36.2	36.6	36.9	37.3	37.6	38.0	38.5

Body density is calculated based on the generalized equation for predicting body density of men developed by A. S. Jackson and M. L. Pollock, *British Journal of Nutrition,* 40 (1978), 497–504. Percent body fat is determined from the calculated body density using the Siri formula.

TABLE 2.12 Recommended Body Composition According to Percent Body Fat

AGE	MALES	FEMALES
≤29	12–20%	17–25%
30–49	13–21%	18–26%
≥50	14–22%	19–27%

▦ High physical fitness standard
▦ Health fitness or criterion referenced standard

lower end of the range constitutes the physical fitness standard; the high end represents the health fitness standard.

Body Mass Index

Another technique scientists use to determine thinness and excessive fatness is the **Body Mass Index (BMI)**. This index incorporates height and weight to estimate critical fat values at which the risk for disease increases. BMI is calculated by dividing the weight in kilograms by the square of the height in meters or multiplying your weight in pounds by 705 and dividing this figure by the square of the height in inches. For example, the BMI for an individual who weighs 172 pounds (78 kg) and is 67 inches (1.7 meters) tall would be 27 [78 ÷ (1.7)^2] or [172 × 705 ÷ (67)^2].

You can compute and record your own BMI and recommended body weight according to BMI guidelines using the form provided in Activity 2.2 (pages 51–52). You also can obtain your BMI for selected weights and heights by looking it up in Table 2.13.

According to the BMI, the lowest risk for chronic disease is in the 22 to 25 range (see Table 2.14). Individuals are classified as overweight if their BMI falls between 25 and 30. BMIs above 30 are defined as obesity and below 18.5 as underweight.

BMI is a useful tool to screen the general population, but, similar to height/weight charts, it fails to differentiate fat from lean body mass or to account for where most of the fat is located (see waist circumference, page 45–46). Using BMI, strength-trained individuals and athletes with a large amount of muscle mass (such as body builders and football players) easily can fall in the moderate or even high-risk categories. Therefore, body composition is a better procedure to determine health risk and recommended body weight.

TABLE **2.13** Body Mass Index

Determine your BMI by looking up the number where your weight and height intersect on the table. According to your results, look up your disease risk in Table 2.14.

Height \ Weight	110	115	120	125	130	135	140	145	150	155	160	165	170	175	180	185	190	195	200	205	210	215	220	225	230	235	240	245	250
5'0"	21	22	23	24	25	26	27	28	29	30	31	32	33	34	35	36	37	38	39	40	41	42	43	44	45	46	47	48	49
5'1"	21	22	23	24	25	26	26	27	28	29	30	31	32	33	34	35	36	37	38	39	40	41	42	43	43	44	45	46	47
5'2"	20	21	22	23	24	25	26	27	27	28	29	30	31	32	33	34	35	36	37	37	38	39	40	41	42	43	44	45	46
5'3"	19	20	21	22	23	24	25	26	27	27	28	29	30	31	32	33	34	35	35	36	37	38	39	40	41	42	43	43	44
5'4"	19	20	21	21	22	23	24	25	26	27	27	28	29	30	31	32	33	33	34	35	36	37	38	39	39	40	41	42	43
5'5"	18	19	20	21	22	22	23	24	25	26	27	27	28	29	30	31	32	32	33	34	35	36	37	37	38	39	40	41	42
5'6"	18	19	19	20	21	22	23	23	24	25	26	27	27	28	29	30	31	31	32	33	34	35	36	36	37	38	39	40	40
5'7"	17	18	19	20	20	21	22	23	23	24	25	26	27	27	28	29	30	31	31	32	33	34	34	35	36	37	38	38	39
5'8"	17	17	18	19	20	21	21	22	23	24	24	25	26	27	27	28	29	30	30	31	32	33	33	34	35	36	36	37	38
5'9"	16	17	18	18	19	20	21	21	22	23	24	24	25	26	27	27	28	29	30	30	31	32	32	33	34	35	35	36	37
5'10"	16	17	17	18	19	19	20	21	22	22	23	24	24	25	26	27	27	28	29	29	30	31	32	32	33	34	34	35	36
5'11"	15	16	17	17	18	19	20	20	21	22	22	23	24	24	25	26	26	27	28	29	29	30	31	31	32	33	33	34	35
6'0"	15	16	16	17	18	18	19	20	20	21	22	22	23	24	24	25	26	26	27	28	28	29	30	31	31	32	33	33	34
6'1"	15	15	16	16	17	18	18	19	20	20	21	22	22	23	24	24	25	26	26	27	28	28	20	30	30	31	32	32	33
6'2"	14	15	15	16	17	17	18	19	19	20	21	21	22	22	23	24	24	25	26	26	27	28	28	29	30	30	31	31	32
6'3"	14	14	15	15	16	16	17	17	18	19	19	20	21	21	22	23	23	24	24	25	26	26	27	28	29	29	30	31	31
6'4"	13	14	15	15	16	16	17	18	18	19	19	20	21	21	22	23	23	24	24	25	26	26	27	27	28	29	29	30	30

TABLE **2.14** Disease Risk According to Body Mass Index (BMI)

BMI	DISEASE RISK	CATEGORY
<18.5	Increased	Underweight
18.5–21.99	Low	Acceptable
22.0–24.99	Very low	Acceptable
25.0–29.99	Increased	Overweight
30.0–34.99	High	Obesity I
35.0–39.99	Very high	Obesity II
>40.0	Extremely high	Obesity III

Waist Circumference

Scientific evidence suggests that the total amount of body fat by itself is not the best predictor of increased risk for disease, but rather the location of the fat. **Android obesity** is seen in individuals who tend to store fat in the trunk or abdominal area (which produces the "apple" shape). **Gynoid obesity** is seen in people who store fat primarily around the hips and thighs (which creates the "pear" shape).

Obese individuals with abdominal fat are clearly at higher risk for heart disease, hypertension, type 2 diabetes ("non-insulin-dependent" diabetes), and stroke than are obese people with similar amounts of body fat stored primarily in the hips and thighs. Evidence also indicates that, among individuals with a lot of abdominal fat, those whose fat deposits are located around internal organs (intra-abdominal or abdominal visceral fat) have an even greater risk for disease than those with fat mainly just beneath the skin (subcutaneous fat).

Complex scanning techniques to identify individuals at risk because of high intra-abdominal fatness are costly, so a simple **waist circumference (WC)** measure, designed by the National Heart, Lung, and Blood

KEY TERMS

Body Mass Index (BMI) An index that incorporates height and weight to estimate critical fat values at which risk for disease increases.

Android obesity Obesity pattern wherein individuals store fat primarily in the trunk or abdominal area.

Gynoid obesity Obesity pattern wherein individuals store fat primarily around the hips and thighs.

Waist circumference (WC) A measurement to assess potential risk for disease based on intra-abdominal fat content.

TABLE 2.15 Disease Risk According to Waist Circumference (WC)

MEN	WOMEN	DISEASE RISK
<35.5	<32.5	Low
35.5–40.0	32.5–35.0	Moderate
>40.0	>35.0	High

TABLE 2.16 Disease Risk According to Body Mass Index (BMI) and Waist Circumference (WC)

CLASSIFICATION	BMI (KG/M²)	DISEASE RISK RELATIVE TO NORMAL WEIGHT AND WC	
		MEN ≥40" (102 CM) WOMEN ≥35" (88 CM)	MEN >40" (102 CM) WOMEN >35" (88 CM)
Underweight	< 18.5	Increased	Low
Normal	18.5–24.9	Very low	Increased
Overweight	25.0–29.9	Increased	High
Obesity Class I	30.0–34.9	High	Very high
Obesity Class II	35.0–39.9	Very high	Very high
Obesity Class III	≥ 40.0	Extremely high	Extremely high

Adapted from: Expert Panel, "Executive Summary of the Clinical Guidelines on the Identification, Evaluation, and Treatment of Overweight and Obesity in Adults," *Archives of Internal Medicine* 158 (1998) 1855–1867.

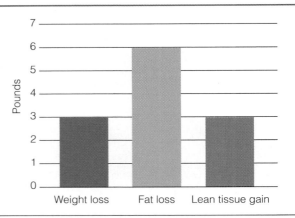

FIGURE 2.6 Effects of a 6-week aerobics program on body composition.

Source: "Fitness Benefits of Aerobic Dance," by W. W. K. Hoeger. Data collected at the University of Texas of The Permian Basin, 1985.

Institute, is used to assess this risk. A waist circumference of more than 40 inches in men and 35 inches in women indicates a higher risk for cardiovascular disease, hypertension, and type 2 diabetes (see Table 2.15). Thus, weight loss is encouraged when individuals exceed these measurements.

WC may even be a better predictor of disease risk than BMI. Thus, BMI in conjunction with WC provides the best combination to identify individuals at higher risk due to excessive body fat. Table 2.16 provides guidelines to identify people at risk according to BMI and WC.

Critical Thinking

How do you feel about your current body weight? What influence does society have on the way you perceive yourself in terms of your weight? Do the results from your body composition measurements make you feel any different about the way you see your current body weight and image?

Effects of Exercise and Diet on Body Composition

If you engage in a diet and exercise program, you should repeat body composition measurements about once a month to monitor changes in lean and fat tissue. This is important because lean body mass is affected by weight-reduction programs as well as by physical activity. A negative caloric balance does lead to a decrease in lean body mass. These effects will be explained in detail in Chapter 6. As lean body mass changes, so will your recommended body weight.

Changes in body composition resulting from a weight control/exercise program are illustrated by a co-ed aerobics course taught during a 6-week summer term. Students participated in aerobic dance routines four times a week, 60 minutes each time. On the first and the last days of class, several physiological parameters, including body composition, were assessed. Students also were given information on diet and nutrition and followed their own weight-control program. At the end of the 6 weeks, the average weight loss for the entire class was only 3 pounds. When body composition was assessed, however, class members were surprised to find that the average fat loss was actually 6 pounds, accompanied by a 3-pound increase in lean body mass (see Figure 2.6).

Calculate your BMI using your height and weight. BMI, which stands for Body Mass Index, is a ratio between weight and height, a mathematical formula that correlates with body fat. BMI is a better predictor of disease risk than is body weight alone. This site also features tools to calculate your ideal weight and your target heart rate.

http://www.halls.md/body-mass-index/bmi.htm

ASSESS YOUR KNOWLEDGE

 Evaluate how well you understand the concepts presented in this chapter using the Assess Your Knowledge and Practice Quizzes options on your Profile Plus CD-ROM.

1. The metabolic profile is used in reference to
   a. insulin sensitivity.
   b. glucose tolerance.
   c. cholesterol levels.
   d. cardiovascular disease.
   e. All of the above are correct choices.

2. Cardiorespiratory endurance is determined by
   a. the amount of oxygen the body is able to utilize per minute of physical activity.
   b. the length of time it takes the heart rate to return to 120 bpm following the 1.5-Mile Run test.
   c. the difference between the maximal heart rate and the resting heart rate.
   d. the product of the heart rate and blood pressure at rest versus exercise.
   e. the time it takes a person to reach a heart rate between 120 and 170 bpm during the 1.0-Mile Walk test.

3. An "excellent" cardiorespiratory fitness rating in ml/kg/min for young male adults is about
   a. 10.
   b. 20.
   c. 30.
   d. 40.
   e. 50.

4. Which of the following parameters is used to estimate maximal oxygen uptake according to the 1.0-Mile Walk Test?
   a. body weight
   b. gender
   c. total 1.0-mile walk time
   d. exercise heart rate
   e. All of the above are used to estimate VO_{2max}.

5. The ability of a muscle to exert submaximal force repeatedly over time is known as
   a. muscular strength.
   b. plyometric training.
   c. muscular endurance.
   d. isokinetic training.
   e. isometric training.

6. A 70 percentile rank places an individual in the _____ fitness category.
   a. excellent
   b. good
   c. average
   d. fair
   e. poor

7. Muscular flexibility is defined as
   a. the capacity of joints and muscles to work in a synchronized manner.
   b. the achievable range of motion at a joint or group of joints without causing injury.
   c. the capability of muscles to stretch beyond their normal resting length without injury to the muscles.
   d. the capacity of muscles to return to their proper length following the application of a stretching force.
   e. the limitations placed on muscles as the joints move through their normal planes.

8. During the starting position of the Modified Sit-and-Reach Test,
   a. the hips, back, and head are placed against a wall.
   b. you measure the distance from the hips to the feet.
   c. you make a fist with the hands.
   d. you stretch forward as far as possible over the reach indicator.
   e. All of the above are correct choices.

(continued)

9. The amount of essential fat in women is
   a. 3 percent.
   b. 5 percent.
   c. 10 percent.
   d. 12 percent.
   e. 17 percent.

10. Which of the following is not a technique used in the assessment of body fat?
    a. hydrostatic weighing
    b. skinfold thickness
    c. body mass index
    d. circumference measurements

Correct answers can be found on page 261.

activity

Personal Fitness Profile: Pre-Test

2.1

Date _____ Course _____ Section _____

Name _____ Age _____ ☐ Male ☐ Female

Body Weight _____

Fitness Component	Test Data	Test Results	Category	Goal
Cardiorespiratory Endurance 1.5-Mile Run	**Time** ____ : ____	VO_{2max} ____ . ____	_____	VO_{2max} ____ . ____
1.0-Mile Walk	**Time** ____ : ____			
	Heart Rate _____	VO_{2max} ____ . ____	_____	VO_{2max} ____ . ____
Muscular Strength/Endurance	**Reps**	**Percentile**		
Bench Jumps	_____	_____	_____	_____
Chair Dips / Modified Push-Ups	_____	_____	_____	_____
Bent-Leg Curl-Ups / Ab. Crunches	_____	_____	_____	_____
Overall Fitness Category			_____	
Muscular Flexibility	**Inches**	**Percentile**		
Modified Sit-and-Reach	_____	_____	_____	_____
Total Body Rotation (R/L)	_____	_____	_____	_____
Overall Fitness Category			_____	
BMI/Body Composition				
Body Mass Index (BMI)	_____		_____	_____
Waist Circumference (WC)	_____ inches		_____	_____
BMI & WC			_____	_____
Chest / Triceps	_____ mm			
Abdominal / Suprailium	_____ mm			
Thigh	_____ mm			
Sum of Skinfolds	_____ mm			
Percent Body Fat		_____	_____	
Lean Body Mass		_____ lbs.		_____

_____ _____
Student Signature Instructor Signature

Personal Fitness Profile: Post-Test

Date _____ Course _____ Section _____

Name _____ Age _____ ☐ Male ☐ Female

Body Weight _____

Fitness Component	Test Data	Test Results	Category	Goal
Cardiorespiratory Endurance	**Time**	VO_{2max}		VO_{2max}
1.5-Mile Run	____ : ____	____ . ____ _____		____ . ____
	Time			
1.0-Mile Walk	____ : ____			
	Heart Rate	VO_{2max}		VO_{2max}
	_____	____ . ____ _____		____ . ____
Muscular Strength/Endurance	**Reps**	**Percentile**		
Bench Jumps	_____	_____	_____	_____
Chair Dips / Modified Push-Ups	_____	_____	_____	_____
Bent-Leg Curl-Ups / Ab. Crunches	_____	_____	_____	_____
Overall Fitness Category			_____	
Muscular Flexibility	**Inches**	**Percentile**		
Modified Sit-and-Reach	_____	_____	_____	_____
Total Body Rotation (R/L)	_____	_____	_____	_____
Overall Fitness Category			_____	
BMI/WC/Body Composition				
Body Mass Index (BMI)	_____		_____	_____
Waist Circumference (WC)	_____ inches		_____	_____
BMI & WC			_____	_____
Chest / Triceps	_____ mm			
Abdominal / Suprailium	_____ mm			
Thigh	_____ mm			
Sum of Skinfolds	_____ mm			
Percent Body Fat		_____ _____		_____
Lean Body Mass		_____ lbs.		_____

_____ _____
Student Signature   Instructor Signature

Computation Form for Recommended Body Weight, Body Mass Index (BMI), and Waist Circumference (WC)

Name _____   Date _____

Course _____   Section _____

Recommended Body Weight According to Percent Body Fat

A. Current Body Weight (BW): _____ lbs

B. Current Percent Fat (%F): _____ %

C. Fat Weight (FW) = BW × %F* = _____ × _____ = _____ lbs

D. Lean Body Mass (LBM) = BW − FW = _____ − _____ = _____ lbs

E. Age: _____

F. Recommended Fat Percent (RFP) Range (see Table 2.12, page 44):

Low End of Recommended Fat Percent Range (LRFP): _____ % (Physical Fitness Standard)

High End of Recommended Fat Percent Range (HRFP): _____ % (Health Fitness Standard)

G. Recommended Body Weight Range:

Low End of Recommended Body Weight Range (LRBW) = LBM ÷ (1.0 − LRFP*)

LRBW = _____ ÷ (1.0 − _____) = _____ lbs

High End of Recommended Body Weight Range (HRBW) = LBM ÷ (1.0 − HRFP*)

HRBW = _____ ÷ (1.0 − _____) = _____ lbs

Recommended Body Weight Range: _____ to _____ lbs

---

*Express percentages in decimal form (e.g., 25% = .25)

Body Mass Index (BMI)*

	Pre-test	Post-test
Date:	_____	_____
Weight (lbs):	_____	_____
Height (inches):	_____	_____
BMI:*	_____	_____
Disease risk: (Table 2.14)	_____	_____

*BMI = [Weight in lbs. $\times$ 705 $\div$ (Height in inches)^2]
  or [Weight in kgs $\div$ (Height in meters)^2]

Waist Circumference (WC)

	Pre-test	Post-test
Date:	_____	_____
Waist (inches):	_____	_____
Disease risk: (Table 2.15)	_____	_____
Disease risk according to BMI and WC (Table 2.16)	_____	_____

Recommended Body Weight According to BMI

RBW based on BMI = Desired BMI $\times$ height (in.) $\times$ height (in) $\div$ 705

RBW at BMI of 25 =   25 $\times$ _____ $\times$ _____ $\div$ 705 = [_____]

RBW at BMI of 22 =   22 $\times$ _____ $\times$ _____ $\div$ 705 = [_____]

Body Composition Conclusions and Goals

Briefly state your feelings about your body composition results and your recommended body weight. Do you plan to reduce your percent body fat and increase your lean body mass? If so, indicate how you plan to achieve these goals.

_____

_____

_____

_____

_____

_____

_____

_____

_____

_____

Exercise is the closest thing we'll ever get to the miracle pill that everyone is seeking. It brings weight loss, appetite control, improved mood and self-esteem, an energy kick, and longer life by decreasing the risk of heart disease, diabetes, stroke, osteoporosis, and chronic disabilities.[1]

© Randy M. Ury/CORBIS

CHAPTER 3

Exercise Prescription

OBJECTIVES

- Determine your readiness to start an exercise program.
- Learn the factors that govern cardiorespiratory exercise prescription: intensity, mode, duration, and frequency.
- Understand the variables that govern development of muscular strength and muscular endurance: mode, resistance, sets, and frequency.
- Understand the factors that contribute to the development of muscular flexibility: mode, intensity, repetitions, and frequency.
- Learn to write personalized cardiorespiratory, strength, and flexibility exercise programs.
- Be introduced to a program for the prevention and rehabilitation of low-back pain.
- Learn some ways to enhance compliance with exercise.
- Be able to write fitness goals.

PROFILE PLUS Check your readiness to begin an exercise program with the clearance for exercise prescription activity on your CD-ROM.

The inspiring story of George Snell from Sandy, Utah, illustrates what fitness can do for a person's health and well-being. At age 45, Snell weighed approximately 400 pounds, his blood pressure was 220/180, he was blind because of diabetes he did not know he had, and his blood glucose (sugar) level was 487. Determined to do something about his physical and medical condition, Snell started a walking/jogging program. After about 8 months of conditioning, he had lost almost 200 pounds, his eyesight had returned, his glucose level was down to 67, and he was taken off medication. Two months later—less than 10 months after initiating his personal exercise program—he completed his first marathon, a running a course of 26.2 miles!

Research results have established that being physically active and participating in a lifetime exercise program contributes greatly to good health, physical fitness, and wellness. Nonetheless, too many individuals who exercise regularly are surprised to find, when they take a battery of fitness tests, that they are not as conditioned as they thought they were. Although these people may be exercising regularly, they most likely are not following the basic principles of exercise prescription. Therefore, they do not reap significant benefits.

To obtain optimal results, all programs must be individualized. Our bodies are not all alike, and fitness levels and needs vary among individuals. The information presented in this chapter provides you with the necessary guidelines to write a personalized cardiorespiratory, strength, and flexibility exercise program to promote and maintain physical fitness and wellness. Information on weight management to achieve recommended body composition (the fourth component of physical fitness) is given in Chapter 6.

Monitoring Daily Physical Activity

Almost half of all adults in the United States do not achieve the recommended daily amount of physical activity. The first step toward becoming more active is to carefully monitor daily physical activity. Other than monitoring actual time engaged in activity, an excellent tool to determine daily physical activity is through the use of a **pedometer**.

Pedometers are small mechanical devices that sense vertical body motion and are used to count footsteps. Wearing a pedometer throughout the day allows a person to determine the total steps taken in a day. Although with less accuracy, some pedometer brands also record distance, calories burned, speeds, and actual time of activity each day.

A pedometer is a great motivational tool to help increase, maintain, and monitor daily physical activity that involves lower body motion (walking, jogging, running). Pedometer use will most likely increase in the next few years to help promote and quantify daily physical activity.

Before purchasing a pedometer, be sure to verify its accuracy. Many of the free or low-cost pedometers provided by corporations for promotion and advertisement purposes are inaccurate, thus discouraging their use. Pedometers also tend to lose accuracy at very slow walking speeds (30 minutes per mile or less) because the vertical movement of the hip is too small to trigger the spring-mounted lever arm inside the pedometer to properly record the steps taken.

You can obtain a good pedometer for about $25, and ratings are available on-line. The most accurate pedometer brands are Yamax, Kenz, New Lifestyles, and Walk4Life. To test the accuracy of a pedometer, follow these steps: clip the pedometer on the waist directly above the knee cap, reset the pedometer to zero, carefully close the pedometer, walk exactly 50 steps at your normal pace, carefully open the pedometer, and look at the number of steps recorded. A reading within 10 percent of the actual steps taken (45 to 55 steps) is acceptable.

The typical male American takes about 6,000 steps per day, whereas women take about 5,300 steps. A general recommendation for adults is 10,000 steps per day, and Table 3.1 provides specific activity ratings based on the number of daily steps taken.

TABLE **3.1** Adult Activity Levels Based on Total Number of Steps Taken per Day

STEPS PER DAY	CATEGORY
<5,000	Sedentary lifestyle
5,000–7,499	Low active
7,500–9,999	Somewhat active
10,000–12,499	Active
≥12,500	Highly active

Source: Tudor-Locke, C. and D. R. Basset. "How Many Steps/Day are Enough? Preliminary Pedometer Indices for Public Health," *Sports Medicine* 34:1–8, 2004.

All daily steps count, but to meet national physical activity recommendations, some of your steps should occur in bouts of at least 10 minutes so you will accumulate 30 minutes of moderate-intensity physical activity in at least three 10-minute activity sessions most days of the week. A 10-minute brisk walk is approximately 1,200 steps (a distance of about a 1,000 yards). A brisk one-mile walk (1,760 yards) is about 2,000 steps. To help users accomplish this amount of activity, new pedometer brands have an "aerobic steps" function that records steps taken in excess of 60 steps per minute over a 10-minute period of time.

The first practical application that you can perform in this course is to determine your current level of daily activity. The log provided in Activity 3.1 (page 75) will help you keep a four-day log of all physical activities that you do on a daily basis. On this log record the time of day, type and duration of the activity/exercise and, if possible, steps taken while engaged in the activity. The results will provide an indication of how active you are and will serve to monitor changes in the next few months and years.

Readiness for Exercise

The research data on the benefits of regular physical activity and exercise is far too impressive to be ignored. All of the benefits of being active, however, do not help unless people carry out a lifetime program of physical activity. Of greater concern, only a small fraction of the population exercises regularly, and of those who exercise, only about 20 percent are able to achieve a high physical fitness standard. More than half of those who start exercising drop out during the first 6 months of the program. Sports psychologists are trying to find out why some people exercise habitually and many do not.

If you are not exercising now, are you willing to give exercise a try? The first step is to decide positively

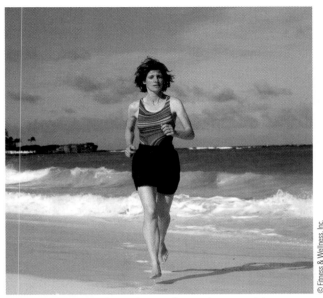

Good cardiorespiratory fitness is essential to enjoy a good quality of life.

© Fitness & Wellness, Inc.

that you will try. To help you make this decision, look at Activity 3.2 (page 77). Make a list of the advantages and disadvantages of incorporating exercise into your lifestyle. Your list of advantages may include things such as:

It will make me feel better.
My self-esteem will improve.
I will lose weight.
I will have more energy.
It will lower my risk for chronic diseases.

Your list of disadvantages may include:

I don't want to take the time.
I'm too out of shape.
There's no good place to exercise.
I don't have the willpower to do it.

When the reasons for exercise outweigh the reasons for not exercising, it will become easier to try.

A questionnaire that may provide answers about your readiness to start an exercise program is also included in Activity 3.2, page 78. Read each statement carefully and circle the number that best describes your feelings. Be completely honest in your answers. You are evaluated in four categories: mastery (self-control), attitude, health, and commitment. The higher you score in any category—mastery, for example—the more important that reason is for you to exercise.

Scores can vary from 4 to 16. A score of 12 and above is a strong indicator that that factor is important to you, whereas 8 and below is low. If you score 12 or

more points in each category, your chances of initiating and sticking to an exercise program are good. If you do not score at least 12 points in three categories, your chances of succeeding at exercise may be slim. You need to be better informed about the benefits of exercise, and retraining may be helpful. Tips on how to enhance commitment to exercise are provided later in the chapter.

Exercise Prescriptions

To better understand how overall fitness can be developed, we have to be familiar with the guidelines that govern exercise prescriptions for cardiovascular endurance, muscular strength and endurance, and body flexibility. A brief summary of these guidelines is provided in the Physical Activity Pyramid given in Figure 3.1, and they will be explained in detail in the next few sections of this chapter.

Cardiorespiratory Endurance

A sound cardiorespiratory endurance program contributes greatly to enhancing and maintaining good health. Of the four health-related physical fitness components, cardiorespiratory endurance is the single most important—except during older age, when strength seems to be more critical. Even though certain levels of muscular strength and flexibility are necessary to perform **activities of daily living**, a person can get by without a lot of strength and flexibility. A person cannot do without a good cardiorespiratory system, though.

Cardiorespiratory Exercise Prescription

The objective of aerobic exercise is to improve the capacity of the cardiorespiratory system. To accomplish this, the heart muscle has to be overloaded like any other muscle in the human body. Just as the biceps muscle in the upper arm is developed through strength training, the heart muscle is exercised to increase in size, strength, and efficiency.

To better understand how the cardiorespiratory system can be developed, we have to be familiar with

K E Y   T E R M S

Pedometer An electronic device that senses body motion and counts footsteps. Some pedometers also record distance, calories burned, speeds, and time spent being physically active.

Activities of daily living Everyday behaviors that people normally do to function in life (cross the street, carry groceries, lift objects, do laundry, sweep floors).

FIGURE **3.1** Physical Activity Pyramid.

Minimize inactivity

Strength and Flexibility: Exercise 2–3 days/week

Cardiorespiratory endurance: Exercise 20–60 minutes 3–5 days/week

Physical activity: Accumulate 60 minutes nearly every day

Photos © Fitness & Wellness, Inc.

four factors involved in aerobic exercise: intensity, mode, duration, and frequency of exercise. The American College of Sports Medicine (ACSM) recommends that a medical exam and a diagnostic exercise stress test be administered prior to **vigorous exercise** by apparently healthy men over age 45 and women over 55.[2]

Intensity of Exercise

Muscles have to be overloaded for them to develop. Just as the training stimulus to develop the biceps muscle can be accomplished with curl-up exercises, the stimulus for the cardiorespiratory system is provided by making the heart pump at a higher rate for a certain period of time.

Cardiorespiratory development occurs when the heart is working between 40 percent/50 percent and 85 percent of heart rate reserve.[3] The 40 percent to 50 percent training intensity should be used by individuals who are quite unfit. Increases in maximal oxygen uptake (VO_{2max}), however, are accelerated when the heart is working closer to 85 percent of **heart rate reserve**. For

this reason, many experts prescribe exercise between 60 percent and 85 percent. **Intensity of exercise** can be calculated easily, and training can be monitored by checking your pulse. To determine the intensity of exercise or **cardiorespiratory training zone**, follow these steps:

1. Estimate your maximal heart rate (MHR) according to the formula MHR = 220 minus age (220 − age)
2. Check your resting heart rate (RHR) some time after you have been sitting quietly for 15 to 20 minutes. You may take your pulse for 30 seconds and multiply by 2, or take it for a full minute. As explained in Chapter 2, you can check your pulse on the wrist by placing two or three fingers over the radial artery or on the neck by placing your fingers over the carotid artery.
3. Determine the heart rate reserve (HRR) by subtracting the resting heart rate from the maximal heart rate (HRR = MHR − RHR).
4. Calculate the training intensities (TI) at 40 percent, 50 percent, 60 percent, and 85 percent. Multiply the heart rate reserve by the respective 40, 50, 60, and

Cardiorespiratory endurance is the ability of the heart, lungs, and blood vessels to deliver adequate amounts of oxygen to the cells to meet the demands of prolonged physical activity.

© Fitness & Wellness, Inc.

85 percentages, and then add the resting heart rate to each of these four values (for example, 85% TI = HRR × .85 + RHR).

Example. The 40%, 50%, 60%, and 85% training intensities for a 20-year-old with a resting heart rate of 68 beats per minute (bpm) would be:

MHR: 220 − 20 = 200 bpm
RHR: = 68 bpm
HRR: 200 − 68 = 132 beats
40% TI = (132 × .40) + 68 = 121 bpm
50% TI = (132 × .50) + 68 = 134 bpm
60% TI = (132 × .60) + 68 = 147 bpm
85% TI = (132 × .85) + 68 = 180 bpm

Therefore, this person's training zones would be as follows:

Low-intensity cardiorespiratory training zone: 121 to 134 bpm
Moderate-intensity cardiorespiratory training zone: 134 to 147 bpm
High-intensity (vigorous) cardiorespiratory training zone: 147 to 180 bpm

When you exercise to improve the cardiorespiratory system, you should maintain the heart rate between the 60 and 85 percent training intensities to obtain adequate development. If you have been physically inactive, you should train at around the 40 to 50 percent intensity during the first 6 to 8 weeks of the exercise program. After the first few weeks, you should exercise at between 60 and 85 percent training intensity.

When determining the training intensity for your own program, you need to consider your personal fitness goals. Individuals who exercise at around the 50 percent training intensity will reap significant health benefits—in particular, improvements in the metabolic profile (see Health Fitness Standard, pages 26–27, and Figure 2.1, page 27). Training at this lower percentage, however, may place you in only the "average" or moderately fit category (see Table 2.2, page 30). Exercising at this lower intensity does lower the risk for cardiovascular mortality (health fitness) but will not allow you to achieve a "good" or "excellent" cardiorespiratory fitness rating (the physical fitness standard). The latter ratings are obtained by exercising closer to the 85 percent threshold.

Following a few weeks of training, you may have a considerably lower resting heart rate (10 to 20 beats fewer in 8 to 12 weeks). Therefore, you should recompute your target zone periodically. You can compute your own cardiorespiratory training zone by using the form in Activity 3.3, page 79. Once you have reached an ideal level of cardiorespiratory endurance, training in the 60 percent to 85 percent range will allow you to maintain your fitness level.

During the first few weeks of an exercise program, you should monitor your exercise heart rate regularly to make sure you are training in the proper zone. Wait until you are about 5 minutes into your exercise session before taking your first reading. When you check your heart rate, count your pulse for 10 seconds and then multiply by 6 to get the per-minute pulse rate. Exercise heart rate will remain at the same level for about 15 seconds following exercise. After 15 seconds, your heart rate will drop rapidly. Do not hesitate to stop during your exercise bout to check your pulse. If the rate is too low, increase the intensity of exercise. If the rate is too high, slow down.

To develop the cardiorespiratory system, you do not have to exercise above the 85 percent rate. From a

KEY TERMS

Vigorous exercise An exercise intensity that is either above 6 METs, 60% of maximal oxygen uptake, or one that provides a "substantial" challenge to the individual.

Heart rate reserve The difference between the maximal heart rate (MHR) and resting heart rate (RHR).

Intensity of exercise How hard a person has to exercise to improve cardiorespiratory endurance.

Cardiorespiratory training zone The range of intensity at which a person should exercise to develop the cardiorespiratory system.

fitness standpoint, training above this percentage will not give extra benefits and actually may be unsafe for some individuals. For unconditioned people and older adults, cardiorespiratory training should be conducted around the 50 percent rate to discourage potential problems associated with high-intensity exercise.

Mode of Exercise

The **mode of exercise** that develops the cardiorespiratory system has to be aerobic in nature. **Aerobic exercise** involves the major muscle groups of the body, and it must be rhythmic and continuous. As the amount of muscle mass involved during exercise increases, so does the effectiveness of the activity in providing cardiorespiratory development.

Once you have established your cardiorespiratory training zone, any activity or combination of activities that will get your heart rate up to that training zone and keep it there for as long as you exercise will give you adequate development. Examples of these activities are walking, jogging, swimming, water aerobics, cross-country skiing, rope skipping, cycling, racquetball, stair climbing, and stationary running or cycling.

The activity you choose should be based on your personal preferences—what you enjoy doing most—and your physical limitations. Low-impact activities greatly decrease the risk for injuries. Most injuries to beginners are related to high-impact activities. For individuals who have been inactive, general strength conditioning also is recommended prior to initiating an aerobic exercise program. Strength conditioning will reduce the incidence of injuries significantly.

The amount of strength or flexibility a person develops through various activities differs, but in terms of cardiorespiratory development, the heart doesn't know whether you are walking, swimming, or cycling. All the heart knows is that it has to pump at a certain rate, and as long as that rate is in the desired range, your cardiorespiratory fitness will improve. From a health fitness point of view, training in the lower end of the cardiorespiratory zone will yield optimal health benefits. The closer the heart rate is to the higher end of the cardiorespiratory training zone, however, the greater will be the improvements in VO_{2max} (high physical fitness).

Duration of Exercise

In terms of **duration of exercise**, the general recommendation is that a person train between 20 and 60 minutes per session. However, for people who have been successful at losing weight, up to 90 minutes of daily moderate-intensity activity may be required to prevent weight regain.

The duration is based on how intensely a person trains. If the training is done at around 85 percent, 20 minutes of exercise is sufficient. At 40 to 50 percent intensity, the individual should train at least 30 minutes. As mentioned in the discussion of intensity of exercise above, unconditioned people and older adults should train at lower percentages; therefore, the activity should be carried out over a longer time.

Although most experts traditionally have recommended 20 to 60 minutes of continuous aerobic exercise per session, more recent evidence suggests that accumulating 30 minutes or more of moderate-intensity physical activity can provide substantial health benefits.[4] Research further indicates that three 10-minute exercise sessions per day (separated by at least 4 hours), at approximately 70 percent of maximal heart rate, also produce fitness benefits.[5] Although the increases in VO_{2max} with this program were not as large (57 percent) as those in a group performing one continuous 30-minute bout of exercise per day, the researchers concluded that moderate-intensity exercise, conducted for 10 minutes three times per day, benefits the cardiorespiratory system significantly.

Results of this study are meaningful because people often mention lack of time as the reason for not taking part in an exercise program. Many think they have to exercise at least 20 continuous minutes to get any benefits at all. Even though 20 to 60 minutes are recommended, short, intermittent exercise bouts also are helpful to the cardiorespiratory system.

For people whose goal is weight management, the Institute of Medicine of the National Academy of Sciences recommends accumulating 60 minutes of moderate-intensity physical activity per day,[6] whereas 60 to 90 minutes of daily moderate-intensity activity is necessary to prevent weight regain.[7] These recommendations are based on evidence that people who maintain healthy weight typically accumulate between 1 and 1½ hours of daily physical activity. Exercise duration should be increased gradually to avoid undue fatigue and exercise-related injuries.

If lack of time is a concern, you should exercise daily at a high intensity for 30 minutes, which can burn as many calories as 60 minutes of moderate-intensity exercise (see "Low-Intensity Versus High-Intensity Exercise for Weight Loss," Chapter 6, page 136)—but only 15 percent of adults in the United States typically exercise at a high-intensity level. Novice and overweight exercisers also need proper conditioning prior to high-intensity exercise to avoid injuries or cardiovascular-related problems.

Exercise sessions always should be preceded by a 5- to 10-minute **warm-up** and followed by a 10-minute

cool-down. The purpose of warm-up is to aid in the transition from rest to exercise. A good warm-up increases muscle and connective tissue extensibility, joint range of motion, and enhances muscular activity. A warm-up consists of general calisthenics, mild stretching exercises, and walking/jogging/cycling for a few minutes at a lower intensity level than the actual target zone. The concluding phase of the warm-up is a gradual increase in exercise intensity to the lower end of the target training zone.

In the cool-down, the intensity of exercise is decreased gradually to help the body return to near resting levels, followed by stretching and relaxation activities. Stopping abruptly causes blood to pool in the exercised body parts, diminishing the return of blood to the heart. This reduced blood return can cause a sudden drop in blood pressure, dizziness and faintness, or even the onset of cardiac abnormalities. The cool-down phase also helps dissipate body heat and aid in the removal of lactic acid produced during high-intensity exercise.

Frequency of Exercise

The recommended **frequency of exercise** for aerobic exercise is three to five days per week. Initially, only three weekly training sessions of 15 to 20 minutes are recommended to avoid musculo-skeletal injuries. You may then increase the frequency so that by the fourth or fifth week you are exercising five times per week for 20 minutes per session in the appropriate heart rate target zone. Thereafter, progressively continue to increase frequency, duration, and intensity of exercise until you have accomplished your goals.

When exercising at 60 to 85 percent of HRR, three 20- to 30-minute exercise sessions per week, performed on nonconsecutive days, are sufficient to improve or maintain VO_{2max}. When training at lower intensities, exercising 30 to 60 minutes more than three days per week are required. If training is conducted more than five days a week, further improvements in VO_{2max} are minimal. Although endurance athletes often train six to seven days per week (often twice per day), their training programs are designed to increase training mileage so they can endure long-distance races (6 to 100 miles) at a high percentage of VO_{2max}.

For individuals on a weight-loss program, the recommendation is 60 to 90 minutes of low- to moderate-intensity activity on most days of the week. Longer exercise sessions increase caloric expenditure for faster weight reduction (see Chapter 6, "Exercise: The Key to Successful Weight Management," pages 133–136).

Although three exercise sessions per week will maintain cardiorespiratory fitness, the importance of regular physical activity in preventing disease and enhancing quality of life has been pointed out clearly by the American College of Sports Medicine, by the U. S. Centers for Disease Control and Prevention, and by the President's Council on Physical Fitness and Sports. These organizations advocate at least 30 minutes of moderate-intensity physical activity almost daily. This routine has been promoted as an effective way to improve health.

These recommendations were subsequently upheld by the U. S. Surgeon General in the 1996 "Report on Physical Activity and Health." The Surgeon General's report states that people can improve their health and quality of life substantially by including moderate amounts of physical activity on most, preferably all, days of the week. Further, it states that no one, including older adults, is too old to enjoy the benefits of regular physical activity.

To enjoy better health and fitness, physical activity must be pursued regularly. According to Dr. William Haskell, from Stanford University: "Physical activity should be viewed as medication, and, therefore, should be taken on a daily basis." Many of the benefits of exercise and activity diminish within 2 weeks of substantially decreased physical activity. These benefits are completely lost within 2 to 8 months of inactivity.

A summary of the cardiorespiratory exercise prescription guidelines according to the American College of Sports Medicine is provided in Figure 3.2. Ideally, to reap both the high-fitness and the health-fitness benefits of exercise, a person needs to exercise a minimum of three times per week in the appropriate target zone for high fitness maintenance, and three to four additional times per week in moderate-intensity activities to enjoy the full benefits of health fitness. All exercise/activity sessions should last about 30 minutes. The form in Activity 3.4 page 83, is provided to help you keep a daily log of your cardiorespiratory (aerobic) activities.

KEY TERMS

Mode of exercise Form of exercise (e.g., aerobic).

Aerobic exercise Activity that requires oxygen to produce the necessary energy to carry out the activity.

Duration of exercise Time exercising per session.

Warm-up A period preceding exercise when exercise begins slowly.

Cool-down A period at the end of an exercise session when exercise is tapered off.

Frequency of exercise How often a person engages in an exercise session.

FIGURE **3.2** Cardiorespiratory exercise prescription guidelines.

Activity:	Aerobic (examples: walking, jogging, cycling, swimming, aerobics, racquetball, soccer, stair climbing)
Intensity:	40%/50%–85% of heart rate reserve
Duration:	20–60 minutes of continuous aerobic activity
Frequency:	3 to 5 days per week

Adapted from: American College of Sports Medicine, *Guidelines for Exercise Testing and Prescription*, (Baltimore: Williams & Wilkins, 2006).

Critical Thinking

Kate started an exercise program last year as a means to lose weight and enhance her body image. She now runs more than 6 miles every day, works out regularly on stair-climbers and elliptical machines, strength-trains daily, participates in step aerobics three times per week, and plays tennis or racquetball twice a week.

Evaluate Kate's program. What suggestions do you have for improvements?

Muscular Strength and Endurance

The capacity of muscle cells to exert force increases and decreases according to demands placed upon the muscular system. If specific muscle cells are overloaded beyond their normal use, such as in strength-training programs, the cells increase in size (hypertrophy), strength, or endurance, or some combination of these. If the demands on the muscle cells decrease, such as in sedentary living or required rest because of illness or injury, the cells decrease in size (atrophy) and lose strength.

Overload Principle

The **overload principle** states that, for strength or endurance to improve, demands placed on the muscle must be increased systematically and progressively over time, and the **resistance** (weight lifted) must be of a magnitude significant enough to produce development. In simpler terms, just like all other organs and systems of the human body, muscles have to be taxed beyond their accustomed loads to increase in physical capacity.

Specificity of Training

Muscular strength is the ability to exert maximum force against resistance. Muscular endurance (also referred to as localized muscular endurance) is the ability of a muscle to exert submaximal force repeatedly over time. Both of these components require **specificity of training**.

As discussed later in this section, a person attempting to increase muscular strength needs a program of few repetitions and near-maximum resistance. To increase muscular endurance, the strength-training program consists primarily of many repetitions at a lower resistance. In like manner, to increase isometric (static) versus dynamic strength (see the next section on Mode of Training), an individual must use the corresponding static or dynamic training procedures to achieve the appropriate results.

In like manner, if a person is trying to improve a specific movement or skill through strength gains, the selected strength-training exercises must resemble the actual movement or skill as closely as possible.

Strength-Training Prescription

Similar to the prescription of cardiorespiratory exercise, several factors or variables have to be taken into account to improve muscular strength and endurance. These are mode, resistance, sets, and frequency of training.

Mode of Training

Two basic training methods are used to improve strength: isometric and dynamic. **Isometric exercise** involves pushing or pulling against immovable objects. **Dynamic exercise** requires movement with the muscle contraction, such as extending the knees with resistance (weight) on the ankles.

Isometric training was used commonly several years ago, but its popularity has waned. Because strength gains with isometric training are specific to the angle of muscle contraction, this type of training remains beneficial in sports such as gymnastics that require regular static contractions during routines.

Dynamic exercise (previously referred to as **isotonic exercise**) can be conducted without weights or with **free weights** (barbells and dumbbells), **fixed-resistance** machines, **variable-resistance** machines, and isokinetic equipment. When performing dynamic exercises without weights (for example, pull-ups, push-ups), with free weights, or with fixed-resistance machines, a constant resistance (weight) is moved through a joint's full range of motion. The greatest resistance that can be lifted equals the maximum weight that can be moved at the weakest angle of the joint, because of changes in muscle

Isometric strength training.

Isokinetic strength training.

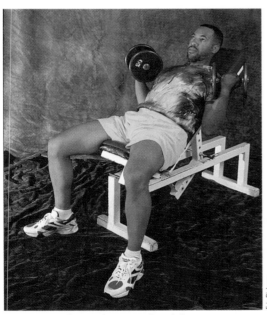

Dynamic strength training.

length and angle of pull as the joint moves through its range of motion.

As strength training became more popular, new strength-training machines were developed. This technology brought about isokinetic and variable-resistance training. These training programs require special machines equipped with mechanical devices that provide differing amounts of resistance, with the intent of overloading the muscle group maximally through the entire range of motion. A distinction of **isokinetic exercise** is that the speed of the muscle contraction is kept constant because the machine provides resistance to match the user's force through the range of motion. Because of the expense of the equipment needed for isokinetic training, this type of program usually is reserved for clinical settings (physical therapy), research laboratories, and certain professional sports.

KEY TERMS

Overload principle Training concept holding that the demands placed on a body system must be increased systematically and progressively over time to cause physiologic adaptation.

Resistance Amount of weight lifted.

Specificity of training A principle holding that, for a muscle to increase in strength or endurance, the training program must be specific to obtain the desired effects.

Isometric exercise Strength training with muscle contraction that produces little or no movement.

Dynamic exercise Strength training with muscle contraction that produces movement.

Isotonic exercise See Dynamic exercise.

Free weights Barbells and dumbbells.

Fixed-resistance training Exercise with strength-training equipment that provides a constant amount of resistance through the range of motion.

Variable-resistance training Exercise that utilizes special equipment with mechanical devices that provide differing amounts of resistance through the range of motion.

Isokinetic exercise Strength training in which the equipment accommodates resistance to match the user's force through the full range of motion.

Dynamic training has two action phases: **concentric** or **positive resistance** and eccentric or **negative resistance**. In the concentric phase, the muscle shortens as it contracts to overcome the resistance. For example, during the bench press exercise, when the resistance is lifted from the chest to full arm extension, the triceps muscle on the back of the upper arm contracts and shortens to extend the elbow. During the **eccentric** phase, the muscle lengthens as it contracts. In the case of the bench press exercise, the same triceps muscle contracts to lower the resistance during elbow flexion, but it lengthens to avoid dropping the resistance.

Eccentric muscle contractions allow us to lower weights in a smooth, gradual, and controlled manner. Without eccentric contractions, weights would be dropped on the way down. Because the same muscles work when you lift and lower a resistance, you should be sure to always execute both actions in a controlled manner. Failure to do so diminishes the benefits of the training program and increases the risk for injuries.

The mode of training depends mainly on the type of equipment available and the specific objective of the training program. Dynamic training is the most popular mode for strength training. Its primary advantage is that strength is gained through the full range of motion. Most daily activities are dynamic in nature. We constantly lift, push, and pull objects, which requires strength through a given range of motion. Another advantage of dynamic exercise is that improvements are measured easily by the amount lifted.

Benefits of isokinetic and variable-resistance training are similar to those of the other dynamic training methods. Theoretically, strength gains should be better because maximum resistance is applied through the entire range of motion. Research, however, has not shown this type of training to be more effective than other modes of dynamic training. A possible advantage is that specific speeds in selected sport skills can be duplicated more closely with isokinetic strength training, which may enhance performance (specificity of training). A disadvantage is that the equipment is not readily available to everyone.

Plate-loaded barbells (free weights) were the most popular weight training equipment available during the first half of the 20th century. Strength training machines were developed in the middle of the century but did not become popular until the 1970s. With the advent of, and subsequent technological improvements to, these machines, a stirring debate surfaced over which of the two training modalities was better.

Free weights require that the individual balance the resistance through the entire lifting motion. Thus, a logical assumption could be made that free weights are a better training modality because of the involvement of additional stabilizing muscles needed to balance the resistance as it is moved through its range of motion. Research, however, has not shown any differences in strength development between the two exercise modalities. Although each modality has pros and cons, the muscles do not know whether the source of a resistance is a barbell, a dumbbell, a Universal Gym machine, a Nautilus machine, or a simple cinder block. What determines the level of a person's strength development is the quality of the program and the individual's effort during the training program itself—not the type of equipment used.

Resistance

Resistance in strength training is the equivalent of intensity in cardiorespiratory exercise prescription. To stimulate strength development, the general recommendation has been to use a resistance of approximately 80 percent of the maximum capacity (1 RM). For example, a person with a 1 RM of 150 pounds should work with about 120 pounds (150 × .80).

The number of repetitions that one can perform at 80 percent of the 1 RM varies among exercises. Data indicates that the total number of repetitions performed at a certain percentage of the 1 RM depends on the amount of muscle mass used (bench press versus triceps extension) and whether it is a single or multi-joint exercise (leg press versus leg curl). In both trained and untrained subjects, the number of repetitions is greater with larger muscle mass involvement and multi-joint exercises.[8]

Because of the time required to constantly determine the 1 RM on each lift to ensure that the person is indeed working around 80 percent, the accepted rule for many years has been that individuals perform between 3 and 12 repetitions maximum (3 to 12 RM) for adequate strength gains. For example, if a person is training with a resistance of 120 pounds and cannot lift it more than 12 times—that is, the person reaches volitional fatigue at or before 12 repetitions—the training stimulus (weight used) is adequate for strength development. Once the person can lift the resistance more than 12 times, the resistance is increased by 5 to 10 pounds and the person again should build up to 12 repetitions. This is referred to as **progressive resistance training**.

Strength development, however, can also occur when working with less than 80 percent of the 1 RM. Although 3 to 12 RM is the most commonly prescribed resistance, benefits do occur when working below 3 or above 12 RM.

At least in the health fitness area, little evidence presently supports the notion that working with a given number of repetitions elicits specific or greater strength, muscular endurance, or **muscular hypertrophy**.[9] Although not precisely to the same extent, muscular strength and endurance are both increased when training within a reasonable amount of repetitions. Thus, the American College of Sports Medicine recommends using a range between 3 and 20 RM. The individual may choose the number of repetitions based on personal preference.

Elite strength athletes typically work between 1 and 6 RM, but often shuffle training with different number of repetitions for selected periods (weeks) of time. Body builders tend to work with moderate resistance levels (60 to 85 percent of the 1 RM) and perform 8 to 20 repetitions to near fatigue. A foremost objective of body building is to increase muscle size. Moderate resistance promotes blood flow to the muscles, "pumping up the muscles" (also known as "the pump") and making them look much larger than they do in a resting state.

From a general fitness point of view, working near a 10-repetition threshold seems to improve overall performance most effectively. We live in a dynamic world in which muscular strength and endurance are both required to lead an enjoyable life. Working around 10 RM produces good results in terms of strength, endurance, and hypertrophy. For older and more frail individuals (50–60 years of age and above), 10 to 15 repetitions to near fatigue may be more appropriate.

We must mention here that a certain resistance (for example, 50 pounds) is seldom the same on two different weight machines, or between free weights and weight machines. The industry has no standard calibration procedure for strength equipment. Consequently, if you lift a certain weight with free weights or a given machine, you may or may not be able to lift the same amount on a different piece of equipment.

Sets

Strength training is done in **sets**. For example, a person lifting 120 pounds eight times performs one set of eight **repetitions** (1/8/120). For general fitness, the recommendation is one to three sets per exercise. Some evidence suggests greater strength gains using multiple sets as opposed to a single set for a given exercise. Other research, however, concludes that similar increases in strength, endurance, and hypertrophy are derived between single- and multiple-set strength training; as long as the single set, or at least one of the multiple sets, is performed to volitional exhaustion (heavy set).[10] Strength gains may be lessened by performing too many sets.

A recommended program for beginners in their first year of training is one or two light warm-up sets per exercise using about 50 percent of the 1 RM (no warm-up sets are necessary for subsequent exercises that use the same muscle group) followed by one to three sets per exercise. Maintaining a resistance and effort that will temporarily fatigue the muscle (volitional exhaustion) in the number of repetitions selected in at least one of the sets is critical to achieve optimal progress. Because of the lower resistances used in body building, four to eight sets can be done for each exercise.

To make the exercise program more time-effective, two or three exercises that require different muscle groups may be alternated. In this way, a person will not have to wait 2 to 3 minutes before proceeding to a new set of a different exercise. For example, the bench press, leg extension, and abdominal curl-up exercises may be combined so the person can go almost directly from one set to the next. Body builders should rest no more than a minute to maximize the "pumping" effect.

To avoid muscle soreness and stiffness, new participants ought to build up gradually to the three sets of maximal repetitions. This can be done by performing only one set of each exercise with a lighter resistance on the first day. During the second session, two sets of each exercise can be done: the first light and the second with the regular resistance. During the third session, three sets could be performed—one light and two heavy sets. After that, a person should be able to do all three heavy sets.

CT Critical Thinking

What role should strength-training have in a fitness program? Should people be motivated for the health fitness benefits, or should they participate to enhance their body image? What are your feelings about individuals (male or female) with large body musculature?

KEY TERMS

Concentric Shortening of a muscle during muscle contraction.

Positive resistance The lifting, pushing, or concentric phase of a repetition during the performance of a strength-training exercise.

Negative resistance The lowering or eccentric phase of a repetition during the performance of a strength-training exercise.

Eccentric Lengthening of a muscle during muscle contraction.

Progressive resistance training A gradual increase of resistance over a period of time.

Muscular hypertrophy An increase in muscle mass or size.

Set The number of repetitions performed for a given exercise.

Repetitions The number of times a movement is performed.

Frequency of Training

Strength training should be done either with a total body workout two or three times per week, or more frequently if using a split-body routine (upper body one day and lower body the next). After a maximum strength workout, the muscles should be rested for about 48 hours to allow adequate recovery. If not recovered completely in 2 or 3 days, the person most likely is overtraining and therefore not reaping the full benefits of the program. In that case, a decrease in the total number of sets or exercises, or both, performed during the previous workout is recommended.

A summary of strength-training guidelines for health fitness purposes is provided in Figure 3.3. Significant strength gains require a minimum of 8 weeks of consecutive training. After achieving the recommended strength level, one training session per week will be sufficient to maintain the new strength level.

Frequency of strength training for body builders varies from person to person. Because they use moderate resistances, daily or even two-a-day workouts are common. The frequency depends on the amount of resistance, number of sets performed per session, and the person's ability to recover from the previous exercise bout (see Table 3.2). The latter often is dictated by level of conditioning.

Strength-Training Exercises

Two strength-training programs, presented in Appendix A, have been developed to provide a complete body workout. Only a minimum of equipment is required for the first program, "Strength-Training Exercises Without Weights" (Exercises 1 through 15). This program can be conducted within the walls of your own home. Your body weight is used as the primary resistance for most exercises. A few exercises call for a friend's help or basic implements from around your home to provide greater resistance.

"Strength-Training Exercises With Weights" (Exercises 16 through 27), requires machines such as those shown in the various photographs. Some of these exercises can also be performed with free weights.

Strength-Training Exercise Guidelines

As you prepare to design your strength-training program, you should keep several guidelines in mind.

1. Select exercises that will involve all major muscle groups: chest, shoulders, back, legs, arms, hips, and trunk.
2. Never lift weights alone. Always have someone work out with you in case you need a spotter or

FIGURE 3.3 Strength training guidelines.

Mode:	8 to 10 dynamic strength-training exercises involving the body's major muscle groups
Resistance:	Sufficient resistance to perform 3 to 20 repetitions to complete or near-complete fatigue (the number of repetitions is optional; you may use 3 to 6, 8 to 12, 12 to 15, or 16 to 20 repetitions)
Sets:	A minimum of 1 set
Frequency:	2 to 3 days per week on nonconsecutive days

Adapted from: American College of Sports Medicine, *Guidelines for Exercise Testing and Prescription*, (Baltimore: Williams & Wilkins, 2006).

TABLE 3.2 Guidelines for Various Strength-Training Programs

STRENGTH-TRAINING PROGRAM	RESISTANCE	SETS	REST BETWEEN SETS*	FREQUENCY (WORKOUTS PER WEEK)**
General fitness	3–20 reps max	1–3	2 min	2–3
Strength athletes	1–6 reps max	3–6	3 min	2–3
Body building	8–20 reps near max	3–8	up to 1 min	4–12

* Recovery between sets can be decreased by alternating exercises that use different muscle groups.

** Weekly training sessions can be increased by using a split-body routine.

help with an injury. When using free weights, one to two spotters are recommended for certain exercises (bench press, squats, overhead press).
3. Warm up properly prior to lifting weights by performing a light- to moderate-intensity aerobic activity (5 to 7 minutes) and some gentle stretches for a few minutes.
4. Exercise larger muscle groups first, such as those in the chest, back, and legs. Then proceed to the smaller muscle groups (arms, abdominals, ankles, neck). The bench press exercise works the chest, shoulders, and back of the upper arms (triceps), whereas the triceps extension works the back of the upper arms only.
5. Exercise opposing muscle groups for a balanced workout. When you work the chest (bench press), work the back (rowing torso). If you work the biceps (arm curl), work the triceps (triceps extension).

6. Perform all exercises in a controlled manner. Avoid fast and jerky movements, and do not throw the entire body into the lifting motion, which would increase the risk of injury and decrease the effectiveness of the exercise. Do not arch the back when lifting a weight.

7. Perform each exercise through the entire possible range of motion.

8. Breathe naturally, and do not hold your breath as you lift the resistance (weight). Inhale during the eccentric phase (bringing the weight down) and exhale during the concentric phase (lifting or pushing the weight up). Practice proper breathing with lighter weights when you are learning a new exercise.

9. Avoid holding your breath while straining to lift a weight. Holding your breath greatly increases the pressure inside the chest and abdominal cavity, making it nearly impossible for the blood in the veins to return to the heart. Although rare, a sudden high intrathoracic pressure may lead to dizziness, a black-out, a stroke, a heart attack, or a hernia.

10. Based on the program selected, allow adequate recovery time between sets of exercises (see Table 3.2).

11. Discontinue training if you experience unusual discomfort or pain. High tension-loads used in strength training can exacerbate potential injuries. Discomfort and pain are signals to stop and determine what's wrong. Be sure to properly evaluate your condition before you continue training.

12. Stretch out for a few minutes at the end of each strength-training workout to help the muscles return to their normal resting length and to minimize muscle soreness and risk of injury.

Core Strength Training

The trunk (spine) and pelvis are referred to as the "core" of the body. Core muscles include the abdominal muscles (rectus, transversus, and internal and external obliques), hip muscles (front and back), and spinal muscles (lower and upper back muscles). These muscle groups are responsible for maintaining the stability of the spine and pelvis.

Many of the major muscle groups of the legs, shoulders, and arms attach to the core. A strong core allows a person to perform activities of daily living with greater ease, improve sports performance through a more effective energy transfer from large to small body parts, and decrease the incidence of low-back pain.

Interest in core strength-training programs has increased recently. A major objective of core training is to exercise the abdominal and lower back muscles in unison. Furthermore, individuals should spend as much time training the back muscles as they do the abdominal muscles. Besides enhancing stability, core training improves dynamic balance, which is often required during participation in physical activity and sports.

Key core-training exercises include the abdominal crunch and bent-leg curl-up, reverse crunch, pelvic tilt, lateral bridge, prone bridge, supine bridge, leg press, lat pull-down, seated back, and back extension (Exercises 4, 11, 12, 13, 14, 15, 19, 21, 25, and 27 in Appendix A) and pelvic clock (Exercise 50 in Appendix C, page 240).

When core training is used in athletic conditioning programs, athletes attempt to mimic the dynamic skills used in their sport. To do so, they use special equipment such as balance boards, stability balls, and foam pads. The use of this equipment allows the athletes to train the core while seeking balance and stability in a sport specific manner.[11]

Designing Your Own Strength-Training Program

The pre-exercise guidelines outlined in the Clearance for Exercise Participation questionnaire (see Activity 1.2, page 23) also apply to strength training. If you have any concerns about whether your present health status will allow you to safely participate in strength training, consult a physician before you start. Strength training is not advised for people with advanced heart disease.

Depending on the facilities available to you, choose one of the two training programs outlined in Appendix A. Once you begin your strength-training, you may use the form provided in Activity 3.4, page 84, to keep a record of your training program.

The resistance, the number of repetitions, and sets you use with your program should be based on your current strength-fitness level and the amount of time that you have for your strength workout. If you are training for reasons other than general health fitness, review Table 3.2, page 64, for a summary of the guidelines.

Muscular Flexibility

Improving and maintaining good joint range of motion throughout life is important in enhancing health and quality of life. Nevertheless, fitness participants generally have underestimated and overlooked flexibility fitness.

The most significant detriments to flexibility are sedentary living and lack of physical activity. As physical activity decreases, muscles lose elasticity, and tendons and ligaments tighten and shorten. Aging also reduces the extensibility of soft tissue, decreasing flexibility.

Generally, flexibility exercises to improve range of motion around the joints are conducted following an aerobic workout. Stretching exercises seem to be most effective when a person is warmed up properly. Cool muscle temperatures decrease joint range of motion. Changes in muscle temperature can increase or decrease flexibility by as much as 20 percent. Because of the effects of muscular temperature on flexibility, many people prefer to do their stretching exercises after the aerobic phase of their workout.

Muscular Flexibility Prescription

The overload and specificity of training principles apply to development of muscular flexibility. To increase the total range of motion of a joint, the specific muscles surrounding that joint have to be stretched progressively beyond their accustomed length. The factors of mode, intensity, repetitions, and frequency of exercise also can be applied to flexibility programs.

Mode of Exercise

Three modes of stretching exercises promote flexibility:

1. Ballistic stretching.
2. Slow-sustained stretching.
3. Proprioceptive neuromuscular facilitation (PNF) stretching.

Although all three types of stretching are effective in developing better flexibility, each has certain advantages. **Ballistic (or dynamic) stretching** exercises provide the necessary force to lengthen the muscles. Although this type of stretching helps to develop flexibility, the ballistic actions may cause muscle soreness and injury as a result of small tears to the soft tissue.

Precautions must be taken not to overstretch ligaments, because they undergo plastic (permanent) elongation. If the stretching force cannot be controlled, as in fast, jerky movements, ligaments can be overstretched easily. This, in turn, leads to excessively loose joints, increasing the risk for injuries, including joint dislocation and subluxation (partial dislocation). Slow, gentle, and controlled ballistic stretching (instead of jerky, rapid, and bouncy movements), however, is effective in developing flexibility and most individuals can perform this safely.

Slow-sustained stretching causes the muscles to relax so greater length can be achieved. This type of stretch causes little pain and has a low risk of injury. Slow-sustained stretching exercises are the most frequently used and recommended for flexibility development programs.

Proprioceptive neuromuscular facilitation (PNF) stretching has become more popular in the last few years. This technique, based on a "contract-and-relax"

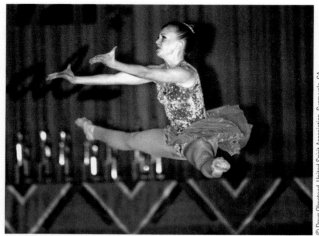
Performance of complex motor skills improves with good flexibility.

© Doug Olmstead, United Spirit Association, Sunnyvale, CA

method, requires the assistance of another person. The procedure is as follows:

1. The person assisting with the exercise provides initial force by pushing slowly in the direction of the desired stretch. The initial stretch does not cover the entire range of motion.
2. The person being stretched then applies force in the opposite direction of the stretch, against the assistant, who tries to hold the initial degree of stretch as closely as possible. An isometric contraction is being performed at that angle.
3. After a few seconds (5–6 seconds) of isometric contraction, the muscles being stretched are relaxed completely. The assistant then increases the degree of stretch slowly to a greater angle.
4. The isometric contraction is repeated, following which the muscle(s) is relaxed again. The assistant then can increase the degree of stretch slowly one more time.
5. Steps 1 through 4 are repeated two to five times, until the exerciser feels mild discomfort. On the last trial, the final stretched position should be held for 15 to 30 seconds.

Theoretically, with the PNF technique, the isometric contraction helps relax the muscle(s) being stretched, which results in longer muscles. Some fitness leaders believe PNF is more effective than slow-sustained stretching.

Another benefit of PNF is an increase in strength of the muscle(s) being stretched. Research has shown approximately 17 and 35 percent increases in absolute strength and muscular endurance in muscles following 12 weeks of PNF stretching. These increases are attributed to the isometric contractions performed during

Proprioceptive neuromuscular facilitation (PNF) stretching technique: (A) isometric phase, (B) stretching phase.

PNF. The disadvantages are that more pain occurs with PNF, a second person is required to assist, and more time is needed to conduct each session.

Intensity of Exercise

When you do flexibility exercises, the **intensity** of each stretch should be only to a point of mild discomfort. Excessive pain is an indication that the load is too high and may lead to injury. All stretching should be done to slightly below the pain threshold. As participants reach this point, they should try to relax the muscle being stretched as much as possible. After completing the stretch, the body part is brought back gradually to the starting point.

Repetitions

The time required for a flexibility exercise session is based on the number of repetitions performed and the length of time each repetition (final stretched position) is held. The general recommendation is that each

---

FIGURE 3.4 Flexibility development guidelines.

Mode:	A static stretching routine that includes every major joint of the body and focuses on joints that have a decreased range of motion
Intensity:	Stretch to end of range of motion to the point of mild discomfort
Repetitions:	2 to 4 repetitions of each stretch and hold the final stretched position for 15 to 30 seconds
Frequency:	A minimum of 3 days per week (ideally 5 to 7 days per week)

Adapted from: American College of Sports Medicine, *Guidelines for Exercise Testing and Prescription*, (Baltimore: Williams & Wilkins, 2006).

---

exercise be done at least four times, holding the final position each time for 15 to 30 seconds. As flexibility increases, a person may gradually increase the time each repetition is held, to a maximum of 1 minute. Individuals who are susceptible to flexibility injuries should limit each stretch to 20 seconds. Pilates exercises are recommended for these individuals, because they increase joint stability (see the discussion on the Pilates exercise system on page 68 in this chapter).

Frequency of Exercise

Flexibility exercises should be conducted a minimum of 2 to 3 days per week, but ideally 5 to 7 days per week. After 6 to 8 weeks of almost daily stretching, flexibility can be maintained with only two or three sessions per week, doing about three repetitions of 15 to 30 seconds each. Figure 3.4 summarizes the flexibility development guidelines.

When To Stretch?

Many people do not differentiate a warm-up from stretching. Warming up means starting a workout slowly with walking, cycling, or slow jogging, followed

K E Y   T E R M S

Ballistic (or dynamic) stretching Exercises performed using jerky, rapid, and bouncy movements.

Slow-sustained stretching Technique whereby the muscles are lengthened gradually through a joint's complete range of motion and the final position is held for several seconds.

Proprioceptive neuromuscular facilitation (PNF) A stretching technique in which muscles are stretched out progressively with intermittent isometric contractions.

Intensity (in flexibility exercise) Degree of stretch.

Photos © Fitness & Wellness, Inc.

by gentle stretching (not through the entire range of motion). Stretching implies movement of joints through their full range of motion and holding the final degree of stretch according to recommended guidelines.

A warm-up that progressively increases muscle temperature and mimics movement that will occur during training enhances performance. For some activities, gentle stretching is recommended in conjunction with warm-up routines. Before steady activities (walking, jogging, cycling), a warm-up of 3 to 5 minutes is recommended. Up to 10 minutes is the recommendation before stop-and-go activities (racquet sports, basketball, soccer) and athletic participation in general (football, gymnastics). Activities that require abrupt changes in direction are more likely to cause muscle strains if they are performed without a proper warm-up that includes mild stretching.

Sports-specific/pre-exercise stretching can improve performance in sports that require greater-than-average range of motion, such as gymnastics, dance, swimming, and figure skating. Some evidence, however, suggests that intense stretching during warm-up can lead to a temporary short-term (up to 60 minutes) decrease in strength. Thus, extensive stretching conducted prior to participation in athletic events that rely on strength and power for peak performance is not recommended.[12]

In terms of preventing injuries, the best time to stretch is controversial. In limited studies on athletic populations, the evidence is unclear as to whether stretching before or after exercise is more beneficial in preventing injury. Additional research is necessary to clarify this issue.

In general, a good time to stretch is after aerobic workouts. Higher body temperature in itself helps to increase the joint range of motion. Muscles also are fatigued following exercise, and a fatigued muscle tends to shorten, which can lead to soreness and spasms. Stretching exercises help fatigued muscles reestablish their normal resting length and prevent unnecessary pain.

Designing a Flexibility Program

To improve body flexibility, each major muscle group should be subjected to at least one stretching exercise. A complete set of exercises for developing muscular flexibility is presented in Appendix B.

You may not be able to hold a final stretched position with some of these exercises (such as lateral head tilts and arm circles), but you still should perform the exercise through the joint's full range of motion. Depending on the number and the length of repetitions, a complete workout will last between 15 and 30 minutes.

Critical Thinking

Carefully consider the relevance of stretching exercises in your personal fitness program throughout the years. How much importance do you place on these exercises? Have any conditions improved through your stretching program or have any specific exercises contributed to your health and well-being?

Pilates Exercise System

Pilates exercises have become increasingly popular in recent years. Previously, Pilates training was used primarily by dancers, but now many fitness participants, rehab patients, models, actors, and even professional athletes are embracing this exercise modality. Pilates studios, college courses, and classes at health clubs now are available nationwide.

The Pilates training system was originally developed in the 1920s by German physical therapist Joseph Pilates. The exercises are designed to help strengthen the body's core by developing pelvic stability and abdominal control—coupled with focused breathing patterns. Pilates exercises are performed either on a mat (floor) or with specialized equipment to help increase strength and flexibility of deep postural muscles. The intent is to improve muscle tone and length (providing a limber body), instead of increasing muscle size (hypertrophy). The exercises are performed in a slow, controlled, precise manner. Properly performed, Pilates exercises require intense concentration. Initial Pilates training should be conducted under the supervision of certified instructors with extensive Pilates teaching experience.

Fitness goals of Pilates programs include improved flexibility, muscle tone, posture, spinal support, body balance, low-back health, sports performance, and mind–body awareness. The Pilates program also is used to help lose weight, increase lean tissue, and manage stress. Although Pilates programs are popular, research is required to corroborate the benefits attributed to the Pilates training system.

Preventing and Rehabilitating Low-Back Pain

Few people make it through life without having low-back pain at some point. An estimated 60 percent to 90 percent of all Americans will suffer from chronic back pain in their lives.[13] On a yearly basis, more than 75 million people report having chronic low-back pain.

Back pain is considered chronic if it persists longer than 3 months. About 80 percent of the time, backache syndrome is preventable and is caused by: (a) physical inactivity, (b) poor postural habits and body mechanics, (c) excessive body weight, and/or (d) psychological stress.

Although people tend to think of back pain as a skeletal problem, the spine's curvature, alignment, and movement are controlled by surrounding muscles. Lack of physical activity is the most common reason for chronic low-back pain. A major contributor to back pain is sitting for long periods, which causes back muscles to shorten, stiffen, and become weaker.

Deterioration or weakening of the abdominal and gluteal muscles, along with tightening of the lower back (erector spinae) muscles, brings about an unnatural forward tilt of the pelvis (Figure 3.5). This tilt puts extra pressure on the spinal vertebrae, causing pain in the lower back. Accumulation of fat around the midsection of the body contributes to the forward tilt of the pelvis, which further aggravates the condition.

Low-back pain is frequently associated with faulty posture and improper body mechanics or body positions in all of life's daily activities, including sleeping, sitting, standing, walking, driving, working, and exercising. Incorrect posture and poor mechanics, as explained in Figure 3.6, increase strain on the lower back as well as many other bones, joints, muscles, and ligaments.

Back pain can be reduced greatly by including some specific stretching and strengthening exercises in the regular fitness program. In most cases, back pain is present only with movement and physical activity. If the pain is severe and persists even at rest, the first step is to consult a physician, who can rule out any disc damage and may prescribe proper bed rest using several pillows under the knees for leg support (see Figure 3.6). This position helps release muscle spasms by stretching the muscles involved. In addition, a physician may prescribe a muscle relaxant or anti-inflammatory medication (or both) and some type of physical therapy.

In most cases of low-back pain, even with severe pain, people feel better within days or weeks without treatment from health care professionals.[14] To relieve symptoms, you may use over-the-counter pain relievers and hot or cold packs. You should also stay active to avoid further weakening of the back muscles. Low-impact activities like walking, swimming, water aerobics, and cycling are recommended. Once you are pain-free in the resting state, you need to start correcting the muscular imbalance by stretching the tight muscles and strengthening the weak ones. Stretching exercises always are performed first.

If there is no indication of disease or injury, such as leg numbness or pain, a herniated disk, or fractures,

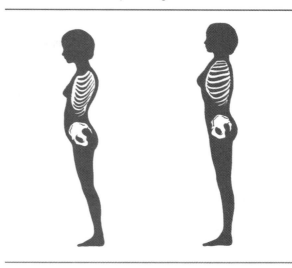

FIGURE **3.5** Incorrect (left) and correct (right) pelvic alignment.

spinal manipulation by a chiropractor or other health care professional can provide pain relief. Spinal manipulation as a treatment modality for low-back pain has been endorsed by the Federal Agency for Health Care Policy and Research. The guidelines suggest that spinal manipulation may help to alleviate discomfort and pain during the first few weeks of an acute episode of low-back pain. Generally, benefits are seen within 10 treatments. People who have had chronic pain for more than 6 months should avoid spinal manipulation until they have been thoroughly examined by a physician.

Several exercises for preventing and rehabilitating the backache syndrome are given in Appendix C, pages 239–240. These exercises can be done twice or more daily when a person has back pain. Under normal circumstances, doing these exercises three to four times a week is enough to prevent the syndrome.

Psychological stress may also lead to back pain.[15] Excessive stress causes muscles to contract. In the case of the lower back, frequent tightening of the muscles can throw the back out of alignment and constrict blood vessels that supply oxygen and nutrients to the back. If you suffer from excessive stress and back pain at the same time, proper stress management (see Chapter 7) should be a part of your comprehensive back-care program.

KEY TERMS

Pilates Exercises that help strengthen the body's core by developing pelvic stability and abdominal control coupled with focused breathing patterns.

FIGURE 3.6 Your back and how to care for it.

HOW TO STAY ON YOUR FEET WITHOUT TIRING YOUR BACK

To prevent strain and pain in everyday activities, it is restful to change from one task to another before fatigue sets in. You can lie down between chores; you should check body position frequently, drawing in the abdomen, flattening the back, bending the knees slightly.

Not this way

Use of a footrest relieves swayback.

Not this way

Bend the knees and hips, not the waist.

Not this way

Hold heavy objects close to you.

Not this way

Never bend over without bending the knees.

HOW TO PUT YOUR BACK TO BED

For proper bed posture, a firm mattress is essential. Bedboards, sold commercially, or devised at home, may be used with soft mattresses. Bedboards, preferably, should be made of 3/4 inch plywood. Faulty sleeping positions intensify swayback and result not only in backache but in numbness, tingling, and pain in arms and legs.

Incorrect:
Lying flat on back makes swayback worse.

Use of high pillow strains neck, arms, shoulders.

Sleeping face down exaggerates swayback, strains neck and shoulders.

Bending one hip and knee does not relieve swayback.

Correct:
Lying on side with knees bent effectively flattens the back. Flat pillow may be used to support neck, especially when shoulders are broad.

Sleeping on back is restful and correct when knees are properly supported.

Raise the foot of the mattress eight inches to discourage sleeping on the abdomen.

Proper arrangement of pillows for resting or reading in bed.

HOW TO SIT CORRECTLY

A back's best friend is a straight, hard chair. If you can't get the chair you prefer, learn to sit properly on whatever chair you get. To correct sitting position from forward slump: Throw head well back, then bend it forward to pull in the chin. This will straighten the back. Now tighten abdominal muscles to raise the chest. Check position frequently.

Use of footrest relieves swayback. Aim is to have knees higher than hips.

Correct way to sit while driving, close to pedals. Use seatbelt or hard backrest, available commercially.

TV slump leads to "dowager's hump," strains neck and shoulders.

If chair is too high, swayback is increased.

Keep neck and back in as straight a line as possible with the spine. Bend forward from hips.

Driver's seat too far from pedals emphasizes curve in lower back.

Strained reading position. Forward thrusting strains muscles of neck and head.

Contraindicated Exercises

Most strength and flexibility exercises are relatively safe to perform, but even safe exercises can be hazardous if they are done incorrectly. Some exercises may be safe for you to perform occasionally but, when executed repeatedly, could cause trauma and injury. Preexisting muscle or joint conditions (old sprains or injuries) can further increase the risk of harm when performing certain exercises. As you develop your exercise program, you are encouraged to follow the exercise descriptions and guidelines given in this book.

A few exercises are not recommended because they pose a potentially high risk for injury. These exercises are sometimes performed in videotaped workouts and some fitness classes. **Contraindicated exercises** may cause harm because of the excessive strain placed on muscles and joints—in particular, the spine, lower back, knees, neck, or shoulders.

Illustrations of contraindicated exercises are presented in Appendix D. Safe alternative exercises are listed below each contraindicated exercise and are illustrated in Appendix A (strength exercises), pages 227–236, and Appendix B (flexibility exercises), pages 237–238. In isolated instances a qualified physical therapist may select one or a few of the contraindicated exercises to treat a certain injury or disability in a carefully supervised setting. Unless you are instructed specifically to use one of these exercises, it is best that you select safe exercises from this book.

Tips to Enhance Compliance with Your Fitness Program

Introducing new behaviors into one's daily routine takes most people months or longer to accomplish. A fitness program is no exception. Adding exercise to a person's lifestyle may require retraining (behavior modification).

Different things motivate different people to start and remain in a fitness program. Regardless of your initial reason for initiating an exercise program, you now need to plan for ways to make your workout fun. The psychology behind it is simple: If you enjoy an activity, you will continue to do it.

The first few weeks probably will be the most difficult, but where there's a will, there's a way. Once you begin to see positive changes, it won't be as hard. Soon you will develop a habit for exercise that will be deeply satisfying and will bring about a sense of self-accomplishment. The following suggestions have been used successfully to help people change their behavior and adhere to a lifetime exercise program.

1. Set aside a regular time for exercise. If you don't plan ahead, it is a lot easier to skip. Every week, using red ink, schedule your exercise time into your day planner. Hold your exercise hour "sacred." Give exercise the same priority as you would give the most important school or business activity of the day. If you are too busy or your schedule too unpredictable, attempt to accumulate 30 minutes of activity daily by doing three separate 10-minute sessions. Read the mail while you walk, take stairs instead of elevators, walk the dog, or ride the stationary bike as you watch the evening news. If you are using physical activity to manage your weight, more planning will be required to ensure that you accumulate 60 to 90 minutes of daily physical activity. (Chapter 6 is devoted to weight management.)
2. Exercise early in the day, when you will be less tired and the chances of something interfering with your workout are minimal; thus, you will be less likely to skip your exercise session.
3. Select aerobic activities you enjoy. Exercise should be as much fun as your favorite hobby. If you pick an activity you don't enjoy, you will be unmotivated and less likely to keep exercising. Don't be afraid to try out a new activity, even if that means learning new skills.
4. Combine different activities. You can train by doing two or three different activities the same week. This **cross-training** may deter the monotony of repeating the same activity every day. Try lifetime sports. Many endurance sports, such as racquetball, basketball, soccer, badminton, roller skating, cross-country skiing, and body surfing (paddling the board), provide a nice break from regular workouts.
5. Wear the proper clothing and use equipment designed for exercise. A poor pair of shoes, for example, can make you more prone to injury, discouraging you from the beginning.
6. Find a friend or group of friends to exercise with. Social interaction will make exercise more fulfilling. Besides, it's harder to skip if someone is waiting to go with you.

KEY TERMS

Contraindicated exercises Exercises that are not recommended because they pose potentially high risk for injury.

Cross-training Using a combination of different aerobic activities to develop or maintain cardiorespiratory endurance.

7. Set goals, and share them with others. Quitting is tougher when someone else knows what you are trying to accomplish. When you reach a targeted goal, reward yourself with a new pair of shoes or a jogging suit.

8. Purchase a pedometer (step counter) and attempt to accumulate 10,000 steps each day. These 10,000 steps may combine all forms of your daily physical activity.

9. Don't become a chronic exerciser. Learn to listen to your body. Overexercising can lead to chronic fatigue and injuries. Exercise should be enjoyable, and in the process you should stop and smell the roses.

10. Exercise in different places and facilities. This will add variety to your workouts.

11. Exercise to music. People who listen to fast-tempo music tend to exercise more vigorously and longer. Using headphones when exercising outdoors, however, can be dangerous. Even indoors, headphones are not advisable. You need to be aware of your surroundings.

12. Conduct periodic assessments. Improving to a higher fitness category is a reward in itself.

13. Listen to your body. Stop exercising if you experience pain or unusual discomfort. Pain and aches are an indication of potential injury. If you do incur an injury, do not return to your regular workouts until you are fully recovered. You may cross-train using activities that do not aggravate your injury (for example, swimming instead of jogging).

14. If a health problem arises, see a physician. When in doubt, it's better to be safe than sorry.

15. Keep a regular record of your activities.

Although fitness testing is important to assess changes in physical capacity, attention must be given to actual program compliance. Regular physical activity is the key to better health and quality of life (see Health Fitness Standard in Chapter 2, page 26). Exercise logs provide the means to carefully document your participation in fitness programs and allow you to monitor your progress and compare it against previous months and years. Activity 3.4, pages 83–86, contains exercise log sheets to monitor your cardiorespiratory endurance, muscular strength, and muscular flexibility programs. You are strongly encouraged to keep a detailed record of all of your activities. Alternatively, you can do this by using the computerized exercise log software available with the CD ROM for this book.

Setting realistic goals will help you design and guide your fitness program.

© Fitness & Wellness, Inc.

Setting Fitness Goals

Before you leave this chapter, consider your fitness goals. In the last few decades we have become accustomed to "quick fixes" with everything from super fast foods to one-hour dry cleaning. Fitness, however, has no quick fix. Fitness takes time and dedication, and only those who are committed and persistent will reap the rewards. As described in Chapter 1, setting realistic fitness goals will guide your program. Activity 3.4, page 83, offers a goal-setting form that will help you determine your fitness goals. Take the time, either by yourself or with your instructor's help, to fill it out.

As you prepare to write realistic fitness goals, base these goals on the results of your initial fitness test (pretest). For instance, if your cardiorespiratory fitness category was "poor" on the pre-test, you should not expect to improve to the "excellent" category in a little more than 3 months. Whenever possible, your fitness goals should be measurable and time-specific. A goal that simply states "to improve my cardiorespiratory endurance" is not as good as a goal that states "to improve to the 'good' fitness category in cardiorespiratory endurance by April 15" or "to run the 1.5-mile course in less than 11 minutes the week of final exams."

After determining each goal, monitor your progress toward your goal regularly. You also will need to write measurable objectives to accomplish that goal. These objectives will be the actual plan of action to accomplish your goal. A sample of objectives to accomplish the previously stated goal for development of cardiorespiratory endurance could be:

1. Use jogging as the mode of exercise.
2. Jog at 10:00 AM five times per week.
3. Jog around the track in the field house.
4. Jog for 30 minutes each exercise session.
5. Monitor heart rate regularly during exercise.
6. Take the 1.5-Mile Run test once a month.

You will not always meet your specific objectives. If so, your goal may be out of reach. Reevaluate your objectives and make adjustments accordingly. If you set unrealistic goals at the beginning of your exercise program, be flexible with yourself and reconsider your plan of action, but do not quit. Reconsidering your plan of action does not mean that you have failed. Failure comes only to those who stop trying, and success comes to those who are committed and persistent.

Strength Training Muscle Map & Explanation. This site provides an anatomical map of the body's muscles. Click on the muscle for exercises designed to specifically strengthen that particular muscle, complete with a video and safety information.
http://www.global-fitness.com/strength/s_map.html

Sport-fitness advisor. This site provides a battery of fitness tests. Click on Flexibility Tests for sit-and-reach test, trunk rotation test or groin flexibility test.
http://www.sport-fitness-advisor.com/fitnesstests.html

ASSESS YOUR KNOWLEDGE

Evaluate how well you understand the concepts presented in this chapter using the Assess Your Knowledge and Practice Quizzes options on your Profile Plus CD-ROM.

1. The optimal or high-intensity cardiorespiratory training zone for a 22-year-old individual with a resting heart rate of 68 bpm is
   a. 120 to 148.
   b. 132 to 156.
   c. 138 to 164.
   d. 146 to 179.
   e. 154 to 188.

2. Which of the following activities does not contribute to the development of cardiorespiratory endurance?
   a. low-impact aerobics
   b. jogging
   c. 400-yard dash
   d. racquetball
   e. All of the activities contribute to its development.

3. The recommended duration for each cardiorespiratory training session is
   a. 10 to 20 minutes.
   b. 15 to 30 minutes.
   c. 20 to 60 minutes.
   d. 45 to 70 minutes.
   e. 60 to 120 minutes.

4. During an eccentric muscle contraction,
   a. the muscle shortens as it overcomes the resistance.
   b. there is little or no movement during the contraction.
   c. a joint has to move through the entire range of motion.
   d. the muscle lengthens as it contracts.
   e. the speed is kept constant throughout the range of motion.

5. The training concept that states that the demands placed on a system must be increased systematically and progressively over time to cause physiological adaptation is referred to as
   a. the overload principle.
   b. positive resistance training.
   c. specificity of training.
   d. variable-resistance training.
   e. progressive resistance.

6. For health fitness, during strength-training each set should be performed between
   a. 1 and 6 reps maximum.
   b. 4 and 10 reps maximum.
   c. 3 and 20 reps maximum.
   d. 8 and 20 reps maximum.
   e. 10 and 30 reps maximum.

7. Which of the following is *not* a mode of stretching?
   a. proprioceptive neuromuscular facilitation
   b. elastic elongation
   c. ballistic stretching
   d. slow-sustained stretching
   e. All are modes of stretching.

8. When you perform stretching exercises, the degree of stretch should be
   a. through the entire arc of movement.
   b. to about 80 percent of capacity.
   c. to the point of mild discomfort.
   d. applied until the muscle(s) start shaking.
   e. progressively increased until the desired stretch is attained.

9. Low-back pain is associated with
   a. physical inactivity.
   b. faulty posture.
   c. excessive body weight.
   d. improper body mechanics.
   e. All are correct choices.

10. A goal is effective when it is
    a. written.
    b. measurable.
    c. time-specific.
    d. monitored.
    e. All are correct choices.

Correct answers can be found on page 261.

Daily Physical Activity Log

activity

3.1

Name _____ Date _____

Course _____ Section _____

Date: [_____] Day of the Week: [_____]

Time of Day	Exercise/ Activity	Duration	Number of Steps	Comments
[ ]	[ ]	[ ]	[ ]	[ ]
[ ]	[ ]	[ ]	[ ]	[ ]
[ ]	[ ]	[ ]	[ ]	[ ]
[ ]	[ ]	[ ]	[ ]	[ ]
[ ]	[ ]	[ ]	[ ]	[ ]
[ ]	[ ]	[ ]	[ ]	[ ]
[ ]	[ ]	[ ]	[ ]	[ ]
Totals:			[ ]	[ ]

Activity category based on steps per day (use Table 3.1, page 54): [_____]

Date: [_____] Day of the Week: [_____]

Time of Day	Exercise/ Activity	Duration	Number of Steps	Comments
[ ]	[ ]	[ ]	[ ]	[ ]
[ ]	[ ]	[ ]	[ ]	[ ]
[ ]	[ ]	[ ]	[ ]	[ ]
[ ]	[ ]	[ ]	[ ]	[ ]
[ ]	[ ]	[ ]	[ ]	[ ]
[ ]	[ ]	[ ]	[ ]	[ ]
[ ]	[ ]	[ ]	[ ]	[ ]
Totals:			[ ]	[ ]

Activity category based on steps per day (use Table 3.1, page 54): [_____]

Date: _____   Day of the Week: _____

Time of Day	Exercise/ Activity	Duration	Number of Steps	Comments
Totals:				

Activity category based on steps per day (use Table 3.1, page 54): _____

Date: _____   Day of the Week: _____

Time of Day	Exercise/ Activity	Duration	Number of Steps	Comments
Totals:				

Activity category based on steps per day (use Table 3.1, page 54): _____

Briefly evaluate your current activity patterns, discuss your feelings about the results, and provide a goal for the weeks ahead.

_____

_____

_____

_____

Exercise Readiness

Name _____ Date _____

Course _____ Section _____

List advantages of starting an exercise program.

1. _____
2. _____
3. _____
4. _____
5. _____
6. _____
7. _____
8. _____
9. _____
10. _____

List disadvantages of starting an exercise program.

1. _____
2. _____
3. _____
4. _____
5. _____
6. _____
7. _____
8. _____
9. _____
10. _____

Exercise Readiness Questionnaire

Instructions

Carefully read each statement and circle the number that best describes your feelings in each statement. Please be completely honest with your answers.

	Strongly Agree	Mildly Agree	Mildly Disagree	Strongly Disagree
1. I can walk, ride a bike (or a wheelchair), swim, or walk in a shallow pool.	4	3	2	1
2. I enjoy exercise.	4	3	2	1
3. I believe exercise can help decrease the risk for disease and premature mortality.	4	3	2	1
4. I believe exercise contributes to better health.	4	3	2	1
5. I have previously participated in an exercise program.	4	3	2	1
6. I have experienced the feeling of being physically fit.	4	3	2	1
7. I can envision myself exercising.	4	3	2	1
8. I am contemplating an exercise program.	4	3	2	1
9. I am willing to stop contemplating and give exercise a try for a few weeks.	4	3	2	1
10. I am willing to set aside time at least three times a week for exercise.	4	3	2	1
11. I can find a place to exercise (the streets, a park, a YMCA, a health club).	4	3	2	1
12. I can find other people who would like to exercise with me.	4	3	2	1
13. I will exercise when I am moody, fatigued, and even when the weather is bad.	4	3	2	1
14. I am willing to spend a small amount of money for adequate exercise clothing (shoes, shorts, leotards, or swimsuit).	4	3	2	1
15. If I have any doubts about my present state of health, I will see a physician before beginning an exercise program.	4	3	2	1
16. Exercise will make me feel better and improve my quality of life.	4	3	2	1

Scoring Your Test:

This questionnaire allows you to examine your readiness for exercise. You have been evaluated in four categories: mastery (self-control), attitude, health, and commitment. Mastery indicates that you can be in control of your exercise program. Attitude examines your mental disposition toward exercise. Health provides evidence of the wellness benefits of exercise. Commitment shows dedication and resolution to carry out the exercise program. Write the number you circled after each statement in the corresponding spaces below. Add the scores on each line to get your totals. Scores can vary from 4 to 16. A score of 12 and above is a strong indicator that that factor is important to you, and 8 and below is low. If you score 12 or more points in each category, your chances of initiating and adhering to an exercise program are good. If you fail to score at least 12 points in three categories, your chances of succeeding at exercise may be slim. You need to be better informed about the benefits of exercise, and a retraining process may be required.

Mastery: 1. _____ + 5. _____ + 6. _____ + 9. _____ = _____

Attitude: 2. _____ + 7. _____ + 8. _____ + 13. _____ = _____

Health: 3. _____ + 4. _____ + 15. _____ + 16. _____ = _____

Commitment: 10. _____ + 11. _____ + 12. _____ + 14. _____ = _____

Exercise Prescription Forms

Name _____ Date _____

Course _____ Section _____

I. Cardiorespiratory Exercise Prescription

Intensity of Exercise

1. Estimate your own maximal heart rate (MHR)

    MHR = 220 minus age (220 − age)

    MHR = ⬚ − ⬚ = ⬚ bpm

2. Resting heart rate (RHR) = ⬚ bpm

3. Heart rate reserve (HRR) = MHR − RHR

    HRR = ⬚ − ⬚ = ⬚ beats

4. Training intensity (TI) = HRR × % TI + RHR

    40% TI = ⬚ × .40 + ⬚ = ⬚ bpm

    50% TI = ⬚ × .50 + ⬚ = ⬚ bpm

    60% TI = ⬚ × .60 + ⬚ = ⬚ bpm

    85% TI = ⬚ × .85 + ⬚ = ⬚ bpm

5. Cardiorespiratory training zone. The recommended cardiorespiratory training zone is found between the 60% and 85% training intensities. Older adults, individuals who have been physically inactive or are in the poor or fair cardiorespiratory fitness categories, however, should follow a 40% to 50% training intensity during the first few weeks of the exercise program.

    Low-intensity cardiorespiratory training zone: ⬚ (40% TI) to ⬚ (50% TI)

    Moderate-intensity cardiorespiratory training zone: ⬚ (50% TI) to ⬚ (60% TI)

    High-intensity cardiorespiratory training zone: ⬚ (60% TI) to ⬚ (85% TI)

Mode of Exercise: List any activity or combination of aerobic activities that you will use in your cardio-respiratory training program:

_____

Duration of Exercise: Indicate the length of your exercise sessions: _____ minutes

Frequency of Exercise: Indicate the days you will exercise: _____

Student's Signature: _____ Date: _____

II. Strength-Training Prescription

Design your own strength-training program using a minimum of eight exercises. Indicate the number of sets, repetitions, and approximate resistance that you will use. Also, state the days of the week, time, and facility that will be used for this program.

Strength-training days: M ☐   T ☐   W ☐   Th ☐   F ☐   Sa ☐   Su ☐

Time of day: [　　　　]   Facility: [　　　　　　　　　　　　　]

Exercise	Sets / Reps / Resistance
1.	
2.	
3.	
4.	
5.	
6.	
7.	
8.	
9.	
10.	
11.	
12.	
13.	
14.	
15.	
16.	

Exercise Prescription Forms
(continued)

Name   Date

Course   Section

III. Muscular Flexibility Prescription

Perform all of the recommended flexibility exercises given on pages 237–238. Use a combination of slow-sustained and proprioceptive neuromuscular facilitation stretching techniques. Indicate the technique(s) used for each exercise and, where applicable, the number of repetitions performed and the length of time that the final degree of stretch was held.

Stretching Schedule (Indicate days, time, and place where you will stretch):

Flexibility-training days: M ☐ T ☐ W ☐ Th ☐ F ☐ Sa ☐ Su ☐ Time of day: ☐

Place: ☐

Stretching Exercises

Exercise	Stretching Technique	Repetitions	Length of Final Stretch
Lateral head tilt			NA*
Arm circles			NA
Side stretch			
Body rotation			
Chest stretch			
Shoulder hyperextension stretch			
Shoulder rotation stretch			NA
Quad stretch			
Heel cord stretch			
Adductor stretch			
Sitting adductor stretch			
Sit-and-reach stretch			
Triceps stretch			

*Not Applicable

IV. Low-Back Conditioning Program

Perform all of the recommended exercises for the prevention and rehabilitation of low back pain given in Appendix C, pages 239–240. Indicate the number of repetitions performed for each exercise.

Exercise	Repetitions
Hip flexors stretch	☐
Single-knee-to-chest stretch	☐
Double-knee-to-chest stretch	☐
Upper and lower back stretch	☐
Sit-and-reach stretch	☐
Gluteal stretch	☐
Back extension stretch	☐
Trunk rotation and lower back stretch	☐
Pelvic tilt	☐
Cat stretch	☐
Abdominal crunch or abdominal curl-up	☐

Proper Body Mechanics

Perform the following tasks using the proper body mechanics given in Figure 3.6 (page 70). Check off each item as you perform the task:

☐ Standing (carriage) position   ☐ Resting position for tired and painful back

☐ Sitting position   ☐ Lifting an object

☐ Bed posture

Behavior Modification

Using Figure 3.6 on page 70, indicate what changes you need to make in daily activities to improve posture and body mechanics and prevent low-back pain.

_____

_____

_____

_____

_____

_____

_____

Goal-Setting Form and Exercise Logs

Name _____   Date _____

Course _____   Section _____

I. Instructions

Indicate your general goal for the four health-related components of fitness and write the specific objectives you will use to accomplish these goals in the next few weeks.

Cardiorespiratory endurance goal: _____

Specific objectives:

1. _____

2. _____

3. _____

Muscular strength/endurance goal: _____

Specific objectives:

1. _____

2. _____

3. _____

Muscular flexibility goal: _____

Specific objectives:

1. _____

2. _____

3. _____

Body composition goal: _____

Specific objectives:

1. _____

2. _____

3. _____

_____   _____
My signature   Witness signature

_____   _____
Today's date   Date of completion

Exercise Logs

Name   Course   Section

II. Aerobic Exercise Log

Date	Body Weight	Exercise Heart Rate	Type of Exercise	Distance in Miles	Time Hrs./Min.	Daily Steps
1						
2						
3						
4						
5						
6						
7						
8						
9						
10						
11						
12						
13						
14						
15						
16						
17						
18						
19						
20						
21						
22						
23						
24						
25						
26						
27						
28						
29						
30						
31						
			Total			

Exercise Logs
(continued)

Name   Course   Section

III. Strength-Training Log

| Date | | | | | | | |
Exercise	St/Reps/Res*	St/Reps/Res*	St/Reps/Res*	St/Reps/Res*	St/Reps/Res*	St/Reps/Res*	St/Reps/Res*

*St/Reps/Res = Sets, Repetitions, and Resistance (e.g., 1/6/125 = 1 set of 6 repetitions with 125 pounds)

Name   Course   Section

III. Strength-Training Log

Date Exercise	St/Reps/Res*	St/Reps/Res*	St/Reps/Res*	St/Reps/Res*	St/Reps/Res*	St/Reps/Res*	St/Reps/Res*

*St/Reps/Res = Sets, Repetitions, and Resistance (e.g., 1/6/125 = 1 set of 6 repetitions with 125 pounds)

© Don Mason/CORBIS

CHAPTER 4

Evaluating Fitness Activities

OBJECTIVES

- Learn the benefits and advantages of selected aerobic activities.
- Learn to rate the fitness benefits of aerobic activities.
- Evaluate the contributions of skill-related fitness activities.
- Understand the sequence of a standard aerobic workout.
- Learn ways to enhance your aerobic workouts.

Evaluate your skill-related fitness levels with the activity on your CD-ROM.

One of the fun aspects of exercise is the sheer variety of activities promoting fitness that are available to you. You can select one or a combination of activities for your program—your choice should be based on personal enjoyment, convenience, and availability. A summary of the most popular physical activities in the United States and the percentage of adults who participate in them are presented in Figure 4.1.

Aerobic Activities

Most people who exercise pick and adhere to a single mode, such as walking, swimming, or jogging. Yet, no single activity develops total fitness. Many activities contribute to cardiorespiratory development, but the extent of contribution to other fitness components is limited and varies among the activities. For total fitness, aerobic activities should be supplemented with strength and flexibility exercises. Cross-training can add enjoyment to the program, decrease the risk of incurring injuries from overuse, and keep exercise from becoming monotonous.

Exercise sessions should be convenient. To enjoy exercise, you should select a time when you will not be rushed and a location that is nearby. People do not enjoy driving across town to get to the gym, health club, track, or pool. If parking is a problem, you may get

FIGURE 4.1 Most popular adult physical activities in the United States.

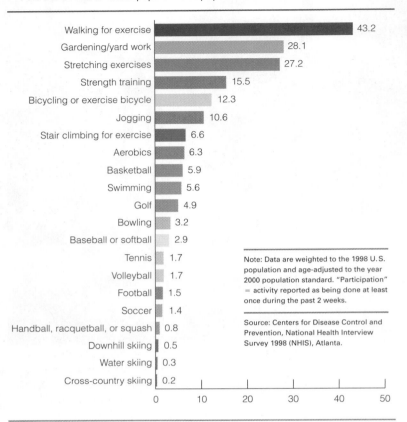

Activity	Value
Walking for exercise	43.2
Gardening/yard work	28.1
Stretching exercises	27.2
Strength training	15.5
Bicycling or exercise bicycle	12.3
Jogging	10.6
Stair climbing for exercise	6.6
Aerobics	6.3
Basketball	5.9
Swimming	5.6
Golf	4.9
Bowling	3.2
Baseball or softball	2.9
Tennis	1.7
Volleyball	1.7
Football	1.5
Soccer	1.4
Handball, racquetball, or squash	0.8
Downhill skiing	0.5
Water skiing	0.3
Cross-country skiing	0.2

Note: Data are weighted to the 1998 U.S. population and age-adjusted to the year 2000 population standard. "Participation" = activity reported as being done at least once during the past 2 weeks.

Source: Centers for Disease Control and Prevention, National Health Interview Survey 1998 (NHIS), Atlanta.

Walking is the most natural aerobic exercise.

discouraged quickly and quit. All of these factors can supply excuses not to stick to an exercise program.

Walking

The most natural, easiest, safest, and least expensive form of aerobic exercise is walking. For years, many fitness practitioners believed that walking was not vigorous enough to improve cardiorespiratory functioning, but brisk walking at speeds of 4 miles per hour or faster does improve cardiorespiratory fitness. From a health-fitness viewpoint, a regular walking program can prolong life significantly (see the discussion of cardiovascular diseases in Chapter 8). Although walking obviously takes longer than jogging, the caloric cost of brisk walking is only about 10 percent lower than jogging the same distance.

Walking is perhaps the best activity to start a conditioning program for the cardiorespiratory system. Inactive people should start with 1-mile walks four or five times per week. Walk times can be increased gradually by 5 minutes each week. Following 3 to 4 weeks of conditioning, a person should be able to walk 2 miles at a 4-mile-per-hour pace, five times per week. Greater aerobic benefits accrue from walking longer and swinging the arms faster than normal. Light hand weights, a backpack (4 to 6 pounds), or tension belts that add load to the upper body (arms) also add to the intensity of walking. Because of the additional load on the cardiorespiratory system, extra weights or loads are not recommended for people who have or are at risk for cardiovascular disease.

Walking in chest-deep water is an excellent form of aerobic activity, particularly for people who have leg and back problems. Because of the buoyancy of water, individuals submerged in water to armpit level weigh only about 10 percent to 20 percent of their weight outside the water. The resistance the water creates as a person walks in the pool adds to the intensity of the activity and provides a good cardiorespiratory workout.

Hiking

Hiking is an excellent activity for the entire family, especially during the summer and on summer vacations.

Many people feel guilty if they are unable to continue their exercise routine during vacations. The intensity of hiking over uneven terrain is greater than walking. An 8-hour hike can burn as many calories as a 20-mile walk or jog.

Another benefit of hiking is the relaxing effects of beautiful scenery. This is an ideal activity for highly

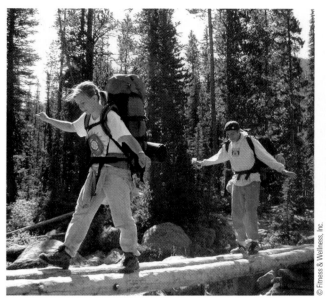

An 8-hour hike can burn as many calories as a 20-mile walk or jog.

Jogging is one of the most popular forms of aerobic exercise.

stressed people who live near woods and hills. A rough day at the office can fade quickly in the peacefulness and beauty of the outdoors.

Jogging

Next to walking, jogging is one of the most accessible forms of exercise. A person can find places to jog almost everywhere. The lone requirement to prevent injuries is a good pair of jogging shoes.

The popularity of jogging in the United States started shortly after publication of Dr. Kenneth Cooper's first *Aerobics* book in 1968. Jim Fixx's *Complete Book of Running* in the mid-1970s contributed further to the phenomenal growth of jogging as a fitness activity in the United States.

Jogging three to five times a week is one of the fastest ways to improve cardiorespiratory fitness. The risk of injury, however—especially in beginners—is higher with jogging than walking. For proper condition-ing, jogging programs should start with 1 to 2 weeks of walking. As fitness improves, walking and jogging can be combined, gradually increasing the jogging segment until it fills the full 20 to 30 minutes.

Many people abuse this activity. People run too fast and too long. Some joggers think that if a little is good, more is better. Not so with cardiorespiratory endurance. As indicated under "Frequency of Exercise" on page 59 in Chapter 3, the aerobic benefit of training more than 30 minutes five times per week is minimal. Further-more, the risk of injury increases greatly as speed

(running instead of jogging) and mileage go up. Jogging approximately 15 miles per week is sufficient to reach an excellent level of cardiorespiratory fitness.

A good pair of shoes is a must for joggers. Many foot, knee, and leg problems originate from improperly fitted or worn-out shoes. A good pair of shoes should offer lateral stability and not lean to either side when placed on a flat surface. The shoe also should bend at the ball of the foot, not at midfoot. Worn-out shoes should be replaced. After 500 miles of use, jogging shoes lose about a third of their shock absorption capabilities. If you suddenly have problems, check your shoes first. It may be time for a new pair.

For safety reasons, joggers should stay away from high-speed roads, not wear headphones, and always run (or walk) against the traffic so they will be able to see all oncoming traffic. At night, joggers should wear reflective clothing or fluorescent material on different parts of the body. Carrying a flashlight is even better, because motorists can see the light from a greater distance than they can see the reflective material. Also, avoid walking or jogging in unfamiliar areas. Always inquire as to safe areas to walk or jog.

An alternative form of jogging, especially for injured people, those with chronic back problems, and over-weight individuals, is deep-water running. This entails running in place while treading water and is almost as strenuous as jogging on land. The running motions used on land are accentuated by pumping the arms and legs hard through the full range of motion. The participant usually wears a flotation vest to help maintain the body in an upright position. Many elite athletes train in water to lessen the wear and tear on the body caused by long-distance running. These athletes have been able to

Aerobics is one of the most popular fitness activities for women in the United States.

Step-aerobics using a resistive-cord belt to enhance upper body work.

maintain high oxygen uptake values through rigorous water running programs.

Aerobics

Aerobics, formerly known as **aerobic dance**, is one of the most common fitness activities for women in the United States. Routines consist of a combination of stepping, walking, jogging, skipping, kicking, and arm swinging movements performed to music. It is a fun way to exercise and promote cardiorespiratory development at the same time.

High-impact aerobics (HIA) is the traditional form of aerobics. The movements exert a great amount of vertical force on the feet as they contact the floor. Proper leg conditioning through other forms of weight-bearing aerobic exercises (brisk walking and jogging), as well as strength training, are recommended prior to participating in HIA.

HIA is an intense activity, and it produces the highest rate of aerobics injuries. Shin splints, stress fractures, low-back pain, and tendinitis are all too common in HIA enthusiasts. These injuries are caused by the constant impact of the feet on firm surfaces. As a result, several alternative forms of aerobics have been developed.

In **low-impact aerobics (LIA)**, the impact is reduced because each foot contacts the surface separately, but the recommended intensity of exercise is more difficult to maintain than with HIA. To help elevate the exercise heart rate, all arm movements and weight-bearing actions that lower the center of gravity should be accentuated. Sustained movement throughout the program is also crucial to keep the heart rate in the target cardiorespiratory zone.

A third aerobics modality is **step aerobics (SA)**, in which participants step up and down from a bench.

Benches range in height from 2 to 10 inches. SA adds another dimension to the aerobics program. As noted previously, variety adds enjoyment to aerobic workouts. SA is considered a high-intensity but low-impact activity. The intensity of the activity can be controlled easily by the height of the bench. Aerobic benches or plates can be stacked together safely to adjust the height of the steps. Beginners are encouraged to use the lowest stepping height and then advance gradually to a higher bench. This will decrease the risk for injury. Even though one foot is always in contact with the floor or bench during step aerobics, this activity is not recommended for individuals with ankle, knee, or hip problems.

Other forms of aerobics include a combination of HIA and LIA, as well as **moderate-impact aerobics (MIA)**. MIA incorporates **plyometric training**. This type of training is used frequently by jumpers (high, long, and triple jumpers) and athletes in sports that require quick jumping ability, such as basketball and gymnastics.

With MIA, one foot is in contact with the ground most of the time. Participants, however, continually try to recover from all lower-body flexion actions. This is done by extending the hip, knee, and ankle joints quickly without allowing the foot (or feet) to leave the ground. These quick movements make the exercise intensity of MIA quite high.

Swimming

Swimming, another excellent form of aerobic exercise, uses many of the major muscle groups in the body. This provides a good training stimulus for the heart and lungs. Swimming is a great exercise option for individuals who cannot jog or walk for extended periods.

Compared to other activities, the risk of injuries from swimming is low. The aquatic medium helps to support the body, taking pressure off bones and joints in

Swimming is a relatively injury-free activity.

© Fitness & Wellness, Inc.

the lower extremities and the back. Maximal heart rates during swimming are approximately 10 to 13 beats per minute (bpm) lower than during running. The horizontal position of the body is thought to aid blood flow distribution throughout the body, decreasing the demand on the cardiorespiratory system. Cool water temperatures and direct contact with the water seem to help dissipate body heat more efficiently, further decreasing the strain on the heart.

Some exercise specialists recommend that this difference in maximal heart rate (10 to 13 bpm) be subtracted prior to determining cardiorespiratory training intensities. For example, the estimated maximal swimming heart rate for a 20-year old would be approximately 187 bpm (220 − 20 − 13). Studies are inconclusive as to whether this decrease in heart rate in water also occurs at submaximal intensities below 70 percent of maximal heart rate.[1] One can argue, nonetheless, that apparently healthy people are able to achieve higher work capacities during land-based activities; thus, the same exercise intensity can be given for water activities. If a lower intensity is used, training benefits may be decreased.

To produce better training benefits during swimming, swimmers should minimize gliding periods such as those in the breast stroke and side stroke. Achieving proper training intensities with these strokes is difficult. The forward crawl is recommended for better aerobic results.

Overweight individuals have to swim fast enough to achieve an adequate training intensity. Excessive body fat makes the body more buoyant, and often the tendency is to just float along. This may be good for reducing stress and relaxing, but it does not greatly increase caloric expenditure to aid with weight loss. Walking or jogging in waist- or armpit-deep water is a better choice for overweight individuals who cannot walk or jog on land for an extended period of time.

With reference to the principle of specificity of training, cardiorespiratory improvements from swimming cannot be measured adequately with a land-based walk/jog test. This is because most of the work with swimming is done by the upper body musculature.

Although the heart's ability to pump more blood improves significantly with any type of aerobic activity, the primary increase in the ability of cells to utilize oxygen (VO_2, or oxygen uptake) with swimming occurs in the upper body and not the lower extremities. Therefore, fitness improvements with swimming are best attained by comparing changes in distance a person swims in a given time, say, 12 minutes.

CT Critical Thinking

Participation in sports is a good predictor of adherence to exercise later in life. What previous experiences have you had with participation in sports? Were these experiences positive, and what effect do they have on your current physical activity patterns?

Water Aerobics

Water aerobics is fun and safe for people of all ages. Besides developing fitness, it provides an opportunity for socialization and fun in a comfortable, refreshing setting.

Water aerobics incorporates a combination of rhythmic arm and leg actions performed in a vertical position while submerged in waist-to-armpit-deep water. The vigorous limb movements against the water's resistance during water aerobics provide the training stimuli for cardiorespiratory development.

KEY TERMS

Aerobic dance A series of exercise routines performed to music; more commonly termed aerobics now.

High-impact aerobics (HIA) Exercises incorporating movements in which both feet are off the ground at the same time momentarily.

Low-impact aerobics (LIA) Exercises in which at least one foot is in contact with the ground or floor at all times.

Step aerobics (SA) A form of exercise that combines stepping up and down from a bench with arm movements.

Moderate-impact aerobics (MIA) Aerobics that include plyometric training.

Plyometric training A form of exercise that requires forceful jumps or springing off the ground immediately after landing from a previous jump.

Photos: Chuck Scheer, Boise State University

Water aerobics offers fitness, fun, and safety for people of all ages.

The popularity of water aerobics as an exercise modality to develop the cardiorespiratory system can be attributed to several factors:

1. Water buoyancy reduces weight-bearing stress on joints and thereby lessens the risk for injuries.
2. Water aerobics is a more feasible type of exercise for overweight individuals and those with arthritic conditions who may not be able to participate in weight-bearing activities such as walking, jogging, and aerobics.
3. Water aerobics is an excellent exercise modality to improve functional fitness in older adults (see Chapter 9, pages 215–217).
4. Heat dissipation in water is beneficial to obese participants, who seem to undergo a higher heat strain than average-weight individuals.
5. Water aerobics is available to swimmers and non-swimmers alike.

The exercises used during water aerobics are designed to elevate the heart rate, which contributes to cardiorespiratory development. In addition, the aquatic medium provides increased resistance for strength improvement with virtually no impact. Because of this resistance to movement, strength gains with water aerobics seem to be better than with land-based aerobic activities. Water exercises also help the joints move through their range of motion, promoting flexibility.

Another benefit is that weight can be reduced without the pain and fear of injuries experienced by many who initiate exercise programs. Water aerobics provides a relatively safe environment for injury-free participation in exercise. The cushioned environment of the water allows patients recovering from leg and back injuries,

individuals with joint problems, injured athletes, pregnant women, and obese people to benefit from water aerobics. In water, these people can exercise to develop and maintain cardiorespiratory endurance while limiting or eliminating the potential for further injury.

Similar to swimming, maximal heart rates achieved during water aerobics are lower than during running. The difference between water aerobics and running is about 10 bpm.[2] Further, research comparing physiologic differences between self-paced treadmill running and self-paced water aerobics exercise showed that even though individuals work at a lower heart rate intensity in water, the oxygen uptake level was the same for both treadmill and water exercise modalities.[3] Apparently healthy people, therefore, can sustain land-based exercise intensities during a water aerobics workout and experience fitness benefits similar to or greater than during land aerobics.[4]

Cycling

Most people learn cycling in their youth. Because it is a non-weight-bearing activity, cycling is a good exercise modality for people with lower-body or lower-back injuries. Cycling helps to develop the cardiorespiratory system, as well as muscular strength and endurance in the lower extremities. With the advent of stationary bicycles, this activity can be performed year-round.

Raising the heart rate to the proper training intensity is more difficult with cycling. As the amount of muscle mass involved during aerobic exercise decreases, so does the demand placed on the cardiorespiratory system. The thigh muscles do most of the work in cycling, making it harder to achieve and maintain a high cardio-respiratory training intensity.

Maintaining a continuous pedaling motion and eliminating coasting periods helps the participant achieve a faster heart rate. Exercising for longer periods also helps to compensate for the lower heart rate intensity during cycling. Comparing cycling to jogging, similar aerobic benefits take roughly three times the distance at twice the speed of jogging. Cycling, however, puts less stress on muscles and joints than jogging does, making the former a good exercise modality for people who cannot walk or jog.

The height of the bike seat should be adjusted so the knee is flexed at about 30 degrees when the foot is at the bottom of the pedaling cycle. The body should not sway from side to side as the person rides. The cycling cadence also is important for maximal efficiency. Bike tension or gears should be set at a moderate level so the rider can achieve about 60 to 100 revolutions per minute.

Safety is a key issue in road cycling. More than a million bicycle injuries occur each year. Proper equipment and common sense are necessary. A well-designed and well-maintained bike is easier to maneuver. Toe clips are recommended to keep feet from sliding and to maintain equal upward and downward force on the pedals.

Skill is important in both road and mountain cycling. Cyclists must be in control of the bicycle at all times. They have to be able to maneuver the bike in traffic, maintain balance at slow speeds, switch gears, apply the brakes, watch for pedestrians and stop lights, ride through congested areas, and overcome a variety of obstacles in the mountains. Stationary cycling, in contrast, does not require special skills. Nearly everyone can do it.

Bike riders must follow the same rules as motorists. Many accidents happen because cyclists run traffic lights and stop signs. Some further suggestions are as follows:

- Select the right bike. Frame size is important. The size is determined by standing flatfooted while straddling the bike. Regular bikes (road bikes) should have a 1- to 2-inch clearance between the groin and the top tube of the frame. On mountain bikes, the clearance should be about 3 inches. The recommended height of the handlebars is about 1 inch below the top of the seat. Upright handlebars are available for individuals with neck or back problems. Hard, narrow seats on road or racing bikes tend to be especially uncomfortable for women. To avoid saddle soreness, use wider and more cushioned seats such as gel-filled saddles.
- Use bike hand signals to let the traffic around you know of your intended actions.

Road cycling requires skill for safety and enjoyment.

© Fitness & Wellness, Inc.

- Don't ride side by side with another rider; single file is safer.
- Be aware of turning vehicles and cars backing out of alleys and parking lots; always yield to motorists in these situations.
- Be on the lookout for storm drains, railroad tracks, and cattle guards, which can cause unpleasant surprises. Front wheels can get caught and riders may be thrown from the bike if these hazards are not crossed at the proper angle (preferably 90 degrees).
- Wear a good helmet, certified by the Snell Memorial Foundation or the American National Standards Institute. Many serious accidents and even deaths have been prevented by the use of helmets. Fashion, aesthetics, comfort, or price should not be a factor when selecting and using a helmet for road cycling. Health and life are too precious to give up because of vanity and thriftiness.
- Wear appropriate clothes and shoes. Clothing should be bright, very visible, lightweight, and not restrict movement. Cycling shorts are recommended to prevent skin irritation. For greater comfort, the shorts have extra padding sewn into the seat and crotch areas. They do not tend to wrinkle and they wick away perspiration from the skin. Shorts should be long enough to keep the skin from rubbing against the seat. Experienced cyclists also wear special shoes with a cleat that snaps directly onto the pedal.
- Take extra warm clothing in a backpack during the winter months in case you have a breakdown and have to walk a long distance for assistance.
- Watch out for ice in cold weather. If you see ice on car windows, expect ice on the road. Be especially careful on and under bridges, because they tend to have ice even when the roads elsewhere are dry.
- Use the brightest bicycle lights you can when riding in the dark, and always keep the batteries well charged.

For additional safety, wear reflectors on the upper torso, arms, and legs, so passing motorists are alerted to you. Stay on streets that have good lighting and plenty of room on the side of the road, even if that means riding an extra few minutes to get to your destination.

• Take a cell phone if you have one, and let someone else know where you are going and when to expect you back.

The stationary bike is one of the most popular pieces of equipment sold by sporting goods stores. Before buying a stationary bike, though, be sure to try the activity for a few days. If you enjoy it, you may want to purchase one. Invest with caution. If you opt to buy a lower priced model, you may be disappointed. Good stationary bikes have comfortable seats, are stable, and provide a smooth and uniform pedaling motion. A sticky bike that is hard to pedal leads to discouragement and ends up being stored in the corner of a basement.

Spinning®

Spinning is a low-impact activity typically performed in a room or studio with dim lights and motivational music, under the direction of a certified instructor and with the noise of many bikes working together. This exercise modality gained immediate popularity upon its introduction in the mid-1990s. Sometimes referred to as studio or indoor cycling, spinning is performed on stationary bicycles developed by world-class cyclist Johnny Goldberg. To bring his rigorous workouts indoors, Goldberg modified his stationary bike into the first Spinner bike. Participants now use specially designed Spinner bikes available at sports equipment stores. The bikes include racing handlebars, pedals with clips, adjustable seats, and a resistance knob to control the intensity of the workout. Use of an exercise heart rate monitor is encouraged to track the intensity at various stages of the workout.

As presently designed, the Spinning program combines five basic movements and five workout stages with the understanding that participants' exercise needs and goals vary. The five exercise movements are:

1. Seated flat—pedaling in the basic seated bike position
2. Seated hill climb—pedaling in the basic seated position but with increased resistance applied
3. Standing running—pedaling while standing up
4. Standing hill climb—pedaling standing up but with a more challenging resistance level
5. Jumping—surging out of the saddle using either

controlled movements and a constant speed or at a fast pace, as during a breakaway in a bike race.

The five workout stages, also known as energy zones, are used to simulate actual cycling training and racing. The workouts are divided into endurance, all terrain, strength, recovery, and advanced training. Cadence, exercise movements, and exercise heart rate dictate the differences between the various zones. Workouts are planned according to each person's fitness level and selected percentages of maximal heart rate during each stage. These workouts provide a challenging program for people of all ages and fitness levels. The social aspect of this activity makes Spinning appealing to many exercisers.

Cross-Training

Cross-training combines two or more activities. This type of training is designed to enhance fitness, provide needed rest for tired muscles, decrease injuries, and eliminate the monotony and burnout of single-activity programs. Cross-training may combine aerobic and non-aerobic activities such as moderate jogging, speed training, and strength training.

Cross-training can produce better workouts than a single activity. For example, jogging develops the lower body and swimming builds the upper body. Rowing contributes to upper-body development and cycling builds the legs. Combining activities such as these provides good overall conditioning and at the same time helps to improve or maintain fitness. Cross-training also offers an opportunity to develop skill and have fun with differing activities.

Speed training often is coupled with cross-training. Faster performance times in aerobic activities (running, cycling) are generated with speed or **interval training**. People who want to improve their running times often run shorter intervals at faster speeds than the actual racing pace. For example, a person wanting to run a 6-minute mile may run four 440-yard intervals at a speed of 1 minute and 20 seconds per interval. A 440-yard walk/jog can become a recovery interval between fast runs.

Strength training is used commonly with cross-training. It helps to condition muscles, tendons, and ligaments. Improved strength enhances overall performance in many activities and sports. For example, although road cyclists in one study who trained with weights showed no improvement in aerobic capacity, the cyclists' riding time to exhaustion improved 33 percent when exercising at 75 percent of their maximal capacity.[5]

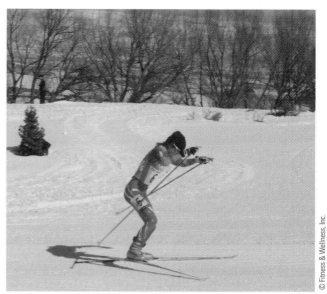

Cross-country skiing requires more oxygen and energy than most other aerobic activities.

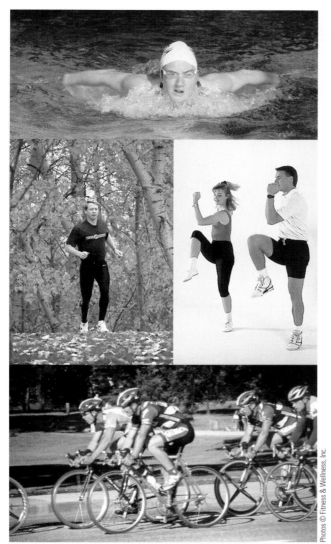

Cross-training enhances fitness, decreases the rate of injuries, and eliminates the monotony of single-activity programs.

Rope Skipping

Rope skipping contributes to cardiorespiratory fitness and also helps to increase reaction time, coordination, agility, dynamic balance, and muscular strength in the lower extremities. At first, rope skipping may seem to be a highly strenuous form of aerobic exercise. Beginners often reach maximal heart rates after only 2 or 3 minutes of jumping. As skill improves, however, the energy demands decrease considerably.

Some people have claimed training benefits equal to a 30-minute jog in only 10 minutes of skipping. Although differences in strength and flexibility development are observed in different activities, 10 minutes of rope skipping at a certain heart rate provide similar cardiorespiratory benefits regardless of the nature of the activity. To obtain an adequate aerobic workout, the duration of exercise must be at least 20 minutes.

As with high-impact aerobics, a major concern of rope skipping is the stress placed on the lower extremities, increasing the risk for injuries. Fitness experts recommend that skipping be used sparingly, and primarily as a supplement to an aerobic exercise program.

Cross-Country Skiing

Many people consider cross-country skiing as the ultimate aerobic exercise because it requires vigorous lower- and upper-body movements. The large amount of muscle mass involved in cross-country skiing makes the intensity of the activity high, yet it places little strain on muscles and joints. One of the highest maximal oxygen uptakes ever measured (85 ml/kg/min) was found in an elite cross-country skier.

In addition to being an excellent aerobic activity, cross-country skiing is soothing. Skiing through the beauty of the snow-covered countryside can be highly enjoyable. Although the need for snow is an obvious limitation, simulation equipment for year-round cross-country training is available at many sporting goods stores.

KEY TERMS

Interval training A repeated series of exercise work bouts (intervals) interspersed with low-intensity or rest intervals.

Some skill is necessary to be proficient at cross-country skiing. Poorly skilled individuals are not able to elevate the heart rate enough to cause adequate aerobic development. Individuals contemplating this activity should seek instruction to be able to fully enjoy and reap the rewards of cross-country skiing.

In-Line Skating

Frequently called blading, in-line skating has become a highly popular fitness activity in recent years. Millions of children and adults participate in this activity. In the early 1990s, stores could not keep up with the demand for in-line skates.

In-line skating has its origin in ice skating. Because warm-weather ice skating was not feasible, wheels replaced blades for summertime participation. Although four-wheel roller skates were invented in the mid-1700s, the activity did not really catch on until the late 1800s. The first in-line skate with five wheels in a row attached to the bottom of a shoe was developed in 1823. The in-line concept took hold in the United States in 1980, when hockey skates were adapted for road-skating.

In-line skating is an excellent activity to develop cardiorespiratory fitness and lower body strength. Intensity of the activity is regulated by how hard you blade. The key to effective cardiorespiratory training is to maintain a constant and rhythmic pattern, using arms and legs, and to minimize the gliding phase of blading. Because blading is a weight-bearing activity, participants also develop superior leg strength.

Instruction is necessary to achieve a minimum level of proficiency in this sport. Bladers commonly encounter hazards—potholes, cracks, rocks, gravel, sticks, oil, street curbs, and driveways. Unskilled bladers are more prone to falls and injuries.

Good equipment will make the activity safer and more enjoyable. Blades range in price from $40 to $500. Recreational participants need not purchase the more costly competitive skates. An adequate blade should provide strong ankle support; soft and flexible boots do not provide enough support. Small wheels offer more stability, and larger wheels enable greater speed. Blades should be purchased from stores that understand the sport and can provide sound advice according to skill level and needs.

Protective equipment is a must for in-line skating. Similar to road cycling, a good helmet that meets the safety standards set by the Snell Memorial Foundation or the American National Standards Institute is important to protect yourself in case of a fall. Wrist guards and knee and elbow pads also are recommended, because the kneecap and the elbows are easily injured in a fall.

In-line skating is a low-impact fitness activity.

Nighttime bladers should wear light-colored clothing and reflective tape.

Rowing

Rowing is a low-impact activity that provides a complete body workout. It mobilizes most major muscle groups, including those in the arms, legs, hips, abdomen, trunk, and shoulders. Rowing is a good form of aerobic exercise and also, because of the nature of the activity (constant pushing and pulling against resistance) promotes strength development.

To accommodate different fitness levels, workloads can be regulated on most rowing machines. Stationary rowing, however, is not among the most popular forms of aerobic exercise. Similar to stationary bicycles, people should try the activity for a few weeks before purchasing a unit.

Stair Climbing

If sustained for at least 20 minutes, stair climbing is a very efficient form of aerobic exercise. Precisely because of the high intensity of stair climbing, many people stay away from stairs and instead take escalators and elevators. Many people dislike living in two-story homes because they have to climb the stairs frequently.

Not too many places have enough flights of stairs to climb continuously for 20 minutes. Stair-climbing machines offer an alternative. In terms of injuries, stair climbing seems to be a relatively safe exercise modality. Because the feet never leave the climbing surface, it is considered a low-impact activity. Joints and ligaments

Stair climbing provides a rigorous aerobic workout.

© StairMaster

Racquet sports require rhythmic and continuous activity to provide cardiorespiratory benefit.

Eric Risberg

are not strained during climbing. The intensity of exercise is controlled easily, because most stair climbing equipment can be programmed to regulate the workload.

Racquet Sports

In racquet sports such as tennis, racquetball, squash, and badminton, the aerobic benefits are dictated by players' skill, the intensity of the game, and the length of time spent playing. Skill is necessary to participate effectively in these sports and also is crucial to sustain continuous play. Frequent pauses during play do not allow people to maintain the heart rate in the appropriate target zone to stimulate cardiorespiratory development.

Many people participate in racquet sports for reasons of enjoyment, social fulfillment, and relaxation. To develop cardiorespiratory fitness, these people supplement the sport with other forms of aerobic exercise such as jogging, cycling, or swimming. If a racquet sport is the main form of aerobic exercise, participants must try to run hard, fast, and as constantly as possible during play—and avoid spending a lot of time retrieving balls, birds, or shuttlecocks. Just as in low-impact aerobics, all movements should be accentuated by reaching out and bending more than usual, for better cardiorespiratory development.

CT Critical Thinking

In your own experience with personal fitness programs throughout the years, what factors have motivated you and helped you the most to stay with a program? What factors have kept you from being physically active, and what can you do to change these factors?

Rating the Fitness Benefits of Aerobic Activities

The fitness contributions of the aerobic activities discussed in this chapter vary according to the specific activity and the individual. As noted previously, the health-related components of physical fitness are cardiorespiratory endurance, muscular strength and endurance, muscular flexibility, and body composition. Although accurately assessing the contributions to each fitness component is difficult, a summary of likely benefits of these activities is provided in Table 4.1. Instead of a single rating or number, ranges are given for some of the categories because the benefits derived are based on the person's effort while participating in the activity.

Regular participation in aerobic activities provides notable health benefits, including an increase in cardiorespiratory endurance, quality of life, and longevity. The extent of cardiorespiratory development (improvement in VO_{2max}) depends on the intensity, duration, and frequency of the activity. The nature of the activity often dictates potential aerobic development. For example, jogging is much more strenuous than walking.

The effort during exercise also influences the amount of physiological development. The training benefits of just going through the motions of a low-impact aerobics routine are less than those of accentuating all motions (see earlier discussion of low-impact aerobics). Table 4.1 includes a starting fitness level for each aerobic activity. Beginners should start with low-intensity activities that have a minimum risk for injuries. In some cases, such as in high-impact aerobics and rope skipping, the risk of injuries remains high despite adequate conditioning. These activities should

TABLE 4.1 Ratings for Selected Aerobic Activities

ACTIVITY	RECOMMENDED STARTING FITNESS LEVEL [1]	INJURY RISK [2]	POTENTIAL CARDIORESPIRATORY ENDURANCE DEVELOPMENT (VO_{2MAX}) [3,4]	UPPER BODY STRENGTH DEVELOPMENT [3]	LOWER BODY STRENGTH DEVELOPMENT [3]	UPPER BODY FLEXIBILITY DEVELOPMENT [3]	LOWER BODY FLEXIBILITY DEVELOPMENT [3]	WEIGHT MANAGEMENT [3]	MET LEVEL [4,5,6]	CALORIC EXPENDITURE (CAL/HOUR) [4,6]
Aerobics										
High-Impact Aerobics	A	H	3–4	2	4	3	2	4	6–12	450–900
Moderate-Impact Aerobics	I	M	2–4	2	3	3	2	3	6–12	450–900
Low-Impact Aerobics	B	L	2–4	2	3	3	2	3	5–10	375–750
Step Aerobics	I	M	2–4	2	3–4	3	2	3–4	5–12	375–900
Cross-Country Skiing	B	M	4–5	4	4	2	2	4–5	10–16	750–1,200
Cross-Training	I	M	3–5	2–3	3–4	2–3	1–2	3–5	6–15	450–1,125
Cycling										
Road	I	M	2–5	1	4	1	1	3	6–12	450–900
Stationary	B	L	2–4	1	4	1	1	3	6–10	450–750
Hiking	B	L	2–4	1	3	1	1	3	6–10	450–750
In-Line Skating	I	M	2–4	2	4	2	2	3	6–10	450–750
Jogging	I	M	3–5	1	3	1	1	5	6–15	450–1,125
Jogging, Deep Water	A	L	3–5	2	2	1	1	5	8–15	600–1,125
Racquet Sports	I	M	2–4	3	3	3	2	3	6–10	450–750
Rope Skipping	I	H	3–5	2	4	1	2	3–5	8–15	600–1,125
Rowing	B	L	3–5	4	2	3	1	4	8–14	600–1,050
Spinning	I	L	4–5	1	4	1	1	4	8–15	600–1,125
Stair Climbing	B	L	3–5	1	4	1	1	4–5	8–15	600–1,125
Swimming (front crawl)	B	L	3–5	4	2	3	1	3	6–12	450–900
Walking	B	L	1–2	1	2	1	1	3	4–6	300–450
Walking, Water, Chest-Deep	I	L	2–4	2	3	1	1	3	6–10	450–750
Water Aerobics	B	L	2–4	3	3	3	2	3	6–12	450–900

[1] B = Beginner, I = Intermediate, A = Advanced

[2] L = Low, M = Moderate, H = High

[3] 1 = Low, 2 = Fair, 3 = Average, 4 = Good, 5 = Excellent

[4] Varies according to the person's effort (intensity) during exercise.

[5] 1 MET represents the rate of energy expenditure at rest (3.5 ml/kg/min). Each additional MET is a multiple of the resting value. For example, 5 METs represents an energy expenditure equivalent to five times the resting value, or about 17.5 ml/kg/min.

[6] Varies according to body weight.

be used only to supplement training and are not recommended for beginners or as the sole mode of exercise.

Physicians who work with cardiac patients frequently use METs to measure activity levels. One **MET** represents the body's energy requirement at rest, or the equivalent of a VO_2 of 3.5 ml/kg/min. A 10-MET activity requires a tenfold increase in the resting energy requirement, or approximately 35 ml/kg/min. MET levels for a given activity vary according to the individual's effort. The harder a person exercises, the higher the MET level. The MET ranges for the various activities is included in Table 4.1.

The various aerobic activities' effectiveness in aiding weight management also is indicated in Table 4.1. As a rule, the greater the muscle mass involved during exercise, the better the results. Rhythmic and continuous activities that involve considerable muscle mass are most effective in burning calories.

Higher-intensity activities burn more calories as well. Increasing exercise time will compensate for lower intensities. If carried out long enough (60 to 90 minutes, five to six times per week), even brisk walking can be a good exercise mode to lose weight. Additional information on a comprehensive weight management program is given in Chapter 6.

Skill-Related Fitness

Skill-related fitness is needed for success in athletics and effective performance of lifetime sports and activities. The components of skill-related fitness, defined in Chapter 1, are agility, balance, coordination, power, speed, and reaction time. All of these are important, to varying degrees, in sports and athletics.

For example, outstanding gymnasts must achieve good skill-related fitness in all components. Significant agility is necessary to perform a double back somersault with a full twist—a skill in which the athlete must rotate simultaneously around one axis and twist around a different one. Static balance is essential for maintaining a handstand or a scale. Dynamic balance is needed to perform many of the gymnastics routines (for example, balance beam, parallel bars, pommel horse).

Coordination is important to successfully integrate into one routine various skills requiring varying degrees of difficulty. Power and speed are needed to propel the body into the air, such as when tumbling or vaulting. Quick reaction time is necessary in determining when to end rotation upon a visual clue, such as spotting the floor on a dismount.

As with the health-related fitness components, the principle of specificity of training applies to skill-related components. According to this principle, the training program must be specific to the type of skill the individual is trying to achieve.

Development of agility, balance, coordination, and reaction time is highly task-specific. To attain a certain skill, the individual must practice the same task many times. There is little crossover learning effect from one skill to another.

For instance, proper practice of a handstand (balance) eventually will lead to successful performance of that skill, but complete mastery of the skill does not ensure that the person will immediately be able to transfer this mastery to other static balance positions in gymnastics. Power and speed may be improved with a specific strength-training program or frequent repetition of the specific task to be improved, or both.

The rate of learning in skill-related fitness varies from person to person, mainly because these components seem to be determined to a large extent by hereditary factors. Individuals with good skill-related fitness tend to do better and learn faster when performing a wide variety of skills. Nevertheless, few individuals enjoy complete success in all skill-related components. Furthermore, though skill-related fitness can be enhanced with practice, improvements in reaction time and speed are limited and seem to be related primarily to genetic endowment.

Although we do not know how much skill-related fitness is desirable, everyone should attempt to develop and maintain a better-than-average level. This type of fitness is crucial for athletes and also is important in leading a better and happier life. Improving skill-related fitness affords an individual more enjoyment and success in a wider variety of lifetime sports (for instance, basketball, tennis, and racquetball) and also can help a person cope more effectively in emergency situations. For example:

1. Good reaction time, balance, coordination, and agility can help you avoid a fall or break a fall and thereby minimize injury.
2. The ability to generate maximum force in a short time (power) may be crucial to ameliorate injury or even preserve life in a situation in which you may be called upon to move a person out of danger or lift a heavy object that has fallen.
3. In our society, with an expanding average lifespan, maintaining speed can be especially important for older adults. Many of them and, for that matter, many unfit and overweight young people no longer have the speed they need to cross an intersection safely before the light changes for oncoming traffic.

Regular participation in a health-related fitness program can heighten performance of skill-related components, and vice versa. For example, significantly overweight people do not have good agility or speed. Because participating in aerobic and strength-training programs helps take off body fat, an overweight individual who loses weight through an exercise program may also improve agility and speed. A sound flexibility program decreases resistance to motion around body joints, which may increase agility, balance, and overall coordination. Improvements in strength definitely help develop power.

KEY TERMS

MET Short for metabolic equivalent, the rate of energy expenditure at rest, or the equivalent of a VO_2 of 3.5 ml/kg/min.

TABLE 4.2 Contributions of Selected Activities to Skill-Related Components

ACTIVITY	AGILITY	BALANCE	COORDINATION	POWER	REACTION TIME	SPEED
Alpine Skiing	4	5	4	2	3	2
Archery	1	2	4	2	3	1
Badminton	4	3	4	2	4	3
Baseball	3	2	4	4	5	4
Basketball	4	3	4	3	4	3
Bowling	2	2	4	1	1	1
Cross-country Skiing	3	4	3	2	2	1
Football	4	4	4	4	4	3
Golf	1	2	5	3	1	3
Gymnastics	5	5	5	4	3	3
Ice Skating	5	5	5	3	3	3
In-line Skating	4	4	4	3	2	4
Judo/Karate	5	5	5	4	5	4
Racquetball	5	4	4	4	5	4
Soccer	5	3	5	5	3	4
Table Tennis	5	3	5	3	5	3
Tennis	4	3	5	3	5	3
Volleyball	4	3	5	4	5	3
Water Skiing	3	4	3	2	2	1
Wrestling	5	5	5	4	5	4

1 = Low, 2 = Fair, 3 = Average, 4 = Good, 5 = Excellent

Similar to the fitness benefits of the aerobic activities discussed previously in this chapter and given in Table 4.1, the contributions of skill-related activities also vary among activities and individuals. The extent to which an activity helps develop each skill-related component varies by the effort the individual makes and, most important, by proper execution (technique) of the skill (correct coaching is highly recommended) and the individual's potential based on genetic endowment. A summary of potential contributions to skill-related fitness for selected activities is provided in Table 4.2.

Team Sports

Choosing activities that you enjoy will greatly enhance your adherence to exercise. People tend to repeat things they enjoy doing. Enjoyment by itself is a reward. Therefore, combining individual activities (such as jogging or swimming) with team sports can deepen your commitment to fitness.

People with good skill-related fitness usually participate in lifetime sports and games, which in turn helps develop health-related fitness. Individuals who enjoyed basketball or soccer in their youth tend to stick to those activities later in life. The availability of teams and community leagues may be all that is needed to stop contemplating and start participating. The social element of team sports provides added incentive to participate. Team sports offer an opportunity to interact with people who share a common interest. Being a member of a team creates responsibility—another incentive to exercise, because you are expected to be there. Furthermore, team sports foster lifetime friendships, strengthening the social and emotional dimensions of wellness.

For those who were not able to participate in youth sports, it's never too late to start (see the discussion of behavior modification and motivation in Chapter 1). Don't be afraid to select a new activity, even if that means learning new skills. The fitness and social rewards will be ample.

Tips to Enhance Your Aerobic Workout

A typical aerobic workout is divided into three parts (see Figure 4.2):

1. A 5- to 10-minute warm-up phase during which the heart rate is increased gradually to the target zone.
2. The actual aerobic workout, during which the heart rate is maintained in the target zone for 20 to 60 minutes.
3. A 10-minute aerobic cool-down, when the heart rate is lowered gradually toward the resting level.

To monitor the target training zone, you will have to check your exercise heart rate. As described in Chapter 2, the pulse can be checked on the radial or the carotid artery. When you check the heart rate, begin with zero and count the number of beats in a 10-second period, then multiply by 6 to get the per-minute pulse rate. You should take your exercise heart rate for 10 seconds rather than a full minute because the heart rate begins to slow down 15 seconds after you stop exercising.

Feeling the pulse while exercising is difficult. Therefore, participants should stop during exercise to check the pulse. If the heart rate is too low, increase the intensity of the exercise. If the rate is too high, slow down. You may want to practice taking your pulse several times during the day to become familiar with the technique.

For the first few weeks of your program, you should monitor your heart rate several times during the exercise session. As you become familiar with your body's response to exercise, you may have to monitor the heart

FIGURE **4.2** Typical aerobic workout pattern.

rate only twice—once at 5 to 7 minutes into the exercise session and a second time near the end of the workout.

Another technique sometimes used to determine your exercise intensity is simply to talk during exercise and then take your pulse immediately after that. Learning to associate the amount of difficulty when talking with the actual exercise heart rate will allow you to develop a sense of how hard you are working. Generally, if you can talk easily, you are not working hard enough. If you can talk but are slightly breathless, you should be close to the target range. If you cannot talk at all, you are working too hard.

If you have difficulty keeping up with your exercise program, you may need to reconsider your objectives and start much more slowly. Behavior modification is a process. From a physiological and psychological point of view, you may not be able to carry out an exercise session for a full 20 to 30 minutes. For the first 2 to 3 weeks, therefore, you may just want to take a few 10-minute daily walks. As your body adapts physically and mentally, you may increase the length and intensity of the exercise sessions gradually.

Most important, learn to listen to your body. At times you will feel unusually fatigued or have much discomfort. Pain is the body's way of letting you know that something is wrong. If you have pain or undue discomfort during or after exercise, you need to slow down or discontinue your exercise program and notify the course instructor. The instructor may be able to pinpoint the reason for the discomfort or recommend that you consult your physician. You also will be able to prevent potential injuries by paying attention to pain signals and making adjustments accordingly.

Let's Get Physical Challenge. This site describes an 8-week, Interactive program designed to help individuals participate in regular, moderate physical activity. This is a fun, noncompetitive program designed to educate people of all ages and abilities. You can do it!
http://www.physicalfitness.org/lgp.html

ASSESS YOUR KNOWLEDGE

Evaluate how well you understand the concepts presented in this chapter using the Assess Your Knowledge and Practice Quizzes options on your Profile Plus CD-ROM.

1. Using a combination of aerobic activities to develop overall fitness is known as
   a. health-related fitness.
   b. circuit training.
   c. plyometric exercises.
   d. cross-training.
   e. skill-related fitness.

2. The best aerobic activity choice for individuals with leg or back injuries is
   a. walking in chest-deep water.
   b. jogging.
   c. step aerobics.
   d. rope skipping.
   e. cross-country skiing.

3. The approximate jogging mileage to reach the excellent cardiorespiratory fitness classification is
   a. 5 miles.
   b. 10 miles.
   c. 15 miles.
   d. 25 miles.
   e. 50 miles.

4. To help elevate the exercise heart rate during low impact aerobics, a person should
   a. accentuate arm movements.
   b. sustain movement throughout the program.
   c. accentuate weight-bearing actions.
   d. All of the above.
   e. None of the above.

5. Achieved maximal heart rates during swimming are approximately _____ beats per minute (bpm) lower than during running.
   a. 2–4
   b. 5–9
   c. 10–13
   d. 14–20
   e. 20–25

6. Which of the following is not a basic movement in spinning?
   a. seated running
   b. standing hill climb
   c. seated flat
   d. jumping
   e. All of the above are exercise movements in spinning.

7. Cross-country skiing
   a. is a high impact activity.
   b. is primarily an anaerobic activity.
   c. places great strain on muscles and joints.
   d. is a low-intensity activity.
   e. All are incorrect choices.

8. A MET represents
   a. the symbol used to indicate that the exercise goal has been met.
   b. a unit of measure that is used to express the value achieved during the Metabolic Exercise Test.
   c. the Maximal Exercise Time achieved.
   d. the rate of energy expenditure at rest.
   e. All choices are incorrect.

9. Which of the following is not a component of skill-related fitness?
   a. mobility
   b. coordination
   c. reaction time
   d. agility
   e. All are skill-related components.

10. When checking exercise heart rate, one should
    a. continue to exercise at the prescribed rate while checking the heart rate.
    b. stop exercising and take the pulse for no longer than 15 seconds.
    c. exercise at a low-to-moderate intensity.
    d. stop exercise and take the heart rate for a full minute.
    e. All choices are valid ways to check exercise heart rate.

Correct answers can be found on page 261.

My Personal Fitness Program

Name _____ Date _____

Course _____ Section _____

I. In the spaces below, provide a list of five activities in which you have participated during the last 6 months. In addition to fitness activities (jogging, aerobics, swimming, strength training), you may list other activities in which you frequently participate that require physical effort (for example, walking, cycling, sweeping, vacuuming, gardening).

According to your own effort of participation, rate each activity for its health-related and motor skill-related benefits (1 = low, 2 = fair, 3 = average, 4 = good, 5 = excellent). Also indicate the frequency and duration of participation (list times per week, month, or 6 months) and add comments regarding your personal feelings related to your participation in the respective activity (liked it, was fun, too hard, got hurt, need more skill, could do it forever, etc.).

	Cardiorespiratory Endurance	Muscular Strength	Muscular Flexibility	Weight Management	Agility	Balance	Coordination	Power	Reaction Time	Speed
1.										

Comments

2.										

Comments

3.										

Comments

4.										

Comments

	Cardiorespiratory Endurance	Muscular Strength	Muscular Flexibility	Weight Management	Agility	Balance	Coordination	Power	Reaction Time	Speed
5.										

Comments

II.   On a separate sheet of paper, keep a 7-day log of all physical activities that you perform. On a daily basis, keep a record of the exact minutes throughout the day that you are active and rate each activity according to its intensity (moderate- or high-intensity). Total your minutes for each day and compute a daily average for all activities. Attach the log to this activity and then answer the following questions:

A.   Did you exercise aerobically at least 3 times per week for 20 to 30 minutes each session?

_____ Yes   _____ No

B.   Did you accumulate an average of 60 minutes of daily physical activity?

_____ Yes   _____ No

C.   What percentage of your total physical activity was moderate intensity,

_____ %

and what percentage was high intensity?

_____ %

III.   According to items I and II above, evaluate your current level of physical activity. State how you feel about your results and indicate if your program is primarily conducive to health fitness or physical fitness (or neither). Do you deem any changes necessary to meet previously stated goals (see Activity 3.4, page 83)?

_____

_____

_____

_____

_____

_____

_____

_____

_____

Nutrition for Wellness

CHAPTER 5

OBJECTIVES

- Define nutrition and describe its relationship to health and well-being.
- Learn the functions of nutrients in the human body.
- Become familiar with nutrients, food groups, and nutrient standards, and learn how to achieve a balanced diet through the use the USDA MyPyramid guidelines.
- Become familiar with eating disorders and with their associated medical problems and behavior patterns.
- Identify myths and fallacies regarding nutrition.
- Learn the 2005 Dietary Guidelines for Americans.

You are what you eat! Analyze your current diet and plan for a healthy change using the activity on your CD-ROM.

Good **nutrition** is clearly linked by scientific studies to overall health and well-being. Proper nutrition means that one's diet supplies all the essential **nutrients** to carry out normal tissue growth, repair, and maintenance. It also implies that the diet will provide enough **substrates** to produce the energy necessary for work, physical activity, and relaxation.

Too much or too little of any nutrient can precipitate serious health problems. The typical U. S. diet is too high in calories, sugar, saturated fat, and sodium, and not high enough in whole grains, fruits, and vegetables. These two factors undermine good health. Food availability is not the problem. The problem is overconsumption.

According to a report on nutrition and health issued by the U. S. Surgeon General, diseases of dietary excess and imbalance are among the leading causes of death in the United States. Similar trends are observed in developed countries throughout the world. In the report, based on more than 2,000 scientific studies, the Surgeon General said that dietary changes can bring better health to all Americans. Other surveys reveal that, on a given day, nearly half of the people in the United States eat no fruit and almost a fourth eat no vegetables.

Diet and nutrition often play a crucial role in the development and progression of chronic diseases. A diet high in saturated fat and cholesterol increases the risk for atherosclerosis and coronary heart disease. In sodium-sensitive individuals, high salt intake has been linked to high blood pressure. As many as 30 percent to 50 percent of all cancers may be diet related. Obesity, diabetes mellitus, and osteoporosis also have been associated with faulty nutrition.

The Essential Nutrients

The **essential nutrients** the human body requires are carbohydrates, fats, protein, vitamins, minerals, and water. Carbohydrates, fats, proteins, and water are termed **macronutrients** because people need to take in proportionately large amounts daily. Nutritionists refer to vitamins and minerals as **micronutrients** because the body requires them in relatively small amounts.

Depending on the amount of nutrients and calories they contain, foods can be classified as high-nutrient density or low-nutrient density. Foods with high-nutrient density contain a low or moderate amount of **calories** but are packed with nutrients. Foods that are high in calories but contain few nutrients are of low-nutrient density and commonly are called "junk food."

Carbohydrates

Carbohydrates are the major source of calories the body uses to provide energy for work, cell maintenance, and heat. They also help regulate fat and metabolize protein. Each gram of carbohydrates provides the human body with 4 calories. The major sources of carbohydrates are breads, cereals, fruits, vegetables, and milk and other dairy products. Carbohydrates are classified as simple carbohydrates and complex carbohydrates.

Simple Carbohydrates

Simple carbohydrates (such as candy, soda, and cakes), commonly denoted as sugars, have little nutritive value. These carbohydrates are divided into two groups:

- monosaccharides (glucose, fructose, and galactose)
- disaccharides (sucrose, lactose, and maltose).

Simple carbohydrates often take the place of more nutritive foods in the diet.

Complex Carbohydrates

Complex carbohydrates are formed when simple carbohydrate molecules are linked together. Three types of complex carbohydrates are:

- starches, found commonly in seeds, corn, nuts, grains, roots, potatoes, and legumes.
- dextrins, formed from the breakdown of large starch molecules exposed to dry heat, such as when bread is baked or cold cereals are manufactured.

High-fiber foods are essential in a healthy diet.

© Fitness & Wellness, Inc.

- glycogen, the animal polysaccharide synthesized from glucose and found in only small amounts in meats. Glycogen constitutes the body's reservoir of glucose. Many hundreds to thousands of glucose molecules are linked to be stored as glycogen in the liver and muscles. When a surge of energy is needed, enzymes in the muscle and the liver break down glycogen and thus make glucose readily available for energy transformation.

Complex carbohydrates provide many valuable nutrients and also are an excellent source of fiber (also called roughage).

Fiber

Fiber is a form of complex carbohydrate. A high-fiber diet gives a person a feeling of fullness without added calories. Dietary fiber is present mainly in plant leaves, skins, roots, and seeds. Processing and refining foods removes almost all of the natural fiber.

In the American diet, the main sources of fiber are whole-grain cereals and breads, fruits, vegetables, and legumes. Fiber is important in the diet because it decreases the risk for cardiovascular disease and cancer. Increased fiber intake also may lower the risk of coronary heart disease because saturated fats often take the place of fiber in the diet, thus increasing the absorption and formation of cholesterol. Other health disorders that have been tied to low intake of fiber are constipation, diverticulitis, hemorrhoids, gallbladder disease, and obesity.

The daily recommended amount of fiber intake for adults 50 years and younger is 25 grams for women and 38 grams for men. Most people in the United States eat only 15 grams of fiber per day, putting them at increased risk for disease. A person can increase fiber intake by

TABLE **5.1** Fiber Content of Selected Foods

FOOD (gm)	SERVING SIZE	DIETARY FIBER
Almonds, shelled	¼ cup	3.9
Apple	1 medium	3.7
Banana	1 small	1.2
Beans (red, kidney)	½ cup	8.2
Blackberries	½ cup	4.9
Beets, red, canned (cooked)	½ cup	1.4
Brazil nuts	1 oz	2.5
Broccoli (cooked)	½ cup	3.3
Brown rice (cooked)	½ cup	1.7
Carrots (cooked)	½ cup	3.3
Cauliflower (cooked)	½ cup	5.0
Cereal		
All Bran	1 oz	8.5
Cheerios	1 oz	1.1
Cornflakes	1 oz	0.5
Fruit and Fibre	1 oz	4.0
Fruit Wheats	1 oz	2.0
Just Right	1 oz	2.0
Wheaties	1 oz	2.0
Corn (cooked)	½ cup	2.2
Eggplant (cooked)	½ cup	3.0
Lettuce (chopped)	½ cup	0.5
Orange	1 medium	4.3
Parsnips (cooked)	½ cup	2.1
Pear	1 medium	4.5
Peas (cooked)	½ cup	4.4
Popcorn (plain)	1 cup	1.2
Potato (baked)	1 medium	4.9
Strawberries	½ cup	1.6
Summer squash (cooked)	½ cup	1.6
Watermelon	1 cup	0.1

Tips to Increase Fiber in the Diet

- Eat more vegetables, either raw or steamed.
- Eat salads daily that include a wide variety of vegetables.
- Eat more fruit, including the skin.
- Choose whole-wheat and whole-grain products.
- Choose breakfast cereals with more than 3 grams of fiber per serving.
- Sprinkle a teaspoon or two of unprocessed bran or 100% bran cereal on your favorite breakfast cereal.
- Add high-fiber cereals to casseroles and desserts.
- Add beans to soups, salads, and stews.
- Add vegetables to sandwiches: sprouts, green and red pepper strips, diced carrots, sliced cucumbers, red cabbage, onions.
- Add vegetables to spaghetti: broccoli, cauliflower, sliced carrots, mushrooms.
- Experiment with unfamiliar fruits and vegetables— collards, kale, broccoflower, asparagus, papaya, mango, kiwi, starfruit.
- Blend fruit juice with small pieces of fruit and crushed ice.
- When increasing fiber in your diet, drink plenty of fluids.

eating more fruits, vegetables, legumes, grains, and cereals. A 6-year study provided strong evidence linking increased fiber intake of 30 grams per day to a significant reduction in heart attacks, cancer of the colon, breast cancer, diabetes, and diverticulitis.[1] Table 5.1 provides the fiber content of selected foods.

Fibers are typically classified according to their solubility in water. Soluble fiber dissolves in water and forms a gel-like substance that encloses food particles. This property allows soluble fiber to bind and excrete fats from the body. Soluble fiber has been shown to decrease blood cholesterol and blood sugar levels. Soluble fibers are found primarily in oats, fruits, barley, and legumes.

Insoluble fiber is not easily dissolved in water, and the body cannot digest it. This fiber is important because it binds water, resulting in a softer and bulkier stool that increases peristalsis (involuntary muscle contractions of intestinal walls), forcing the stool onward, and allows

KEY TERMS

Nutrition The science that studies the relationship of foods to optimal health and performance.

Nutrients Substances found in food that provide energy, regulate metabolism, and help with growth and repair of body tissues.

Substrates Foods that are used as energy sources (carbohydrates, fat, protein).

Essential nutrients Carbohydrates, fats, protein, vitamins, minerals, and water—the nutrients the human body requires for survival.

Macronutrients The nutrients the body needs in proportionately large amounts; carbohydrates, fats, proteins, and water are examples.

Micronutrients The nutrients the body needs in small quantities —vitamins and minerals—that serve specific roles in transformation of energy and body tissue synthesis.

Calorie The amount of heat necessary to raise the temperature of 1 gram of water 1° Centigrade; used to measure the energy value of food and the cost of physical activity.

Carbohydrates Compounds composed of carbon, hydrogen, and oxygen that the body uses as its major source of energy.

Fiber Plant material that human digestive enzymes cannot digest.

food residues to pass through the intestinal tract more quickly. Speeding the passage of food residues through the intestines seems to lower the risk for colon cancer, mainly because cancer-causing agents are not in contact as long with the intestinal wall. Insoluble fiber also is thought to bind with carcinogens (cancer-producing substances), and more water in the stool may dilute the cancer-causing agents, lessening their potency. Sources of insoluble fiber include wheat, cereals, vegetables, and skins of fruits.

Fats

Fats, or **lipids**, are the most concentrated source of energy. Each gram of fat supplies 9 calories to the body. Fats, also part of the cell structure, are used as stored energy and as an insulator to preserve body heat. They absorb shock, supply essential fatty acids, and carry the fat-soluble vitamins A, D, E, and K. The main sources of dietary fat are milk and other dairy products, and meats and alternates. Fats are classified into simple, compound, and derived fats.

Simple Fats

Simple fats consist of a glyceride molecule linked to one, two, or three units of fatty acids. According to the number of fatty acids attached, simple fats are divided into monoglycerides (one fatty acid), diglycerides (two fatty acids), and triglycerides (three fatty acids). More than 90 percent of the weight of fat in foods and more than 95 percent of the stored fat in the human body is in the form of triglycerides.

The length of the carbon atom chain and the amount of hydrogen saturation in fatty acids vary. Based on the extent of saturation, fatty acids are said to be saturated or unsaturated. Unsaturated fatty acids are classified further into monounsaturated and polyunsaturated fats. Saturated fatty acids are mainly of animal origin. Unsaturated fats are found mostly in plant products.

In saturated fatty acids, the carbon atoms are fully saturated with hydrogens; only single bonds link the carbon atoms on the chain. These saturated fatty acids are more commonly known as saturated fats. Examples of foods high in saturated fatty acids are meats, meat fat, lard, whole milk, cream, butter, cheese, ice cream, hydrogenated oils (a process that makes oils saturated), coconut oil, and palm oils. Saturated fats tend to be solids that typically do not melt at room temperature. Coconut and palm oils are exceptions. In general, saturated fats raise the blood cholesterol level. The jury on coconut and palm oils is still out, because recent research indicates that these oils may be neutral in

terms of their effects on cholesterol and may actually provide some health benefits.

In unsaturated fatty acids (unsaturated fats), double bonds form between the unsaturated carbons. Monounsaturated fatty acids (MUFA) have only one double bond along the chain. Examples are olive, canola, rapeseed, peanut, and sesame oils. Polyunsaturated fatty acids (PUFA) contain two or more double bonds between unsaturated carbon atoms along the chain. Corn, cottonseed, safflower, walnut, sunflower, and soybean oils are high in polyunsaturated fatty acids. Unsaturated fats are usually liquid at room temperature.

Compound Fats

Compound fats are a combination of simple fats and other chemicals. Examples are phospholipids, glucolipids, and lipoproteins.

Derived Fats

Derived fats combine simple and compound fats. Sterols are an example. Although sterols contain no fatty acids, they are considered lipids because they do not dissolve in water. The most often mentioned sterol is cholesterol, which is found in many foods and is manufactured from saturated fats in the body.

Proteins

Proteins are used to build and repair tissues including muscles, blood, internal organs, skin, hair, nails, and bones. They are a part of hormones, enzymes, and antibodies, and help maintain a normal balance of body fluids. Proteins can also be used as a source of energy, but only if not enough carbohydrates are available. The primary sources are meats, meat alternates, milk, and other dairy products.

Proteins are composed of **amino acids**, containing nitrogen, carbon, hydrogen, and oxygen. Because the body cannot produce them, 9 of the 20 amino acids are called essential amino acids. The other 11, termed nonessential amino acids, can be manufactured in the body if food proteins in the diet provide enough nitrogen. For normal body function, all amino acids must be present in the diet.

A deficiency in protein is not a problem in the usual American diet. Two glasses of skim milk combined with about 4 ounces of poultry or fish meet the daily protein requirement. Protein deficiency, however, could be a concern in some vegetarian diets (see discussion on vegetarianism, pages 115–116).

Vitamins

Vitamins function as **antioxidants** and as coenzymes (primarily the B complex), which regulate the work of enzymes; and vitamin D even functions as a hormone.

Based on their solubility, vitamins are classified into two types: fat-soluble vitamins (A, D, E, and K) and water-soluble vitamins (B complex and C). The body cannot manufacture vitamins; they can be obtained only through a well-balanced diet. Additional information on the importance of vitamins is presented later in this chapter.

Minerals

Minerals serve several important functions. They are constituents of all cells, especially those in hard parts of the body (bones, nails, teeth). They are crucial in maintaining water balance and the acid–base balance. They are essential components of respiratory pigments, enzymes, and enzyme systems, and they regulate muscular and nervous tissue excitability.

Water

Water, the most important nutrient, is involved in almost every vital body process. Water is used in digesting and absorbing food, in the circulatory process, in removing waste products, in building and rebuilding cells, and in transporting other nutrients.

Water is contained in almost all foods, but primarily in liquid foods, fruits, and vegetables. Although for decades the recommendation was to consume at least 8 cups of water per day, a panel of scientists of the Institute of Medicine of the National Academy of Sciences indicated in 2004 that people are getting enough water from the liquids (milk, juices, sodas, coffee) and the moisture content of solid foods. Caffeine-containing drinks are also acceptable as a water source because data indicate that people who regularly consume such beverages do not have a greater 24-hour urine output than those who don't.

Most Americans and Canadians remain well-hydrated simply by using thirst as their guide. An exception to this practice, however, is when an individual exercises in the heat or does so for an extended time. Water lost under these conditions must be replenished regularly, without waiting for the onset of thirst.

Nutrition Standards

Nutritionists use a variety of nutrient standards. The most widely known is the Recommended Dietary Allowances (RDA). This is not the only standard, though. Nutrition standards include the Dietary Reference Intakes and the Daily Values on food labels. Each standard has a different purpose and utilization in dietary planning and assessment.

Dietary Reference Intakes

To help people meet dietary guidelines, the National Academy of Sciences has developed a set of dietary nutrient intakes for healthy people in the United States and Canada, the **Dietary Reference Intakes (DRIs)**. The DRIs are based on a review of the most current research on adequate amounts and maximum safe nutrient intakes of healthy people. The DRI reports are written by the Food and Nutrition Board of the Institute of Medicine in cooperation with scientists from Canada.

Within the umbrella of DRI are four types of reference values for planning and assessing diets:

1. Estimated Average Requirements (EAR)
2. Recommended Dietary Allowances (RDA)
3. Adequate Intakes (AI)
4. Tolerable Upper Intake Levels (UL).

The type of reference value used for a given nutrient and a specific age/gender group is determined according to available scientific information and the intended use of the dietary standard.

The **Estimated Average Requirements (EAR)** is the amount of nutrient that is estimated to meet the nutrient requirement of half the healthy people in specific age and gender groups. At this nutrient intake level, the nutritional requirements of the upper 50 percent of the people are not met.

KEY TERMS

Fats (lipids) A class of nutrients that the body uses as a source of energy.

Proteins A class of nutrients that the body uses to build and repair body tissues.

Amino acids The basic building blocks of protein.

Vitamins Organic substances essential for normal bodily metabolism, growth, and development.

Antioxidants Compounds that prevent oxygen from combining with other substances it might damage.

Minerals Inorganic elements needed by the body.

Dietary Reference Intakes (DRIs) Four types of nutrient standards that are used to establish adequate amounts and maximum safe nutrient intakes in the diet: Estimated Average Requirements (EAR), Recommended Dietary Allowances (RDA), Adequate Intakes (AI), and Tolerable Upper Intake Levels (UL).

Estimated Average Requirements (EAR) The amount of a nutrient that meets the dietary needs in half the people.

TABLE **5.2** Recommended Dietary Allowances and Adequate Intakes for Selected Nutrients

	RECOMMENDED DIETARY ALLOWANCES (RDA)														ADEQUATE INTAKES (AI)					
	Thiamin (mg)	Riboflavin (mg)	Niacin (mg NE)	Vitamin B$_6$ (mg)	Folate (mcg DFE)	Vitamin B$_{12}$ (mcg)	Phosphorus (mg)	Magnesium (mg)	Vitamin A (mcg)	Vitamin C (mg)	Vitamin E (mg)	Selenium (mcg)	Iron (mcg)		Calcium (mg)	Vitamin D (mcg)	Fluoride (mg)	Pantothenic acid (mg)	Biotin (mg)	Choline (mg)
Males																				
14–18	1.2	1.3	16	1.3	400	2.4	1,250	410	900	75	15	55	11		1,300	5	3	5.0	25	550
19–30	1.2	1.3	16	1.3	400	2.4	700	400	900	90	15	55	8		1,000	5	4	5.0	30	550
31–50	1.2	1.3	16	1.3	400	2.4	700	420	900	90	15	55	8		1,000	5	4	5.0	30	550
51–70	1.2	1.3	16	1.7	400	2.4	700	420	900	90	15	55	8		1,200	10	4	5.0	30	550
>70	1.2	1.3	16	1.7	400	2.4	700	420	900	90	15	55	8		1,200	15	4	5.0	30	550
Females																				
14–18	1.0	1.0	14	1.2	400	2.4	1,250	360	700	65	15	55	15		1,300	5	3	5.0	25	400
19–30	1.1	1.1	14	1.3	400	2.4	700	310	700	75	15	55	18		1,000	5	3	5.0	30	425
31–50	1.1	1.1	14	1.3	400	2.4	700	320	700	75	15	55	18		1,000	5	3	5.0	30	425
51–70	1.1	1.1	14	1.5	400	2.4	700	320	700	75	15	55	8		1,200	10	3	5.0	30	425
>70	1.1	1.1	14	1.5	400	2.4	700	320	700	75	15	55	8		1,200	15	3	5.0	30	425
Pregnant	1.4	1.4	18	1.9	600	2.6	*	+40	750	85	15	60	27		*	*	3	6.0	30	450
Lactating	1.5	1.6	17	2.0	500	2.8	*	*	1,300	120	19	70	10		*	*	3	7.0	35	550

* Values for these nutrients do not change with pregnancy or lactation. Use the value listed for women of comparable age.

Source: Adapted with permission from *Recommended Dietary Allowances,* 10th Edition, and the *Dietary Reference Intakes* series. Copyright © 1989 and 2002, respectively, by the National Academy of Sciences. Courtesy of the National Academies Press, Washington, DC.

The **Recommended Dietary Allowances (RDA)** set forth the daily amount of a nutrient considered adequate to meet the known nutrient needs of nearly all healthy people in the United States. The RDAs for selected nutrients are presented in Table 5.2. Because the committee must decide what level of intake to recommend for everybody, the RDA is set well above the EAR and covers about 98 percent of the population. Stated another way, the RDA recommendation for any nutrient is well above almost everyone's actual requirement.

The RDA could be considered a goal for adequate intake. The process for determining the RDA depends on being able to set an EAR. RDAs are statistically determined from the EAR values. If an EAR cannot be set, no RDA can be established.

When data are insufficient or inadequate to set an EAR, an **Adequate Intakes (AI)** value is determined instead of the RDA. The AI value is derived from approximations of observed nutrient intakes by a group or groups of healthy people. The AI value for children and adults is expected to meet or exceed the nutritional requirements of a specific healthy population.

The **Tolerable Upper Intake Levels (UL)**, which eventually will be available for all nutrients, establishes the highest level of nutrient intake that seems to be safe for most healthy people and beyond which there is an increased risk of adverse effects. As intakes increase above the UL, so does the risk for adverse effects. Generally speaking, the optimum nutrient range for healthy eating is between the RDA and the UL. The established ULs for selected nutrients are presented in Table 5.3.

Daily Values

The **Daily Values (DVs)** are reference values for nutrients and food components for use on commercial food labels. The DVs are based on a 2,000-calorie diet and may therefore require adjustments depending on an individual's daily **Estimated Energy Requirement (EER)** in calories.

TABLE **5.3** Tolerable Upper Intake Levels (UL) of Selected Nutrients for Adults (19–70 years)

NUTRIENT	UL PER DAY
Calcium	2.5 gr
Phosphorus	4.0 gr*
Magnesium	350 mg
Vitamin D	50 mcg
Fluoride	10 mg
Niacin	35 mg
Iron	45 mg
Vitamin B_6	100 mg
Folate	1,000 mcg
Choline	3.5 gr
Vitamin A	3,000 mcg
Vitamin C	2,000 mg
Vitamin E	1,000 mg
Selenium	400 mcg

* 3.5 gr per day for pregnant women.

For example, on a 2,000-calorie diet (EER), recommended carbohydrate intake is about 300 grams (about 60 percent of EER), and fat is less than 65 grams (about 30 percent of EER) (see Figure 5.1). The vitamin, mineral, and protein DVs were adapted from the RDAs. The DVs are also not as specific for age and gender groups as are the DRIs.

The food label is a good guide for planning a daily diet. For example, if the DV for carbohydrates in a given meal adds up to only 35 percent, you know that several additional high-carbohydrate food items are required throughout that day to reach the 100 percent DV. Further, if the DV for fat from another food item is 60 percent or 70 percent, you should limit your fat intake during the rest of that day.

Both the DRIs and the DVs apply only to healthy adults. They are not intended for people who are ill and may require additional nutrients or dietary adjustments.

CT Critical Thinking

What do the nutrition standards mean to you? How much of a challenge would it be to apply those standards in your daily life?

Dietary Guidelines

Most people would like to live life to its fullest, have good health, and lead a productive life. One of the ways

FIGURE **5.1** Food label using Daily Values.

Nutrition Facts

Serving Size 1 cup (240 ml)
Servings Per Container 4

Amount Per Serving

Calories 120   Calories from Fat 45

	% Daily Value*
Total Fat 5g	**8%**
Saturated Fat 3g	**15%**
Trans Fat 1g	
Cholesterol 20mg	**7%**
Sodium 120mg	**5%**
Total Carbohydrate 12g	**4%**
Dietary Fiber 0g	**0%**
Sugars 12g	
Protein 8g	

Vitamin A 10%	•	Vitamin C 4%
Calcium 30%	•	Iron 0%

* Percent Daily Values are based on a 2,000 calorie diet. Your daily values may be higher or lower depending on your calorie needs:

		Calories	2,000	2,500
Total Fat	Less than	65g	80g
Sat Fat	Less than	20g	25g
Cholesterol	Less than	300mg	300mg
Sodium	Less than	2,400mg	2,400mg
Total Carbohydrate		300g	375g
Fiber		25g	30g

Calories per gram:
Fat 9 • Carbohydrate 4 • Protein 4

KEY TERMS

Recommended Dietary Allowances (RDA) The daily amount of a nutrient (statistically determined from the EARs) considered adequate to meet the known nutrient needs of almost 98 percent of all healthy people in the United States.

Adequate Intakes (AI) The recommended amount of a nutrient intake when sufficient evidence is not available to calculate the EAR and subsequent RDA.

Tolerable Upper Intake Levels (UL) The highest level of nutrient intake that appears to be safe for most healthy people without an increased risk of adverse effects.

Daily Values (DVs) Reference values for nutrients and food components used in food labels.

Estimated energy requirement (EER) The average dietary energy (caloric) intake that is predicted to maintain energy balance in a healthy adult of defined age, gender, weight, height, and level of physical activity, consistent with good health.

TABLE 5.4 Current and Recommended Intake of Carbohydrate, Fat, and Protein Expressed as a Percentage of Total Calories

	CURRENT %	RECOMMENDED %*
Carbohydrates	50%	45–65%
Simple	26%	Less than 25%
Complex	24%	20–40%
Fat	34%	20–35%**
Monounsaturated	11%	Up to 20%
Polyunsaturated	10%	Up to 10%
Saturated	13%	Less than 7%
Protein	16%	10–35%

* 2002 recommended guidelines by the National Academy of Sciences.

** Less than 30% recommended by most health organizations. A higher amount may be indicated for people with metabolic syndrome.

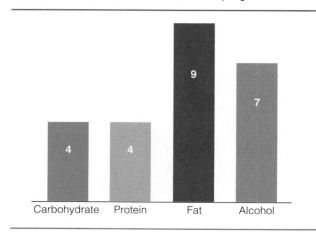

FIGURE 5.2 Caloric value (calories) per gram of food.

to do this is through a well-balanced diet. As illustrated in Table 5.4, the recommended guidelines by the National Academy of Sciences (NAS) in 2002 state that daily caloric intake should be distributed so that 45 to 65 percent of the total calories come from carbohydrates (mostly complex carbohydrates and less than 25 percent from sugar), 20 to 35 percent from fat, and 10 to 35 percent from protein.[2] These ranges offer greater flexibility in planning diets according to individual health and physical activity needs.

In addition to the macronutrients, the diet must include all of the essential vitamins and minerals. The source of fat calories is also critical. The National Cholesterol Education Program recommends that saturated fat constitute less than 7 percent, polyunsaturated fat up to 10 percent, and monounsaturated fat up to 20 percent of total calories. Rating a given diet accurately is difficult without a complete nutrient analysis. You have an opportunity to perform this analysis in Activity 5.1, page 125.

The 2002 NAS guidelines are in sharp contrast to those of major national health organizations, which recommend 50 to 60 percent of total calories from carbohydrates, less than 30 percent from fat, and about 15 percent from protein. The most drastic difference appears in the NAS-allowed range of fat intake, up to 35 percent of total calories. This higher percentage was included to accommodate individuals with metabolic syndrome (see Chapter 8, page 182) who have an abnormal insulin response to carbohydrates and may need additional fat in the diet.

The NAS recommendations will be effective only if people consistently replace saturated and trans fatty acids with unsaturated fatty acids. The latter will require dramatic changes in the typical "unhealthy" American diet, which is generally high in red meats, whole dairy

products, and fast foods—all of which are high in saturated and/or trans fatty acids.

Determining Fat Content in the Diet

As illustrated in Figure 5.2, each gram of carbohydrates and protein supplies the body with 4 calories, and fat provides 9 calories per gram consumed (alcohol yields 7 calories per gram). In this regard, just looking at the total amount of grams consumed for each type of food can be misleading.

For example, a person who consumes 160 grams of carbohydrates, 100 grams of fat, and 70 grams of protein has a total intake of 330 grams of food. This indicates that 30 percent of the total grams of food is in the form of fat (100 grams of fat ÷ 330 grams of total food × 100).

Almost half of this diet, however, consists of fat calories. In the diet, 640 calories are derived from carbohydrates (160 grams × 4 calories/gram), 280 calories from protein (70 grams × 4 calories/gram), and 900 calories from fat (100 grams × 9 calories/gram), for a total of 1,820 calories. If 900 calories are derived from fat, you can see that almost half of the total caloric intake is in the form of fat (900 ÷ 1,820 × 100 = 49.5 percent).

Realizing that each gram of fat provides 9 calories is a useful guideline when figuring the fat content of individual foods. As shown in Figure 5.3, all you have to do is multiply the grams of fat by 9 and divide by the total calories in that specific food. Multiply that number by 100 to get the percentage. For example, if a food label lists a total of 20 calories and 7 grams of fat, the fat content is 53 percent of total calories (7 × 9 ÷ 120 × 100). This simple guideline can help you decrease fat in your diet.

FIGURE **5.3** Determining percent calories from fat in food.

Serving = 120 calories   Fat = 5 g

Percent Fat Calories = (g of fat $\times$ 9)
$\div$ calories per serving $\times$ 100

5 g of fat $\times$ 9 calories per g of fat =
45 calories from fat

45 calories from fat $\div$ 120 calories per
serving $\times$ 100 = 38% fat

Balancing the Diet

Achieving and maintaining a balanced diet is not as difficult as most people think. The MyPyramid healthy eating guide in Figure 5.4 (page 114) contains five major food groups and oils. The food groups are grains, vegetables, fruits, milk, and meats and beans.

Whole grains, vegetables, fruits, and low-fat milk (and byproducts) provide the nutritional base for a healthy diet. If you increase the intake of these food groups, remember to decrease the intake of low-nutrient-dense foods to effectively balance caloric intake with energy needs.

Whole grains are a major source of fiber as well as other nutrients. Whole grains contain the entire grain kernel (the bran, germ, and endosperm). Examples include whole-wheat flour, whole cornmeal, oatmeal, cracked wheat (bulgur), and brown rice.

Refined grains have been milled, a process that removes the bran and germ. The process also removes fiber, iron, and many B vitamins. Refined grains include white flour, white bread, white rice, and degermed cornmeal. Refined grains are often enriched to add back B vitamins and iron. Fiber, however, is not added back.

Prevention of Disease

An entirely new field of research with promising results in disease prevention, especially in the fight against cancer, is in the area of **phytochemicals** ("phyto" comes from the Greek word for plant). The main function of phytochemicals in plants is to protect them from sunlight. In humans, phytochemicals seem to have a powerful ability to block the formation of cancerous tumors. Their actions are so diverse that, at almost every stage of cancer, phytochemicals have the ability to block, disrupt, slow down, or even reverse the process (also see Chapter 8).

These compounds are not found in pills. The message here is to eat a diet with ample fruits and vegetables. The daily recommended amount of fruits and vegetables has absolutely no substitute. People can't expect to eat a poor diet, pop a few pills, and derive the same benefits.

Milk and milk products (select low-fat or non-fat) can decrease the risk of low bone mass (osteoporosis) throughout life. Besides calcium, milk is also a good source of potassium, vitamin D, and protein, and may aid with body weight management.

The recommendation for poultry, fish, or meat is to eat 3 ounces—and no more than 6 ounces—daily. All visible fat and skin should be trimmed off meats and poultry before cooking.

The difficult part for most people is retraining themselves to adopt a lifetime healthy nutrition plan. You can achieve a balanced diet if you: (a) avoid excessive fats, oils, sweets, sodium (salt), and alcohol, (b) increase your fiber intake, and (c) eat the minimum number of servings recommended for each of the five major groups in MyPyramid.

Nutrient Analysis

To aid you in balancing your diet, Activity 5.1, page 125, provides a form for you to record your daily food intake. First, make as many copies as the number of days you wish to analyze. Whenever you eat something, record the food and the amount eaten. Doing this immediately after each meal will enable you to keep track of your actual food intake more easily.

At the end of each day, consult the list of foods in Appendix E and record the number of calories for all foods consumed. Referring to Activity 5.1, page 125, record the amount and calories under the respective food groups. If you eat twice the amount of a standard serving, double the calories and the amount.

You can evaluate your diet by checking Figure 5.4 to see if you ate the minimum required daily amount for each food group. If you meet the minimum amounts at the end of each day, you are doing quite well in balancing your diet.

In addition to meeting the daily amount guidelines, a complete nutrient analysis is recommended to rate your diet accurately. A nutrient analysis can pinpoint potential problem areas in your diet, such as too much

KEY TERMS

Phytochemicals Compounds found in vegetables and fruits with cancer-fighting properties.

FIGURE 5.4 MyPyramid: Steps to a healthier you.

The colors of the pyramid illustrate variety: each color represents one of the five food groups, plus one for oils. Different band widths suggest the proportional contribution of each food group to a healthy diet.

A person climbing steps reminds consumers to be physically active each day.

The narrow slivers of color at the top imply moderation in foods rich in solid fats and added sugars.

The broad bases at the bottom represent nutrient-dense foods that should make up the bulk of the diet.

Greater intakes of grains, vegetables, fruit, and milk are encouraged by the broad bases of orange, green, red, and blue.

MyPyramid
STEPS TO A HEALTHIER YOU
MyPyramid.gov

GRAINS VEGETABLES FRUITS OIL MILK MEAT & BEANS

SOURCE: USDA, 2005.

GRAINS

In general: 1 slice of bread, 1 cup of ready-to-eat cereal, ½ cup of cooked rice, cooked pasta, or cooked cereal can be considered as 1 oz equivalent of grains. Look for "whole" before the grain name on the list of ingredients and make at least half your grains whole.

VEGETABLES

In general: 1 cup of raw or cooked vegetables or vegetable juice, or 2 cups of raw leafy greens can be considered as 1 cup from the vegetable group. Try to eat more dark green and orange veggies, as well as dry beans and peas.

FRUITS

In general: 1 cup of fruit or 100% fruit juice, or ½ cup of dried fruit can be considered as 1 cup from the fruit group. Eat a variety of fruit, including fresh, frozen, canned, or dried fruit. Go easy on fruit juices.

OILS

Measured in teaspoons of either oils or solid fats. Most sources should come from fish, nuts, and vegetable oils. Limit solid fats such as butter, stick margarine, shortening, and lard.

MILK

In general: 1 cup of milk or yogurt, 1½ oz of natural cheese, or 2 oz of processed cheese can be considered as 1 cup from the milk group. Go low-fat or fat free. If you can't consume milk, choose lactose-free products or other calcium sources.

MEATS & BEANS

In general: 1 oz of meat, poultry, or fish, ¼ cup cooked dry beans, 1 egg, 1 tbsp of peanut butter, or ½ oz of nuts or seeds can be considered as 1 oz equivalent from the Meats & Beans group.

Recommended Daily Amounts from Each Food Group

FOOD GROUP	1600 cal	1800 cal	2000 cal	2200 cal	2400 cal	2600 cal	2800 cal	3000 cal
Fruits	1½ c	1½ c	2 c	2 c	2 c	2 c	2½ c	2½ c
Vegetables	2 c	2½ c	2½ c	3 c	3 c	3½ c	3½ c	4 c
Grains	5 oz	6 oz	6 oz	7 oz	8 oz	9 oz	10 oz	10 oz
Meat and legumes	5 oz	5 oz	5½ oz	6 oz	6½ oz	6½ oz	7 oz	7 oz
Milk	3 c	3 c	3 c	3 c	3 c	3 c	3 c	3 c
Oils	5 tsp	5 tsp	6 tsp	6 tsp	7 tsp	8 tsp	8 tsp	10 tsp
Discretionary calorie allowance	132 cal	195 cal	267 cal	290 cal	362 cal	410 cal	426 cal	512 cal

*Discretionary calorie allowance: At each calorie level, people who consistently choose calorie-dense foods may be able to meet their nutrient needs without consuming their full allotment of calories. The difference between the calories needed to supply nutrients and those needed for energy is known as the *discretionary calorie allowance.*

Source: http://mypyramid.gov/ Additional information on MyPyramid can be obtained at this site, including an online individualized MyPyramid eating plan based on your age, gender, and activity level.

fat, saturated fat, cholesterol, sodium, and the like. A complete nutrient analysis can be an educational experience, because most people do not realize how detrimental and non-nutritious many common foods are.

You can do the analysis with the aid of the computer software available with this book and using the information you have recorded already on the form provided in Activity 5.1. Up to 7 days may be analyzed when using the software. Before running the software, fill out the information at the top of the form (age, weight, height, gender, and activity rating), and make sure the foods are recorded by the standard amounts given in the list of selected foods in Appendix E. The software also accommodates vegetarianism.

Vegetarianism

More than 12 million people in the United States follow vegetarian diets. **Vegetarians** rely primarily on foods from the bread, cereal, rice, pasta, and fruit and vegetable groups and avoid foods from animal sources including the milk, yogurt, and cheese and meat groups.

The five basic types of vegetarians are:

1. Vegans: those who eat no animal products at all.
2. Ovovegetarians: those who allow eggs in the diet.
3. Lactovegetarians: those who allow foods from the milk group.
4. Ovolactovegetarians: those who include egg and milk products in the diet.
5. Semivegetarians: those who do not eat red meat but include fish and poultry in addition to milk products and eggs in their diets.

Well-planned vegetarian diets are healthful, are consistent with the Dietary Guidelines for Americans, and can meet the DRIs for nutrients. Vegetarians who do not select their food combinations properly, however, can develop nutritional deficiencies of protein, vitamins, minerals, and even calories. Even more attention should be paid when planning vegetarian diets for infants and children. Without careful planning, a strictly plant-based diet will prevent proper growth and development.

Protein deficiency is a concern in some vegetarian diets. Vegans in particular must be careful to eat foods that provide a balanced distribution of essential amino acids, such as grain products and legumes. Strict vegans also need a supplement of vitamin B_{12}. This vitamin is not found in plant foods; its only source is animal foods. A deficiency of this vitamin can lead to anemia and nerve damage.

The key to a healthful vegetarian diet is to eat foods with complementary proteins. Most plant-based products lack one or more essential amino acids in adequate amounts. For example, both grains and legumes are good protein sources, but neither provides all the essential amino acids. Grains and cereals are low in the amino acid lysine, and legumes lack methionine. Combining foods from these two groups, such as tortillas and beans, rice and beans, rice and soybeans, or wheat bread and peanuts, will complement each other. These complementary proteins may be consumed over the course of the day, but it is best if they are consumed during the same meal.

MyPyramid can also be used as a guide for vegetarians. The key is food variety. Most vegetarians today consume dairy products and eggs. Meat can be replaced with legumes, nuts, seeds, eggs, and meat substitutes (tofu, tempeh, soy milk, and commercial meat replacers such as veggie burgers and soy hot dogs). For additional MyPyramid healthy eating tips for vegetarians and ways to get enough of the previously mentioned nutrients, go to http://mypyramid.gov/.

Consumption of nuts and soy foods, commonly used in vegetarian diets, has received considerable attention in recent years. Although nuts are 70 to 90 percent fat, most of it is unsaturated fat. And research indicates that people who eat nuts several times a week have a lower incidence of heart disease. Eating 2 to 3 ounces (about one-half cup) of almonds, walnuts, or macadamia nuts a day may decrease high blood cholesterol by about 10 percent.

Heart-health benefits are attributed to the unsaturated fats and also to other nutrients found in nuts, such as vitamin E and folic acid. Nuts are also packed with additional B vitamins, calcium, copper, potassium, magnesium, fiber, and phytochemicals. Many of these nutrients are cancer- and cardio-protective.

Nuts do have a drawback: They are high in calories. A handful of nuts provides as many calories as a piece of cake. Therefore, you should avoid using nuts as a snack. Nuts are recommended for use in place of high-protein foods such as meats, bacon, eggs, or as part of a meal in fruit or vegetable salads, homemade bread, pancakes, casseroles, yogurt, and oatmeal. Peanut butter is also healthier than cheese or some cold cuts in sandwiches.

The increasing popularity of soy foods is attributed primarily to Asian research that points to less heart disease and fewer hormone-related cancers in people who regularly consume soy foods. The benefits of soy lie in its high protein content and plant chemicals, known as isoflavones, that act as antioxidants and may protect

KEY TERMS

Vegetarians Individuals whose diet is of vegetable or plant origin.

against estrogen-related cancers (breast, ovarian, and endometrial). Soy consumption also has been linked to a lower risk for prostate cancer.

In addition, soy protein can lower blood cholesterol to a greater extent than would be expected just from its low-fat and high-fiber content. The evidence of heart-protecting benefits from soy foods is so strong that the Food and Drug Administration allows the following claim on food labels: "25 grams of soy proteins a day, as part of a diet low in saturated fat and cholesterol, may reduce the risk of heart disease." One to two cups of soy milk, ½ cup of tofu, 1½ tablespoons of soy protein isolate, or ¼ cup of soy flour provide about 10 grams of soy protein.

Those who are interested in vegetarian diets should consult other resources. A thorough discussion on such diets cannot be covered adequately in a few paragraphs.

Nutrient Supplementation

Approximately half of all adults in the United States take daily nutrient **supplements**. Nutrient requirements for the body normally can be met by consuming as few as 1,200 calories per day, as long as the diet contains the recommended amounts of food from the different food groups.

Most supplements do not seem to provide additional benefits for healthy people who eat a balanced diet. They do not help people run faster, jump higher, relieve stress, improve their sexual prowess, cure a common cold, or boost energy levels. Some of the special cases are discussed below.

People should not take **megadoses** of vitamins and minerals. For some nutrients, a dose of five times the RDA taken over several months may create problems. For others, such a dose may not pose any threat to human health. Vitamin and mineral intake should not exceed the ULs. For nutrients that do not have an established UL, a person should not take a dosage higher than three times the RDA.

Among the populations that may benefit from supplementation are those with nutrient deficiencies (including low calcium intake), alcoholics and street-drug users who do not have a balanced diet, smokers, vegans (strict vegetarians), individuals on extremely low-calorie diets (fewer than 1,200 calories per day), older adults who don't eat balanced meals regularly, newborn infants (usually given a single dose of vitamin K to prevent abnormal bleeding), and people who have disease-related disorders or who are taking medications that interfere with proper absorption of nutrients.

Iron

Iron deficiency (determined through blood testing) is more common in women than men. Iron supplementation is frequently recommended for women who have a heavy menstrual flow. Some pregnant and lactating women also may require supplements. The average pregnant woman who eats an adequate amount of a variety of foods should take a low dose of iron supplement daily. Women who are pregnant with more than one baby may need additional supplements.

Antioxidants

Much research and discussion is taking place regarding the effectiveness of antioxidants in thwarting several chronic diseases. Although foods probably contain more than 4,000 antioxidants, the four more studied antioxidants are vitamins C, E, and beta-carotene (a precursor to vitamin A), and the mineral selenium (see Table 5.5).

Oxygen is utilized during metabolism to change carbohydrates and fats into energy. During this process oxygen is transformed into stable forms of water and carbon dioxide. A small amount of oxygen, however, ends up in an unstable form, referred to as oxygen free radicals. A free radical molecule has a normal proton nucleus with a single unpaired electron.

Having only one electron makes the free radical extremely reactive, and it looks constantly to pair the electron with an electron from another molecule. When a free radical steals the second electron from another molecule, that other molecule in turn becomes a free radical. This chain reaction goes on until two free radicals meet to form a stable molecule.

Free radicals attack and damage proteins and lipids, in particular cell membranes and DNA. This damage is thought to contribute to the development of conditions such as cardiovascular disease, cancer, emphysema, cataracts, Parkinson's disease, and premature aging. Environmental factors that seem to encourage the formation of free radicals include solar radiation, cigarette smoke, air pollution, radiation, some drugs, injury or infection, and chemicals (such as pesticides), among others.

The body's own defense systems typically neutralize free radicals so they don't cause any damage. When free radicals are produced faster than the body can neutralize them, however, they can damage the cells. Antioxidants are found abundantly in food, especially in fruits and vegetables. Unfortunately, most Americans do not eat the minimum daily recommended amounts of fruits and vegetables.

TABLE 5.5 Antioxidant Nutrients, Sources, and Functions

NUTRIENT	GOOD SOURCES	ANTIOXIDANT EFFECT
Vitamin C	Citrus fruit, kiwi fruit, cantaloupe, strawberries, broccoli, green or red peppers, cauliflower, cabbage	Appears to inactivate oxygen-free radicals.
Vitamin E	Vegetable oils, yellow and green leafy vegetables, margarine, wheat germ, oatmeal, almonds, whole-grain breads, cereals	Protects lipids from oxidation.
Beta-carotene	Carrots, squash, pumpkin, sweet potatoes, broccoli, green leafy vegetables	Soaks up oxygen-free radicals.
Selenium	Seafood, Brazil nuts, meat, whole grains	Helps prevent damage to cell structures.

Antioxidant Nutrients

Some researchers believe that taking antioxidant supplements further prevents free-radical damage. Controversy, however, surrounds the need to take antioxidants in supplement form. The benefits of antioxidants are obtained from food sources themselves. People who consume nine servings of fresh fruits and vegetables daily could get their daily vitamin C and beta-carotene requirements through their diet. Small dietary adjustments can also ensure that both vitamin E and selenium are adequate in the daily diet.

Vitamin C may offer benefits against heart disease, cancer, and cataracts. Antioxidant recommendations for vitamin C over the years have ranged from 250 to 500 mg per day (the RDA is 75 to 90 mg). People who consume the recommended amounts of daily fruits and vegetables, nonetheless, need no supplementation because they obtain their daily vitamin C requirements through the diet alone.

Vitamin C is water-soluble, and the body eliminates it in about 12 hours. For best results, consume vitamin C-rich foods twice a day. High intake of a vitamin C supplement, above 500 mg per day, is not recommended. The body absorbs very little vitamin C beyond the first 200 mg per serving or dose.

Beta-carotene supplementation was encouraged in the early 1990s. It is better, however, to obtain the daily recommended dose of beta-carotene (20,000 IU) from food sources rather than supplements. Clinical trials have found that beta-carotene supplements did not offer protection against heart disease or cancer or provide any other health benefits. Therefore, it is recommended that you "skip the pill and eat the carrot." One medium raw carrot contains about 20,000 IU of beta-carotene.

Based on earlier recommendations, people were encouraged to take between 200 to 800 IU of daily Vitamin E supplementation. Disappointing follow-up reviews of hundreds of studies, however, has led to the withdrawal of this recommendation.[3] Although no evidence suggests that Vitamin E supplementation below the upper limit of 1,000 mg per day is harmful, little or no clinical research supports any health benefits. Nuts, seeds, vegetable oils, whole grains, and leafy greens are good sources of Vitamin E (see Table 5.6). You should try to incorporate these foods regularly in the diet to obtain the RDA.

Adequate intake of the mineral selenium is encouraged. Individuals who take 200 mcg of selenium daily seem to decrease their risk of acquiring prostate cancer by 63 percent, colorectal cancer by 58 percent, and lung cancer by 46 percent.[4] Data also point to decreased risks of acquiring cancers of the breast, liver, and digestive tract. According to Dr. Edward Giovannucci of the Harvard Medical School, the evidence for benefits of selenium in reducing prostate cancer risk is so strong that public health officials should recommend that people increase selenium intake now.[5]

One Brazil nut (unshelled) that you crack yourself provides about 100 mcg of selenium. Shelled nuts found in supermarkets average only about 20 mcg each. Based on the current body of research, a dose of 100 to 200 mcg per day seems to provide the necessary amount of antioxidant for this nutrient. There is no reason to take more than 200 mcg daily. In fact, the UL for selenium has been set at 400 mcg. Too much selenium can damage cells rather than protect them. If you choose to take supplements, take an organic form of selenium from yeast and not selenium selenite. The selenium content of various foods is provided in Table 5.6.

KEY TERMS

Supplements Tablets, pills, capsules, liquids, or powders that contain vitamins, minerals, amino acids, herbs, or fiber that are taken to increase the intake of these substances.

Megadoses For most vitamins, 10 times the RDA or more; for vitamins A and D, five and two times the RDA, respectively.

TABLE 5.6 Antioxidant Content of Selected Foods

BETA-CAROTENE	IU
Apricot (1 medium)	675
Broccoli (½ cup, frozen)	1,740
Broccoli (½ cup, raw)	680
Cantaloupe (1 cup)	5,160
Carrot (1 medium, raw)	20,255
Green peas (½ cup, frozen)	535
Mango (1 medium)	8,060
Mustard greens (½ cup, frozen)	3,350
Papaya (1 medium)	6,120
Spinach (½ cup, frozen)	7,395
Sweet potato (1 medium, baked)	24,875
Tomato (1 medium)	1,395
Turnip greens (½ cup, boiled)	3,960

VITAMIN E	IU	mg*
Almond oil (1 tbsp)		5.3
Almonds (1 oz)	10.1	
Canola oil (1 tbsp)		9.0
Cottonseed oil (1 tbsp)		5.2
Hazelnuts (1 oz)	4.4	
Kale (1 cup)	15.0	
Margarine (1 tbsp)		2.0
Peanuts (1 oz)	3.0	
Shrimp (3 oz, boiled)	3.1	
Sunflower seeds (1 oz, dry)	14.2	
Sunflower seed oil (1 tbsp)		6.9
Sweet potato (1 medium, baked)	7.2	
Wheat germ oil (1 tbsp)		20.0

VITAMIN C	mg
Acerola (1 cup, raw)	1,640
Acerola juice (8 oz)	3,864
Cantaloupe (½ melon, medium)	90
Cranberry juice (8 oz)	90
Grapefruit (½, medium, white)	52
Grapefruit juice (8 oz)	92
Guava (1 medium)	165
Kiwi (1 medium)	75
Lemon juice (8 oz)	110
Orange (1 medium)	66
Orange juice (8 oz)	120
Papaya (1 medium)	85
Pepper (½ cup, red, chopped, raw)	95
Strawberries (1 cup, raw)	88

SELENIUM	mcg
Brazil nuts (1)	100
Bread, whole wheat enriched (1 slice)	15
Beef (3 oz)	33
Cereals (3½ oz)	20
Chicken breast, roasted, no skin (3 oz)	24
Cod, baked (3 oz)	57
Egg, hard boiled (1 large)	15
Fruits (3½ oz)	1
Noodles, enriched, boiled (1 cup)	50
Oatmeal, cooked (1 cup)	23
Red snapper (3 oz)	150
Rice, long grain, cooked (1 cup)	20
Salmon, baked (3 oz)	35
Spaghetti w/meat sauce (1 cup)	36
Tuna, canned, water, drained (3 oz)	68
Turkey breast, roasted, no skin (3 oz)	28
Walnuts, black, chopped (¼ cup)	5
Vegetables (3½ oz)	1

* Vitamin E values for oils are commonly expressed in milligrams (mg). One mg is almost equal to 1 IU (international unit).

Multivitamins

Although much interest has been generated by the previously mentioned supplements, multivitamins are still the preferred supplement of the American people. A multivitamin complex that provides 100 percent of the DV for most nutrients can help fill in certain dietary deficiencies.[6] Some evidence suggests that regular intake decreases the risk for cardiovascular disease and colon cancer and improves immune function.

Multivitamins, however, are not magic pills. They may help, but they don't provide a license to eat carelessly. Multivitamins don't provide energy, fiber, or phytochemicals.

Folate

A folate (a B vitamin) supplement has been recommended for all premenopausal women. In particular, folate supplements are encouraged prior to and during pregnancy. This includes women who might become pregnant. Studies have shown that high folate intake (400 mcg per day) during early pregnancy can prevent serious birth defects. Folate also seems to offer protection against colon and cervical cancers. In all the above instances, supplements should be taken under a physician's supervision.

Increasing evidence indicates that taking 400 mcg of folate along with vitamins B_6 and B_{12} prevents heart attacks by reducing homocysteine levels in the blood (see Chapter 8). High concentrations of homocysteine accelerate the process of plaque formation (atherosclerosis) in the arteries. Five servings of fruits and vegetables per day usually meet the needs for these nutrients. Currently, close to 9 in 10 adults in the United States do not meet the recommended 400 mcg of folate per day. Because of the critical role of folate in preventing heart disease, some experts also recommend a daily vitamin B complex that includes 400 mcg of folate.

Benefits of Foods

Even though you may consider taking some supplements, fruits and vegetables are the richest sources of antioxidants and phytochemicals. Researchers at the U. S. Department of Agriculture compared the antioxidant effects of vitamins C and E with those of various common fruits and vegetables. The results indicated that three-fourths cup of cooked kale (which contains only 11 IU of vitamin E and 76 mg of vitamin C) neutralized as many free radicals as approximately 800 IU of vitamin E or 600 mg of vitamin C supplements. Other excellent sources of antioxidants found by these researchers include blueberries, strawberries, spinach, Brussels sprouts, plums, broccoli, beets, oranges, and grapes.

Many people who eat unhealthy diets think they need supplementation to balance their diet. This is fallacy about nutrition. The problem here is not necessarily a lack of vitamins and minerals, but a diet too high in calories, saturated fat, and sodium. Vitamin, mineral, and fiber supplements do not supply all of the nutrients and other beneficial substances present in food and needed for good health.

Wholesome foods contain vitamins, minerals, carbohydrates, fiber, proteins, fats, phytochemicals, and other substances not yet discovered. Researchers do not know if the protective effects are caused by the antioxidants alone, or in combination with other nutrients (such as phytochemicals), or by some other nutrients in food that have not been investigated yet. Many nutrients work in synergy, enhancing chemical processes in the body.

Supplementation will not offset poor eating habits. Pills are no substitute for common sense. If you think your diet is not balanced, you first need to conduct a nutrient analysis (see Activity 5.1 on page 125) to determine which nutrients you lack in sufficient amounts. Eat more of them, as well as foods that are high in antioxidants and phytochemicals. After you perform a nutrient assessment, a **registered dietitian** can help you decide what supplement(s), if any, might be necessary.

If you take supplements in pill form, look for products that meet the USP (U. S. Pharmacopoeia) disintegration standards on the bottle. The USP symbol suggests that the supplement should completely dissolve in 45 minutes or less. Supplements that do not dissolve, of course, cannot get into the bloodstream.

Critical Thinking

Do you take supplements? If so, for what purposes are you taking them—and do you think you could restructure your diet so you could do without them?

Eating Disorders

Eating disorders are medical illnesses that involve critical disturbances in eating behaviors thought to stem from some combination of environmental pressures. These disorders are characterized by an intense fear of becoming fat, which does not disappear even after the individual has lost extreme amounts of weight. The two most common types of eating disorders are **anorexia nervosa** and **bulimia nervosa**, although **binge-eating**, also known as compulsive overeating, is recognized as an eating disorder as well.

Most people who have eating disorders are afflicted by significant family and social problems. They may lack fulfillment in many areas of their lives. The eating disorder then becomes the coping mechanism to avoid dealing with these problems. Taking control over their own body weight helps them feel that they are restoring some sense of control over their lives.

Anorexia nervosa and bulimia nervosa are common in industrialized nations where society encourages low-calorie diets and thinness. Although frequently seen in

---

KEY TERMS

Synergy   A reaction in which the result is greater than the sum of its two parts.

Registered dietitian (RD)   A person with a college degree in dietetics who meets all certification and continuing education requirements of the American Dietetic Association or Dietitians of Canada.

Anorexia nervosa   An eating disorder characterized by self-imposed starvation to lose and then maintain very low body weight.

Bulimia nervosa   An eating disorder characterized by a pattern of binge eating and purging.

Binge-eating disorder   An eating disorder characterized by uncontrollable episodes of eating excessive amounts of food within a relatively short time.

young women, the majority seeking treatment are between the ages of 25 and 50. Surveys, nonetheless, indicate that as many as 40 percent of college-age women are struggling with an eating disorder.

Eating disorders are not limited to women. Every one in 10 cases exists in men. But because the role of men in society and their body image are viewed differently, these cases often go unreported.

Individuals who have clinical depression and obsessive compulsive behavior are more susceptible. About half of all people with eating disorders have some sort of chemical dependency (alcohol and drugs), and a majority of them come from families with alcohol and drug-related problems. Of reported cases of eating disorders, a large number are individuals who are, or have been, victims of sexual molestation.

Eating disorders develop in stages. Typically, individuals who are already dealing with significant issues in life start a diet. At first they feel in control and are happy about the weight loss even if they are not overweight. Encouraged by the prospect of weight loss and the control they can exert over their own weight, the individual takes dieting to an extreme and often combines it with exhaustive exercise and the overuse of laxatives and diuretics.

Although a genetic predisposition may contribute, most cases are environmentally related. The syndrome typically emerges following emotional issues or a stressful life event and the uncertainty about the ability to cope efficiently. Life experiences that can trigger the syndrome might be gaining weight, starting the menstrual period, beginning college, losing a boyfriend, having poor self-esteem, being socially rejected, starting a professional career, or becoming a wife or a mother.

The eating disorder now takes on a life of its own and becomes the primary focus of attention for the individuals afflicted with it. Their self-worth revolves around what the scale reads every day, their relationship with food, and their perception of how they look each day.

Anorexia Nervosa

An estimated 1 percent of the population in the United States is anorexic. Anorexic individuals seem to fear weight gain more than death from starvation. Furthermore, they have a distorted image of their body and think of themselves as being fat, even when they are emaciated.

Anorexics commonly develop obsessive and compulsive behaviors and emphatically deny their condition. They are preoccupied with food, meal planning, and grocery shopping, and they have unusual eating habits. As they lose weight and their health begins to deteriorate, anorexics feel weak and tired. They might

realize they have a problem, but they will not stop the starvation and refuse to consider the behavior abnormal.

Once they have lost a lot of weight and malnutrition sets in, physical changes become more visible. Typical changes are **amenorrhea** (stopping menstruation), digestive problems, extreme sensitivity to cold, hair and skin problems, fluid and electrolyte abnormalities (which may lead to an irregular heartbeat and sudden stopping of the heart), injuries to nerves and tendons, abnormalities of immune function, anemia, growth of fine body hair, mental confusion, inability to concentrate, lethargy, depression, dry skin, lower skin and body temperature, and osteoporosis.

Diagnostic criteria for anorexia nervosa are:[7]

- Refusal to maintain body weight over a minimal normal weight for age and height (weight loss leading to maintenance of body weight less than 85 percent of that expected or failure to make expected weight gain during periods of growth, leading to body weight less than 85 percent of that expected).
- Intense fear of gaining weight or becoming fat, even though underweight.
- Disturbance in the way in which one's body weight, size, or shape is perceived; undue influences of body weight or shape on self-evaluation; or denial of the seriousness of the current low body weight.
- In postmenarcheal females, amenorrhea (absence of at least three consecutive menstrual cycles). (A woman is considered to have amenorrhea if her periods occur only following estrogen therapy.)

Many of the changes induced by anorexia nervosa can be reversed. Individuals with this condition can get better with professional therapy, turn to bulimia nervosa, or they may die from the disorder. Twenty percent of anorexics die as a result of their condition. Anorexia nervosa has the highest mortality rate of all psychosomatic illnesses today. The disorder, however, is 100 percent curable. But treatment almost always requires professional help, and the sooner it is started, the better the chances for reversibility and cure.

Therapy consists of a combination of medical and psychological techniques to restore proper nutrition, prevent medical complications, and modify the environment or events that triggered the syndrome.

Seldom can anorexics overcome the problem by themselves. They strongly deny their condition. They are able to hide it and deceive friends and relatives. Based on their behavior, many of them meet all of the characteristics of anorexia nervosa, but it goes undetected because both thinness and dieting are socially acceptable. Only a well-trained clinician is able to diagnose anorexia nervosa.

Bulimia Nervosa

Bulimia nervosa is more prevalent than anorexia nervosa. As many as one in every five women on college campuses may be bulimic, according to some estimates. Bulimia nervosa also is more prevalent than anorexia nervosa in males, although bulimia is still much more prevalent in females.

Bulimics usually are healthy-looking people, well-educated, and near recommended body weight. They seem to enjoy food and often socialize around it. In actuality, they are emotionally insecure, rely on others, and lack self-confidence and self-esteem. Recommended weight and food are important to them.

The binge–purge cycle usually occurs in stages. As a result of stressful life events or the simple compulsion to eat, bulimics engage periodically in binge eating that may last an hour or longer.

With some apprehension, bulimics anticipate and plan the cycle. Next they feel an urgency to begin, followed by large and uncontrollable food consumption, during which they may eat several thousand calories (up to 10,000 calories in extreme cases). After a short period of relief and satisfaction, feelings of deep guilt, shame, and intense fear of gaining weight ensue. Purging seems to be an easy answer, as the bingeing cycle can continue without fear of gaining weight.

The diagnostic criteria for bulimia nervosa are:[8]

- Recurrent episodes of binge eating. An episode of binge eating is characterized by both of the following:
  — Eating in a discrete period of time (for example, within any 2-hour period), an amount of food that is definitely more than most people would eat during a similar period and under similar circumstances.
  — A sense of lack of control over eating during the episode (a feeling that one cannot stop eating or control what or how much one is eating).
- Recurring inappropriate compensatory behaviors to prevent weight gain, such as self-induced vomiting; misuse of laxatives, diuretics, enemas, or other medications; fasting; or excessive exercise.
- The binge eating and inappropriate compensatory behaviors both occur, on average, at least twice a week for 3 months.
- Self-evaluation is unduly influenced by body shape and weight.

The most typical form of purging is self-induced vomiting. Bulimics, too, frequently ingest strong laxatives and emetics. Near-fasting diets and strenuous bouts of exercise are common. Medical problems associated with bulimia nervosa include cardiac arrhythmias, amenorrhea, kidney and bladder damage, ulcers, colitis, tearing of the esophagus or stomach, tooth erosion, gum damage, and general muscular weakness.

Unlike anorexics, bulimics realize their behavior is abnormal and feel great shame about it. Fearing social rejection, they pursue the binge–purge cycle in secrecy and at unusual hours of the day.

Bulimia nervosa can be treated successfully when the person realizes that this destructive behavior is not the solution to life's problems. A change in attitude can prevent permanent damage or death.

Binge-Eating Disorder

Binge-eating disorder is probably the most common of the three eating disorders. About 2 percent of American adults are afflicted with binge-eating disorder in a 6-month period. Although most people think they overeat from time to time, eating more than one should now and then does not mean the individual has a binge-eating disorder. The disorder is slightly more common in women than in men; three women for every two men have the disorder.

Binge-eating disorder is characterized by uncontrollable episodes of eating excessive amounts of food within a relatively short time. The causes of binge-eating disorder are unknown, although depression, anger, sadness, boredom, and worry can trigger an episode. Unlike bulimics, binge eaters do not purge; thus, most people with this disorder are either overweight or obese. Typical symptoms of binge-eating disorder include:

- Eating what most people think is an unusually large amount of food
- Eating until uncomfortably full
- Eating out of control
- Eating much faster than usual during binge episodes
- Eating alone because of embarrassment of how much food is being consumed
- Feeling disgusted, depressed, or guilty after overeating

Treatment

Treatment for eating disorders is available on most school campuses through the school's counseling center or the health center. Local hospitals also offer treatment for these conditions. Many communities have support groups, frequently led by professional personnel and often free of charge. All information and the identity of the individual are kept confidential so the person need

KEY TERMS

Amenorrhea Cessation of regular menstrual flow.

not fear embarrassment or repercussion when seeking professional help.

2005 Dietary Guidelines for Americans

The 2005 Dietary Guidelines for Americans (Figure 5.5) provide science-based advice to promote health and to reduce risk for major chronic diseases through diet and physical activity. The recommendations are to the general public age 2 years and older and based on the preponderance of scientific and medical knowledge that is current at the time of publication of the committee's report. The extensive review of the evidence has led to the development of the following recommendations:[9]

1. Consume a variety of foods within and among the basic food groups while staying within energy needs.
2. Control calorie intake to manage body weight.
3. Be physically active every day.
4. Increase daily intake of fruits and vegetables, whole grains, and non-fat or low-fat milk and milk products.
5. Choose fats wisely for good health.
6. Choose carbohydrates wisely for good health.
7. Choose and prepare foods with little salt.
8. If you drink alcoholic beverages, do so in moderation.
9. Keep food safe to eat.
10. Clean hands, contact surfaces, and fruits and vegetables. (This does not apply to meat and poultry, which should not be washed.)
11. Separate raw, cooked, and ready-to-eat foods while shopping, preparing, or storing.
12. Cook foods to a safe temperature.
13. Chill (refrigerate) perishable foods promptly.
14. Avoid higher-risk foods (e.g., deli meats and frankfurters that have not been reheated to a safe temperature and may therefore contain *Listeria* bacteria).

Additional information on these guidelines are posted at www.health.gov/dietaryguidelines.

A Lifetime Commitment to Wellness

Proper nutrition, a sound exercise program, and quitting smoking (for those who smoke) are the three factors that do the most for health, longevity, and quality of life. Achieving and maintaining a balanced diet is not as difficult as most people would think. The difficult part for most people is retraining themselves to follow a lifetime healthy nutrition plan; that is, one that:

● Emphasizes fruits, vegetables, whole grains, and fat-free or low-fat milk and milk products.

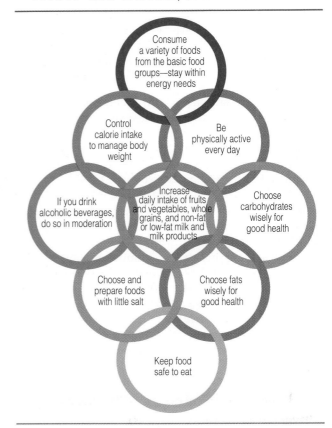

FIGURE **5.5** 2005 Dietary Guidelines for Americans.

● Includes lean meats, poultry, fish, beans, eggs, and nuts (in moderation).
● Is low in saturated fats, trans fatty acids, cholesterol, salt (sodium), and added sugars.

A well-balanced diet contains a variety of foods from all food groups, including wise selection of foods from animal sources. No single food can provide all the necessary nutrients and other beneficial substances in the amounts the body needs. For good nutrition, you should meet the recommended daily amounts of food from the different food groups in MyPyramid. Within each food group, choose a variety of foods. Food items vary, and each item provides different combinations of nutrients and other substances needed for good health.

CT Critical Thinking

What factors in your life and the environment have contributed to your current dietary habits? Do you need to make changes? What may prevent you from doing so?

In spite of ample scientific evidence linking poor dietary habits to early disease and mortality rates, many people are not willing to change their eating patterns. Even when faced with obesity, elevated blood lipids, hypertension, and other nutrition-related conditions, many people do not change. They remain in the precontemplation stage of change (see the discussion of behavior modification in Chapter 1).

The motivating factor to change one's eating habits seems to be a major health breakdown, such as a heart attack, a stroke, or cancer. An ounce of prevention is worth a pound of cure. The sooner you implement the dietary guidelines presented in this chapter, the better will be your chances of preventing chronic diseases and reaching a higher state of wellness.

The Mayo Clinic Web Site. This very informative site will show you how to balance your dietary intake with your physical activity to maintain healthy weight. To find your healthy weight, go to Program & Tools and click Healthy Weight. You provide personal information regarding your age, gender, height, weight, and activity level and the Mayo Clinic provides you with a healthy diet plan to meet your goals. It's fun and educational.
http://www.mayoclinic.com

The Nutrition Analysis Web Site. This interactive site allows you to enter a variety of foods to receive a complete nutritional review of your diet based on the Recommended Dietary Allowances for your age and gender.
http://nat.crgq.com

ASSESS YOUR KNOWLEDGE

Evaluate how well you understand the concepts presented in this chapter using the Assess Your Knowledge and Practice Quizzes options on your Profile Plus CD-ROM.

1. The science of nutrition studies the relationship of
   a. vitamins and minerals to health.
   b. foods to optimal health and performance.
   c. carbohydrates, fats, and proteins to the development and maintenance of good health.
   d. the macronutrients and micronutrients to physical performance.
   e. kilocalories to calories in food items.

2. Faulty nutrition often plays a crucial role in the development and progression of which disease?
   a. cardiovascular disease
   b. cancer
   c. osteoporosis
   d. diabetes
   e. All are correct choices.

3. According to MyPyramid, daily vegetable consumption is measured in
   a. servings.
   b. ounces.
   c. cups.
   d. calories.
   e. All of the above are correct.

4. The daily recommended amount of fiber intake for adults 50 years and younger is
   a. 10 grams per day for women and 12 grams for men.
   b. 21 grams per day for women and 30 grams for men.
   c. 28 grams per day for women and 35 grams for men.
   d. 25 grams per day for women and 38 grams for men.
   e. 45 grams per day for women and 50 grams for men.

5. Unhealthy fats include
   a. unsaturated fatty acids.
   b. monounsaturated fats.
   c. polyunsaturated fatty acids.
   d. saturated fats.
   e. alpha-linolenic acid.

6. The daily recommended carbohydrate intake is
   a. 45 to 65 percent of the total calories.
   b. 10 to 35 percent of the total calories.
   c. 20 to 35 percent of the total calories.
   d. 60 to 75 percent of the total calories.
   e. 35 to 50 percent of the total calories.

7. The amount of a nutrient that is estimated to meet the nutrient requirement of half the healthy people in specific age and gender groups is known as the
   a. Estimated Average Requirement.
   b. Recommended Dietary Allowance.
   c. Daily Value.
   d. Adequate Intake.
   e. Dietary Reference Intake.

8. The percent fat intake for an individual who on a given day consumes 2,385 calories with 106 grams of fat is
   a. 44 percent of total calories.
   b. 17.7 percent of total calories.
   c. 40 percent of total calories.
   d. 31 percent of total calories.
   e. 22.5 percent of total calories.

9. Treatment of anorexia nervosa
   a. almost always requires professional help.
   b. is often accomplished in the home.
   c. is most successful when friends take the initiative to help.
   d. requires that the individual be placed in the environment where the disorder started.
   e. is best done under the supervision of a physician.

10. Which of the following is *not* a goal of the 2005 Dietary Guidelines for Americans?
   a. Increase daily intake of fruits and vegetables, whole grains, and non-fat or low-fat milk and milk products.
   b. Be physically active each day.
   c. Choose carbohydrates wisely for good health.
   d. Control calorie intake to manage body weight.
   e. All are correct choices.

Correct answers can be found on page 261.

Nutrient Analysis

Name   Date

Course   Section

Age   Weight   Height   Gender   M   F   (Pregnant—P, Nursing—N)

Activity Rating for computer
software use (check one):

○ Sedentary
○ Lightly active
○ Moderately active
○ Very active
○ Extremely active

No.	Food	Amount	Calories*	Grains	Vegetables	Fruits	Milk	Meat and Beans
								Food Groups
1								
2								
3								
4								
5								
6								
7								
8								
9								
10								
11								
12								
13								
14								
15								
16								
17								
18								
19								
20								
21								
22								
23								
24								
25								
26								
27								
28								
29								
30								
Totals								
Recommended amounts***			**	6–11	3–5	2–4	2–3	2–3
Deficiencies								

* See list of nutritive value of selected foods in Appendix E.

** Determine your estimated energy requirement (EER) using Table 6.1, page 137.

*** Use Figure 5.4 to determine the recommended amounts based on your EER or go to http://mypyramid.gov/

Nutrient Analysis

Name _____   Date _____

Course _____   Section _____

Age _____ Weight _____ Height _____   Gender   M   F   (Pregnant—P, Nursing—N)

Activity Rating for computer software use (check one):

○ Sedentary
○ Lightly active
○ Moderately active
○ Very active
○ Extremely active

No.	Food	Amount	Calories*	Grains	Vegetables	Fruits	Milk	Meat and Beans
1								
2								
3								
4								
5								
6								
7								
8								
9								
10								
11								
12								
13								
14								
15								
16								
17								
18								
19								
20								
21								
22								
23								
24								
25								
26								
27								
28								
29								
30								
Totals								
Recommended amounts***			**	6–11	3–5	2–4	2–3	2–3
Deficiencies								

Food Groups

* See list of nutritive value of selected foods in Appendix E.
** Determine your estimated energy requirement (EER) using Table 6.1, page 137.
*** Use Figure 5.4 to determine the recommended amounts based on your EER or go to http://mypyramid.gov/

CHAPTER 6

Weight Management

OBJECTIVES

- Recognize myths and fallacies regarding weight management.
- Understand the physiology of weight control.
- Become familiar with the effects of diet and exercise on resting metabolic rate.
- Recognize the role of a lifetime exercise program in a successful weight management program.
- Learn to write and implement weight reduction and weight maintenance programs.
- Identify behavior modification techniques that help a person adhere to a lifetime weight maintenance program.

Chronicle your daily activities using the exercise log on your CD-ROM.

A good physical fitness program will include achieving and maintaining recommended body weight as a major objective. Two terms commonly used with reference to the condition of weighing more than recommended are **overweight** and **obesity**. Obesity levels are established at a point at which excess body fat can lead to significant health problems.

Obesity is a health hazard of epidemic proportions in most developed countries around the world. According to the World Health Organization, an estimated 35 percent of the adult population in industrialized nations is obese. Obesity has been established at a Body Mass Index (BMI) of 30 or higher.

In the United States, 63 percent of men and 55 percent of women are overweight (BMI greater than 25), and 21 percent of men and 27 percent of women are obese.[1] An estimated 97 million people are overweight and 30 million are obese. Between 1960 and 2000, the overall (men and women combined) prevalence of adult obesity increased from about 13 percent to 24 percent. Most of this increase occurred in the 1990s. The prevalence of obesity is even higher in ethnic groups, especially African Americans and Hispanic Americans.

As illustrated in Figure 6.1, the U. S. obesity epidemic continues to escalate. In 1990, not a single state reported an obesity rate above 20 percent of the state's total population. By the year 2004, 33 states had an obesity rate between 20 and 24 percent; and nine states had reached a rate above 25 percent.

FIGURE **6.1** Incidence of obesity in the United States (based on BMI > 30 or 30 pounds overweight), 1990 and 2004.

Percentages of the total number of people in the respective state who are obese.

○ No data   ● 10%–14%   ● 20–24%
● <10%   ● 15%–19%   ● ≥25%

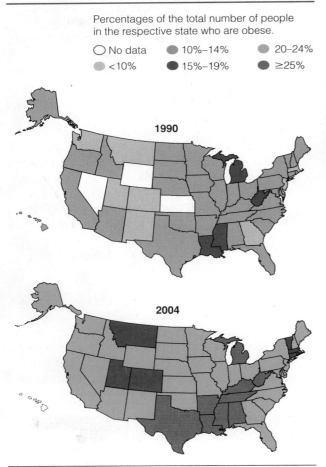

Source: *Obesity Trends Among U. S. Adults Between 1985 and 2004* (Atlanta: Centers for Disease Control and Prevention, 2004).

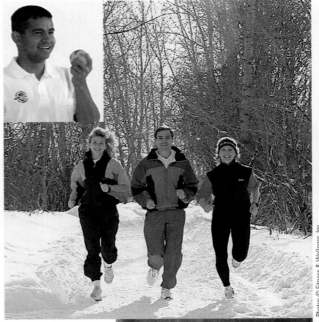

Achieving and maintaining a high physical fitness percent body fat requires a lifetime commitment to regular physical activity, exercise, and proper nutrition.

Most of the blame for the alarming increase in obesity lies in the amount of food we eat and our lack of physical activity. According to the U. S. Department of Agriculture, the average daily caloric intake in the United States increased from 3,100 calories per person in the 1960s to 3,700 calories in the 1990s. Further, as the nation continues to evolve into a more mechanized and automated society (relying on escalators, elevators, remote controls, computers, electronic mail, cell phones, automatic-sensor doors), the amount of required daily physical activity continues to decrease. We are being lulled into a high-risk, sedentary lifestyle.

About 44 percent of all women and 29 percent of all men are on a diet at any given moment. People spend about $40 billion yearly attempting to lose weight. More than $10 billion goes to memberships in weight reduction centers and another $30 billion to diet food sales.

Furthermore, according to the National Institutes of Health, the total cost attributable to obesity-related disease is approximately $100 billion per year.

As the second leading cause of preventable death in the United States, excessive body weight and physical inactivity cause more than 112,000 deaths each year.[2] Furthermore, obesity is more prevalent than smoking (19 percent), poverty (14 percent), and problem drinking (6 percent).[3] Obesity and unhealthy lifestyle habits are the most critical public health problems that we face in the 21st century.

The American Heart Association has identified obesity as one of the six major risk factors for coronary heart disease. Obesity is associated with poor health status and is a risk factor for hypertension, congestive heart failure, high blood lipids, atherosclerosis, stroke, thromboembolitic disease, varicose veins, type 2 diabetes, osteoarthritis, gallbladder disease, sleep apnea, asthma, ruptured intervertebral disks, and arthritis. Estimates also indicate that 14 percent of all cancer deaths in men and 20 percent in women are related to current overweight and obesity patterns in the United States.[4] Furthermore, obesity is implicated in psychological maladjustment and a higher accidental death rate. Extremely obese people have worse mental health related to quality of life.

A primary objective of overall physical fitness and enhanced quality of life is to attain recommended body composition. Individuals at recommended body weight are able to participate in a wide variety of moderate to vigorous activities without functional limitations. These people have the freedom to enjoy most of life's recreational activities and reach their fullest potential. Excessive body weight does not afford an individual the fitness level to enjoy vigorous lifetime activities such as basketball, soccer, racquetball, surfing, mountain cycling, and mountain climbing. Maintaining high fitness and recommended body weight gives a person a degree of independence throughout life that the majority of people in developed nations no longer enjoy.

Critical Thinking

Do you consider yourself overweight? If so, how long have you had a weight problem, what attempts have you made to lose weight, and what has worked best for you?

Tolerable Weight

Many people want to lose weight so they will look better. That's a noteworthy goal. The problem, however, is that they often have a distorted image of what they would really look like if they were to reduce to what they think is their ideal weight. Hereditary factors play a big role, and only a small fraction of the population has the genes for a "perfect body." **Tolerable weight** is a more realistic goal. This is a realistic standard that is not "ideal" but is "acceptable." It is likely to be closer to the health-fitness standard than the physical-fitness standard for many people.

The media have a great influence on people's perception of what constitutes ideal body weight. Most people rely on fashion, fitness, and beauty magazines to determine what they should look like. The "ideal" body shapes, physiques, and proportions shown in these magazines are rare and are achieved through airbrushing and

medical reconstruction.[5] Many individuals, primarily young women, go to extremes in an attempt to achieve these unrealistic body shapes. Failure to attain a "perfect body" often leads to eating disorders.

When people set their own target weight, they should be realistic. Attaining the "high physical fitness" percent body fat standard shown in Table 2.12 (page 44) is extremely difficult for some. It is even more difficult to maintain, unless the person makes a commitment to a vigorous lifetime exercise program and permanent dietary changes. Few people are willing to do that. The "Moderate" percent body fat category is more realistic for many people.

A question you should ask yourself is: Am I happy with my weight? Part of enjoying a higher quality of life is being happy with yourself. If you are not, you either need to do something about it or learn to live with it.

If your percent of body fat is higher than the health-fitness standard shown in Table 2.12, page 44 (or a BMI above 25), you should try to reach and stay in this category, for health reasons. This is the category that seems to pose no detriment to health.

If you have achieved the health-fitness standard but would like to be more fit, ask yourself a second question: How badly do I want it? Enough to implement lifetime exercise and dietary changes? If you are not willing to change, you should stop worrying about your weight and deem the health-fitness standard tolerable for you.

Fad Dieting

Only about 10 percent of all people who begin a traditional weight loss program (without exercise) are able to lose the desired weight. Worse, less than 5 percent of this group is able to keep the weight off for a significant time. Traditional diets have failed in helping people keep the weight off because few diet programs incorporate lifetime changes in food selection and overall increases in daily physical activity and exercise as the keys to successful weight loss and maintenance.

Fad diets continue to deceive people. Capitalizing on hopes that the latest diet to hit the market will really work this time, fad diets continue to appeal to people of

KEY TERMS

Overweight Excess body weight when compared to a given standard such as height or recommended percent body fat.

Obesity A chronic disease characterized by an excessively high amount of body fat (about 20 percent above recommended weight or a BMI at 30 or above).

Tolerable weight A realistic body weight that is close to the health fitness percent body fat standard.

How to Recognize Fad Diets

Fad diets have characteristics in common. These diets typically

- are nutritionally unbalanced.
- are based on testimonials.
- were developed according to "confidential research."
- promote rapid and "painless" weight loss.
- promise miraculous results.
- restrict food selection.
- require the use of selected products.
- use liquid formulas instead of foods.
- misrepresent salespeople as individuals qualified to provide nutrition counseling.
- fail to provide information on risks associated with weight loss and use of the diet.
- do not involve physical activity.
- do not encourage healthy behavioral changes.
- are not supported by the scientific community or national health organizations.
- fail to provide information for weight maintenance upon completion of diet phase.

FIGURE **6.2** Effects of three forms of diet on fat loss.

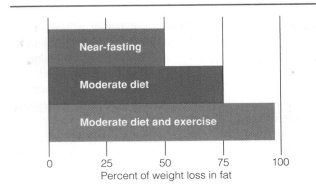

Adapted from *Alive Man: The Physiology of Physical Activity* by R. J. Shephard (Springfield, IL: Charles C. Thomas, 1975): 484–488.

all shapes and sizes. These diets may work for a while, but their success is usually short-lived. Most of these diets are low in calories and deprive the body of certain nutrients, generating a metabolic imbalance that in extreme cases may result in death. With these diets a lot of the weight lost is in the form of water and protein, not fat.

On a crash diet, close to half of the weight loss is in lean (protein) tissue (see Figure 6.2). When the body uses protein instead of a combination of fats and carbohydrates as a source of energy, the individual loses weight as much as 10 times faster. This is because a gram of protein produces less than half the amount of energy than fat does. In the case of muscle protein, one-fifth of protein is mixed with four-fifths of water. Each pound of muscle yields only one-tenth the amount of energy as a pound of fat. As a result, most of the weight loss is in the form of water, which on the scale, of course, looks good.

Among the popular diets on the market in recent years are the low-carbohydrate/high protein (LCHP) diet plans. Although variations exist among them, in general, "low-carb" diets limit the intake of carbohydrate-rich foods. Examples of these diets are the Atkins Diet, The Zone, Protein Power, the Scarsdale Diet, The Carb Addict's Diet, and Sugar Busters.

Rapid weight loss occurs during LCHP diets because the low carbohydrate intake forces the liver to produce glucose. The source for most of this glucose is body proteins. As mentioned, protein is mostly water; thus, weight is lost rapidly. When a person terminates the diet, the body rebuilds some of the protein tissue and the person quickly regains some weight.

Two studies in the *New England Journal of Medicine* indicated that individuals on a LCHP diet for 6 months lost about twice as much weight as those on a low-fat diet.[6] After a year, however, participants in the LCHP diet had regained more weight than those on the low-fat diet plan.

Years of research will be required to determine the extent to which long-term adherence to LCHP diets increases the risk for heart disease, cancer, and kidney or bone damage. LCHP diets are contrary to the nutrition advice of most national leading health organizations (which recommend a diet low in animal fat and saturated fat and high in complex carbohydrates). Without fruits, vegetables, and whole grains, high-protein diets lack many vitamins, minerals, phytochemicals, and fiber—all dietary factors that protect against an array of ailments and diseases.

The major risk associated with long-term adherence to LCHP diets might be the increased risk of heart disease, because high-protein foods are also high in fat content. Low-carbohydrate intake also produces loss of vitamin B, calcium, and potassium. Side effects commonly associated with these diets are weakness, nausea, bad breath, constipation, irritability, lightheadedness, and fatigue. Potential bone loss can further accentuate the risk for osteoporosis. Long-term adherence to an LCHP diet also can increase the risk for cancer. If you choose to go on an LCHP diet for longer than a few weeks, let your physician know so that he or she may

Are Low-Carb/High-Protein Diets More Effective?

A few studies suggest that, at least over the short term, low-carb/high-protein (LCHP) diets are more effective than carbohydrate-based diets in producing weight loss. These results are preliminary and controversial. In LCHP diets,

- much of the weight loss is water and muscle protein, not body fat. Some of this weight is regained quickly upon resuming regular dietary habits.

- few people are able to stay on the diet for more than a few weeks at a time. Most stop dieting before achieving their target weight.

- participants are rarely found on a national weight-loss registry of people who have lost 30 pounds and kept off the weight for a minimum of 6 years.

- food choices are severely restricted. With less variety available, individuals tend to eat less (800–1,200 calories/day) and thus lose more weight.

- the allowed foods may promote heart disease, cancer, and increase the risk of osteoporosis.

- the allowed foods are fundamentally high in fat (about 60 percent fat calories).

- the food program carries high risks for people with diabetes, high blood pressure, heart disease, or kidney disease.

- participants are given no information about long-term healthy eating patterns.

monitor your blood lipids, bone density, and kidney function.

Some diets allow only certain specialized foods. If people would realize that no "magic" foods provide all the necessary nutrients, that a person has to eat a variety of foods to be well nourished, the diet industry would not be as successful. Most of these diets create a nutritional deficiency, which can be detrimental to health. Some people eventually get tired of eating the same thing day in and day out and start eating less—which results in weight loss. If they achieve the lower weight without making permanent dietary changes, however, they gain back the weight quickly if they return to their old eating habits.

A few diets recommend exercise along with caloric restrictions—the best method for weight reduction, of course. People who adhere to these programs will succeed, so the diet has achieved its purpose. Unfortunately, if the people do not change their food selection and activity level permanently, they gain back the weight once they discontinue dieting and exercise.

Principles of Weight Management

Only a few years ago, the principles governing a weight loss and maintenance program seemed to be fairly clear. Now we realize that the final answers are not in yet. Traditional concepts related to weight control have centered on three assumptions:

1. Balancing food intake against output allows a person to achieve recommended weight.
2. Fat people just eat too much.
3. The human body doesn't care how much (or little) fat is stored.

Although these statements contain some truth, they still are open to much debate and research. We now know that the causes of obesity are complex and combine genetic, behavior, and lifestyle factors.

Energy-Balancing Equation

In keeping with the **energy-balancing equation**, if caloric intake exceeds output, the person gains weight; when caloric output is more than intake, the individual loses weight. Each pound of fat equals 3,500 calories. Therefore, theoretically, to increase body fat (weight) by 1 pound, a person would have to consume an excess of 3,500 calories. Equally, to lose 1 pound, the individual would have to decrease caloric intake by 3,500 calories. This principle seems straightforward, but the human body is not quite that simple.

The genetic instinct to survive tells the body that fat storage is vital, and, therefore, the **setpoint** sets an acceptable fat level for each person. This setpoint remains somewhat constant or may climb gradually because of poor lifestyle habits.

Diet and Metabolism

Under strict calorie reduction (fewer than 800 calories per day), the body makes compensatory metabolic adjustments in an effort to maintain its fat storage. The **basal metabolic rate (BMR)** may drop dramatically against a consistent negative caloric balance, and the

K E Y   T E R M S

Energy-balancing equation A body weight formula stating that when caloric intake equals caloric output, weight remains unchanged.

Setpoint Body weight and body fat percentage unique to each person that is regulated by genetic and environmental factors.

Basal metabolic rate (BMR) Lowest level of caloric intake necessary to sustain life.

© 2001 PhotoDisc, Inc.

A wide variety of foods is required to maintain a well-nourished body.

person may be on a plateau for days or even weeks without losing much weight. When the dieter goes back to the normal or even below-normal caloric intake, at which the weight may have been stable for a long time, he or she quickly regains the fat lost as the body strives to restore a comfortable fat level.

These findings were substantiated by research conducted at Rockefeller University in New York,[7] which showed that the body resists maintaining altered weight. Obese and lifetime nonobese individuals were used in the investigation. Following a 10 percent weight loss, in an attempt to regain the lost weight, the body compensated by burning up to 15 percent fewer calories than expected for the new reduced weight (after accounting for the 10 percent loss). The effects were similar in the obese and nonobese participants. These results imply that after a 10 percent weight loss, a person would have to eat less or exercise more to account for the estimated deficit of about 200 to 300 daily calories.

In this same study, when the participants were allowed to increase their weight to 10 percent above their "normal" body weight (pre-weight loss), the body burned 10 percent to 15 percent more calories than expected. This indicates an attempt by the body to waste energy and return to the preset weight. The study provides another indication that the body is highly resistant to weight changes unless the person incorporates additional lifestyle changes to ensure successful weight management. (Methods to manage weight will be discussed later in this chapter.)

This research shows why most dieters regain the weight they lose through dietary means alone. Let's use

a practical illustration: Jim would like to lose some body fat and assumes that he has reached a stable body weight at an average daily caloric intake of 2,500 calories (no weight gain or loss at this daily intake). In an attempt to lose weight rapidly, he now goes on a strict low-calorie diet (or, even worse, a near-fasting diet). Immediately the body activates its survival mechanism and readjusts its metabolism to a lower caloric balance.

After a few weeks of dieting at under 800 calories per day, the body now can maintain its normal functions at 2,000 calories per day. Having lost the desired weight, Jim terminates the diet but realizes the original intake of 2,500 calories per day will have to be lower to maintain the new lower weight. To adjust to the new lower body weight, he restricts his intake to about 2,200 calories per day. Jim is surprised to find that even at this lower daily intake (300 fewer calories), his weight comes back at a rate of about 1 pound every 2 to 3 weeks. After the diet ends, this new lowered metabolic rate may take several months to kick back up to its normal level.

From this explanation, individuals clearly should not go on very low-calorie diets. Doing so will decrease the resting metabolic rate and also will deprive the body of basic daily nutrients required for normal function. Very low-calorie diets should be used only in conjunction with dietary supplements and under proper medical supervision.[8] Furthermore, research indicates that people who go on very low-calorie diets are not as effective in keeping the weight off once they terminate the diet.

Under no circumstances should a person go on a diet that calls for below 1,200 and 1,500 calories, respectively, for women and men. Weight (fat) is gained over months and years, not overnight. Equally, weight loss should be gradual, not abrupt. A daily caloric intake of 1,200 to 1,500 calories provides the necessary nutrients if properly distributed over the various food groups (meeting the minimum daily required servings from each group). Of course, the individual has to learn which foods meet the requirements and yet are low in fat, sugar, and calories.

Furthermore, when a person tries to lose weight by dietary restrictions alone, **lean body mass** (muscle protein, along with vital organ protein) decreases. The amount of lean body mass lost depends entirely on the caloric limitation. When a person goes on a near-fasting diet, up to half of the weight lost can be lean body mass and the other half, actual fat loss. If the diet is combined with exercise, close to 100 percent of the weight loss is in the form of fat, and lean tissue actually may increase (see Figure 6.2, page 130). Loss of lean body mass is not good, because it weakens the organs and muscles and slows the metabolism.

Reduction in lean body mass is common in people on severely restricted diets. No diet with caloric intakes below 1,200 to 1,500 calories will prevent loss of lean body mass. Even at this intake level, some loss is inevitable unless the diet is combined with exercise. Although many diets claim they do not alter the lean component, the simple truth is that, regardless of what nutrients may be added to the diet, caloric restrictions always prompt a loss of lean tissue.

Too many people go on low-calorie diets again and again. Every time they do, the metabolic rate slows as more lean tissue is lost. People in their 40s and older who weigh the same as they did when they were 20 often think they are at recommended body weight. During this span of 20 years or more, however, they may have dieted too many times without exercising. Shortly after terminating each diet, they regain the weight, but much of that gain is in fat. Maybe at age 20 they weighed 150 pounds, of which only 15 percent was fat. Now, at age 40, even though they still weigh 150 pounds, they might be 30 percent fat (see Figure 6.3, and also Figure 2.2, page 39). At recommended body weight, they wonder why they are eating so little and still having trouble staying at that weight.

Further, data indicates that diets high in fat and refined carbohydrates, near-fasting diets, and perhaps even artificial sweeteners, keep people from losing weight and, in reality, contribute to fat gain. The only practical and sensible way to lose fat weight is to combine exercise and a sensible diet high in complex carbohydrates and low in fat and sugar.

Because of the effects of proper food management on body weight, most of the successful dieter's effort should be spent in retraining eating habits, increasing the intake of complex carbohydrates and high-fiber foods, and decreasing the consumption of refined carbohydrates (sugars) and fats. This change in eating habits will bring about a decrease in total daily caloric intake. Because 1 gram of carbohydrates provides only 4 calories, as contrasted with 9 calories per gram of fat, you could eat twice the volume of food (by weight) when substituting carbohydrates for fat. Some fat, however, is recommended in the diet—preferably, polyunsaturated and monounsaturated fats. These so-called good fats do more than help protect the heart, they help delay hunger pangs.

A "diet" cannot be viewed as a temporary tool to aid in weight loss but, instead, as a permanent change in eating behaviors to ensure weight management and better health. The role of increased physical activity also must be considered because successful weight loss and recommended body composition seldom are attainable without a moderate reduction in caloric intake combined with a regular exercise program.

FIGURE 6.3 Effects of constant dieting without exercise on body weight, percent body fat, and lean body mass.

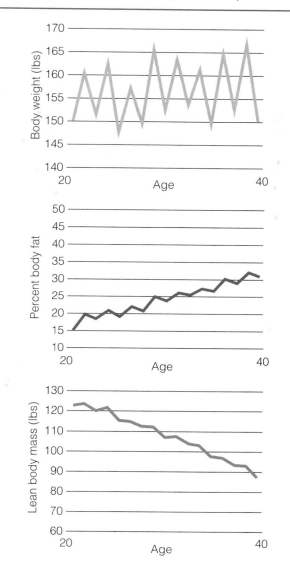

Exercise: The Key to Successful Weight Management

A more effective way to tilt the energy-balancing equation in your favor is by burning calories through physical activity. Exercise also seems to exert control over how

KEY TERMS

Lean body mass Nonfat component of the human body.

much a person weighs. If, starting at age 25, a person gains 1 pound of weight per year, this represents a simple energy surplus of under 10 calories per day (10 × 365 = 3,650). In many cases, most of the additional weight accumulated in middle age comes from people becoming less physically active and not resulting from increased caloric intake. Dr. Jack Wilmore, a leading exercise physiologist and expert weight management researcher, stated:[9]

> Physical inactivity is certainly a major, if not the primary, cause of obesity in the United States today. A certain minimal level of activity might be necessary for us to accurately balance our caloric intake to our caloric expenditure. With too little activity, we appear to lose the fine control we normally have to maintain this incredible balance. This fine balance amounts to less than 10 calories per day, or the equivalent of one potato chip.

Exercise enhances the rate of weight loss and is vital in maintaining the weight loss. Not only will exercise maintain lean tissue, but advocates of the setpoint theory say that exercise resets the fat thermostat to a new, lower level.

A few individuals can lose weight by participating in 30 minutes of exercise per day, but most people need 60 to 90 minutes of daily physical activity for proper weight management (the 30 minutes of exercise are included as part of the 60 to 90 minutes of physical activity).

Although 30 minutes of moderate-intensity activity per day provides substantial health benefits, the Institute of Medicine of the National Academy of Sciences recommends that people trying to manage their weight accumulate 60 minutes of moderate-intensity physical activity most days of the week.[10] The evidence shows that people who maintain recommended weight typically accumulate an hour or more of daily physical activity.

As illustrated in Figure 6.4, greater weight loss can be achieved by combining a diet with an exercise program. Of even greater significance, however, only the individuals who remain physically active for over 60 minutes per day are able to keep the weight off (see Figure 6.5).[11]

Further, data from the National Weight Control Registry (http://www.nwcr.ws/) indicates that individuals who have lost at least 30 pounds and kept them off for a minimum of 6 years typically accumulate 90 minutes of daily activity. Those who are less active gradually regain the lost weight. Individuals who completely stop physical activity regain almost 100 percent of the weight within 18 months of discontinuing the weight loss program (see Figure 6.5). Thus, if weight management is *not* a consideration, 30 minutes of daily activity

FIGURE **6.4** The roles of diet and exercise in weight loss.

Legend:
- Exercise (MI ≤ 30 min/day)*
- Exercise (HI = 30 min/day)
- Exercise (MI ≥ 60 min/day)
- Diet
- Diet & Exercise (MI ≥ 60 min/day)

* Exercise with no change in daily caloric intake
MI = moderate intensity
HI = high intensity
Diet: 1,200–1,500 calories/day

provides health benefits. To prevent weight gain, 60 minutes of daily activity are recommended; to maintain substantial weight loss, 90 minutes may be required.

A combination of aerobic and strength-training exercises works best in weight-loss programs. Aerobic exercise is the best to offset the setpoint, and the continuity and duration of these types of activities cause many calories to be burned in the process. Unfortunately, of those individuals who are attempting to lose weight, only 19 percent of women and 22 percent of men decrease their caloric intake and exercise above an average of 25 or more minutes per day.[12]

Strength training is critical in helping maintain lean body mass. Although the increase in BMR (basal metabolic rate) through increased muscle mass is presently being debated in the literature and merits further research, data indicate that each additional pound of muscle tissue raises the BMR in the range of 6 to 35 calories per day.[13]

To examine the effects of even a small increase in BMR on long-term body weight, let's use a low estimate of 10 calories per pound of muscle per day. For an individual who adds 3 pounds of muscle tissue as a result of strength training, the increase in BMR would be 30 calories per day (10 × 3). Such an increase would burn an additional 10,950 calories per year (30 × 365) or the equivalent of 3.1 pounds of fat (10,950 ÷ 3,500). This

FIGURE **6.5** Effects of daily energy expenditure on percent of weight regained following a weight reduction program.

- No physical activity
- Physical activity = 20 min/day
- Physical activity/exercise = 30 min/day
- Physical activity/exercise ≥ 60 min/day

Regular participation in a combined lifetime aerobic and strength-training exercise program is the key to successful weight management.

increase in BMR would more than offset the typical adult weight gain of 1 to 2 pounds per year.

This figure of 10,950 calories per year does not include the actual energy cost of the strength-training workout. If we use an energy expenditure of only 150 calories per strength-training session, done twice per week, over a year's time it would represent 15,600 calories (150 × 2 × 52) or the equivalent of another 4.5 pounds of fat (15,600 ÷ 3,500).

Although size (inches) and percent body fat both decrease when sedentary individuals begin an exercise program, body weight often remains the same or might even increase during the first couple of weeks after beginning the program. Exercise helps to increase muscle tissue, connective tissue, blood volume (as much as 500 ml, or the equivalent of 1 pound, following the first week of aerobic exercise), enzymes and other structures within the cell, and glycogen (which binds water). All of these changes lead to a higher functional capacity of the human body. With exercise, most of the weight loss becomes apparent after a few weeks of training, when the lean component has stabilized.

The Myth of Spot-Reducing

Research has revealed the fallacy of spot-reducing or losing cellulite, as some people call the fat deposits that bulge out in certain areas of the body. These deposits are nothing but enlarged fat cells from accumulated body fat. Merely doing several sets of sit-ups daily will not get rid of fat in the midsection of the body. When fat comes off, it does so throughout the entire body, not just in the exercised area. Although the greatest proportion of fat may come off the biggest fat deposits, the caloric output of a few sets of sit-ups has almost no effect on reducing total body fat. A person has to exercise much longer to really see results.

Exercise Restrictions

Dieting never has been fun and never will be. People who are overweight and are serious about losing weight will have to make exercise a regular part of their daily life, along with proper food management and a sensible cut in caloric intake. Some precautions are in order, because excessive body fat is a risk factor for cardiovascular disease. Depending on the extent of the weight problem, a medical examination and possibly a stress

ECG may be necessary before undertaking the exercise program. A physician should be consulted in this regard.

Significantly overweight individuals also may have to choose activities in which they will not have to support their own body weight but still will be effective in burning calories. Injuries to joints and muscles are common in overweight individuals who participate in weight-bearing exercises such as walking, jogging, and aerobics. Better alternatives for overweight people are riding a bicycle (either road or stationary), water aerobics, walking in a shallow pool, or running in place in deep water (treading water). The latter three modes of exercise are gaining quickly in popularity because little skill is required to participate. These activities seem to be just as effective as other forms of aerobic activity in helping individuals lose weight without the pain and the fear of injuries.

One final benefit of exercise for weight control is that it allows fat to be burned more efficiently. Both carbohydrates and fats are sources of energy. When the glucose levels begin to drop during prolonged exercise, more fat is used as energy substrate. Equally important is that fat-burning enzymes increase with aerobic training.

Fat is lost primarily by burning it in muscle. Therefore, as the concentration of the enzymes increases, so does the ability to burn fat.

Low-Intensity Versus High-Intensity Exercise for Weight Loss

Some individuals promote low-intensity exercise over high-intensity exercise for the purpose of losing weight. Compared with high-intensity exercise, a greater proportion of calories burned during low-intensity exercise is derived from fat. The lower the intensity of exercise, the higher the percentage of fat utilization as a source of energy. In theory, if you are trying to lose fat, this principle makes sense, but in reality it is misleading. The bottom line when you are trying to lose weight is to burn more calories. When your daily caloric expenditure exceeds your intake, you lose weight. The more calories you burn, the more fat you lose.

During low-intensity exercise, up to 50 percent of the calories burned may be derived from fat (the other 50 percent from glucose [carbohydrates]). With intense exercise, only 30 percent to 40 percent of the caloric expenditure comes from fat. Overall, however, you can burn twice as many (or more) calories during high-intensity exercise, and subsequently more fat as well.

Let's look at a practical illustration. If you exercise for 30 minutes at a moderate intensity and burn 200 calories, about 100 of those calories (50 percent) would come from fat. If you exercise at high intensity during those same 30 minutes, you may burn 400 calories with

120 to 160 of the calories (30 percent to 40 percent) coming from fat. Thus, if you exercise at a low intensity, you have to do so twice as long to burn the same number of calories.

Moreover, high-intensity exercise by itself seems to trigger greater fat loss than low-intensity exercise. Research conducted at Laval University in Quebec, Canada, showed that subjects who performed a high-intensity, intermittent-training program lost more body fat than a low- to moderate-intensity continuous aerobic endurance group.[14] Even more surprisingly, this finding occurred despite the fact that the high-intensity group burned fewer total calories per exercise session. The results support the notion that vigorous exercise is more conducive to weight loss than is low- to moderate-intensity exercise.

Before you start high-intensity exercise sessions, a word of caution is in order: Be sure that it is medically safe for you to participate in such activities and that you build up gradually to that level. If you are cleared to participate in high-intensity exercise, do not attempt to do too much too quickly, as you may suffer injuries and discouragement. You must allow your body a proper conditioning period of 8 to 12 weeks, or even longer for those with a moderate to serious weight problem. Also, high intensity does not mean high impact. High-impact activities are the most common cause of exercise-related injuries (see the discussion on Aerobics in Chapter 4, page 90, and on acute sports injuries in Chapter 9, page 203).

This discussion of high-intensity versus low-intensity exercise does not mean that low intensity is not effective. Low-intensity exercise provides substantial health benefits, and people who initiate exercise programs are more willing to participate and stay with low-intensity programs. Low-intensity exercise does promote weight loss, but it is not as effective as higher-intensity exercise. You will have to exercise longer to obtain the same results.

Designing Your Own Weight-Loss Program

In addition to exercise and food management, sensible adjustments in caloric intake are recommended. Most research finds that a negative caloric balance is required to lose weight. Perhaps the only exception is with people who are eating too few calories. A nutrient analysis often reveals that "faithful" dieters are not consuming enough calories. These people actually need to increase their daily caloric intake (combined with an exercise program) to get their metabolism to kick back up to a normal level.

TABLE **6.1** Estimated Energy Requirement (EER) Based on Age, Body Weight, and Height (includes activities of independent living only and no moderate physical activity or exercise)

Men: EER = $662 - (9.53 \times \text{Age}) + (15.91 \times \text{BW}) + (539 \times \text{HT})$
Women: EER = $354 - (6.91 \times \text{Age}) + (9.36 \times \text{BW}) + (726 \times \text{HT})$

BW = body weight in kilograms (divide BW in pounds by 2.2046), HT = height in meters (multiply HT in inches by .0254).

Source: National Academy of Sciences, Institute of Medicine, *Dietary Reference Intakes for Energy, Carbohydrates, Fiber, Fat, Protein and Amino Acids (Macronutrients)* (Washington, DC: National Academy Press, 2002).

Estimating Your Caloric Intake

With Activity 6.1 (page 145) and Tables 6.1 and 6.2, you can estimate your daily energy (caloric) requirement. Because this is only an estimated value, individual adjustments related to many of the factors discussed in this chapter may be necessary to establish a more precise value. Nevertheless, the estimated value does offer a beginning guideline for weight control or reduction.

The **estimated energy requirement (EER)** without additional planned activity and exercise is based on age, total body weight, and gender. Individuals who hold jobs that require a lot of walking or heavy manual labor burn more calories during the day than those who have sedentary jobs (such as working behind a desk). To estimate your EER, refer to Table 6.1. For example, the EER computation for a 20-year-old man, 71 inches tall, who weighs 160 pounds, would be as follows:

1. Body weight in kilograms = 72.6 kg (160 lbs ÷ 2.2046)
   Height in meters = 1.8 mts (71 × 0.0254)
2. EER = $662 - (9.53 \times \text{Age}) + (15.91 \times \text{BW}) + (539 \times \text{Ht})$
   EER = $662 - (9.53 \times 20) + (15.91 \times 72.6) + (539 \times 1.8)$
   EER = $662 - 190.6 + 1155 + 970$
   EER = 2596

Thus, the EER to maintain body weight for this individual would be 2,596 calories per day.

The second step is to determine the average number of calories this man burns daily as a result of exercise. To get this number, he must figure out the total number of minutes he exercises weekly and then figure the daily average exercise time. For instance, if he cycles at 10 miles per hour five times a week, 60 minutes each time, he exercises 300 minutes per week (5 × 60). The average daily exercise time is 42 minutes (300 ÷ 7, rounded off to the lowest unit).

Next, from Table 6.2, find the energy requirement for the activity (or activities) he has chosen for the exercise program. In the case of cycling (10 miles per hour), the requirement is .05 calories per pound of body weight per minute of activity (cal/lb/min). With a body weight of 160 pounds, this man would burn 8 calories each minute (body weight × .05, or 160 × .05). In 42 minutes, he burns approximately 336 calories (42 × 8).

Calcium and Weight Management

Eating calcium-rich foods—especially from dairy products—may help control or reduce body weight. Individuals with a high calcium intake gain less weight and less body fat than those with a lower intake. Women on low-calcium diets more than double the risk of becoming overweight.

These data indicate that, even in the absence of caloric restriction, obese people with high dietary calcium intake (the equivalent of 3 to 4 cups of milk per day) lose body fat and weight. Furthermore, dieters who consume calcium-rich dairy foods lose more fat and less lean body mass than those who consume less dairy products.

Researchers believe that

- calcium regulates fat storage inside the cell.
- calcium helps the body break down fat or causes fat cells to produce less fat.
- high calcium intake converts more calories into heat rather than fat.
- adequate calcium intake contributes to a decrease in intra-abdominal (visceral) fat.

The data also seem to indicate that calcium from dairy sources is more effective in attenuating weight and fat gain and accelerating fat loss than calcium obtained from other sources. Most likely, other nutrients found in dairy products may enhance the weight-regulating action of calcium.

Although additional research is needed, the best recommendation at this point is that if you are attempting to lose or maintain weight loss, do not eliminate dairy foods from your diet. Substitute non-fat (skim milk) or low-fat dairy products for other drinks and foods in your diet to help you manage weight and total daily caloric intake.

Sources: M. B. Zemel, "Role of Dietary Calcium and Dairy Products in Modulating Adiposity," *Lipids* 38 (2): 139–146, 2003; "A Nice Surprise from Calcium," *University of California Berkeley Wellness Letter*, 19, no. 11 (August 2003): 1.

KEY TERMS

Estimated energy requirement (EER) The average dietary energy (caloric) intake that is predicted to maintain energy balance in a healthy adult of defined age, gender, weight, height, and level of physical activity, consistent with good health.

TABLE **6.2** Caloric Expenditure of Selected Physical Activities

ACTIVITY*	CAL/LB/MIN	ACTIVITY*	CAL/LB/MIN	ACTIVITY*	CAL/LB/MIN
Aerobics		Gymnastics		Stationary Cycling	
Moderate	0.065	Light	0.030	Moderate	0.055
Vigorous	0.095	Heavy	0.056	Vigorous	0.070
Step aerobics	0.070	Handball	0.064	Strength Training	0.050
Archery	0.030	Hiking	0.040	Swimming (crawl)	
Badminton		Judo/Karate	0.086	20 yds/min	0.031
Recreation	0.038	Racquetball	0.065	25 yds/min	0.040
Competition	0.065	Rope Jumping	0.060	45 yds/min	0.057
Baseball	0.031	Rowing (vigorous)	0.090	50 yds/min	0.070
Basketball		Running (on a level surface)		Table Tennis	0.030
Moderate	0.046	11.0 min/mile	0.070	Tennis	
Competition	0.063	8.5 min/mile	0.090	Moderate	0.045
Bowling	0.030	7.0 min/mile	0.102	Competition	0.064
Calisthenics	0.033	6.0 min/mile	0.114	Volleyball	0.030
Cycling (on a level surface)		Deep water**	0.100	Walking	
5.5 mph	0.033	Skating (moderate)	0.038	4.5 mph	0.045
10.0 mph	0.050	Skiing		Shallow pool	0.090
13.0 mph	0.071	Downhill	0.060	Water Aerobics	
Dance		Level (5 mph)	0.078	Moderate	0.050
Moderate	0.030	Soccer	0.059	Vigorous	0.070
Vigorous	0.055	Stairmaster		Wrestling	0.085
Golf	0.030	Moderate	0.070		
		Vigorous	0.090		

* Values are for actual time engaged in the activity.   ** Treading water

Adapted from:
P. E. Allsen, J. M. Harrison, and B. Vance, *Fitness for Life: An Individualized Approach* (Dubuque, IA: Wm. C. Brown, 1989).
C. A. Bucher and W. E. Prentice, *Fitness for College and Life* (St. Louis: Times Mirror/Mosby College Publishing, 1989).
C. F. Consolazio, R. E. Johnson, and L. J. Pecora, *Physiological Measurements of Metabolic Functions in Man* (New York: McGraw-Hill, 1963).
R. V. Hockey, *Physical Fitness: The Pathway to Healthful Living* (St. Louis: Times Mirror/Mosby College Publishing, 1989).
W. W. K. Hoeger et al., Research conducted at Boise State University, 1986–1993.

The third step is to obtain the estimated total caloric requirement, with exercise, needed to maintain body weight. To do this, add the typical daily requirement (without exercise) and the average calories burned through exercise. In our example, it is 2,932 calories (2,596 + 336).

Therefore, this man has to consume fewer than 2,932 calories daily to lose weight. Because of the many factors that play a role in weight control, this is only an estimated daily requirement. Furthermore, to lose weight, we cannot predict that he will lose exactly 1 pound of fat in 1 week if he cuts his daily intake by 500 calories (500 × 7 = 3,500 calories, or the equivalent of 1 pound of fat).

The daily energy requirement is only a target guideline for weight control. Periodic readjustments are necessary because individuals differ and the estimated daily cost changes as you lose weight and modify your exercise habits.

To determine the target caloric intake to lose weight, multiply your current weight by 5 and subtract this amount from the total daily energy requirement (3,166 in our example) with exercise. For our moderately active male example, this would mean consuming only 2,366 calories per day to lose weight (160 × 5 = 800 and 2,932 − 800 = 2,132 calories).

This final caloric intake to lose weight never should be below 1,200 calories for women and 1,500 for men. If distributed properly over the various food groups, these figures are the lowest caloric intakes that provide the necessary nutrients the body needs. In terms of percentages of total calories, the daily distribution should be approximately 60 percent carbohydrates (mostly complex carbohydrates), less than 30 percent fat, and about 12 percent protein.

The time of day when food is consumed also may play a part in losing weight. When a person is attempting to lose weight, intake should consist of a minimum of 25 percent of the total daily calories for breakfast, 50 percent for lunch, and 25 percent or less at dinner. Breakfast, in particular, is a critical meal. Many people skip breakfast because it's the easiest meal to skip. Evidence, however, indicates that people who skip breakfast are hungrier later in the day and end up consuming more total daily calories than those who eat breakfast. Furthermore, regular breakfast eaters have less of a weight problem, lose weight more effectively, and have less difficulty maintaining lost weight.

If most of the daily calories are consumed during one meal (as in the typical evening meal) the body may perceive that something is wrong and will slow down the metabolism so it can store more calories in the form of fat. Also, eating most of the calories during one meal causes a person to go hungry the rest of the day, making it more difficult to adhere to the diet.

Monitoring Your Diet Through Daily Food Logs

To help you monitor and adhere to your diet plan, you may use the daily food intake record form in Activity 6.2, page 147. First make a master copy so you can make copies as needed in the future. Guidelines are provided for 1,200-, 1,500-, 1,800-, and 2,000-calorie diet plans. These plans have been developed based on the MyPyramid food plan and the Dietary Guidelines for Americans to meet the Recommended Dietary Allowances. The objective is to meet (not exceed) the number of servings allowed for each diet plan. Each time you eat a serving of any food, record it in the appropriate box. Evidence indicates that people who monitor daily caloric intake are more successful at weight loss than those who don't self-monitor.

To lose weight, you should use the diet plan that most closely approximates your target caloric intake. The plan is based on the following caloric allowances for these food groups:

- Grains: 80 calories per serving.
- Fruits: 60 calories per serving.
- Vegetables: 25 calories per serving.
- Milk (use low-fat products): 120 calories per serving.
- Meat and beans: Use low-fat (300 calories per serving) frozen entrees or an equivalent amount if you prepare your own main dish (see the following discussion).

As you start your diet plan, pay particular attention to food serving sizes. Take care with cup and glass sizes. A standard cup is 8 ounces, but most glasses nowadays contain between 12 and 16 ounces. If you drink 12 ounces of fruit juice, in essence you are getting two servings of fruit because a standard serving is ¾ cup of juice.

Read food labels carefully to compare the caloric value of the serving listed on the label with the caloric guidelines provided above. Here are some examples:

- One slice of standard white bread has about 80 calories. A plain bagel may have 200 to 350 calories. Although it is low in fat, a 350-calorie bagel is equivalent to almost 4 servings in the bread, cereal, rice, and pasta group.
- The standard serving size listed on the food label for most cereals is 1 cup. As you read the nutrition information, however, you will find that for the same cup of cereal, one type of cereal has 120 calories and another cereal has 200 calories. Because a standard serving in the bread, cereal, rice, and pasta group is 80 calories, the first cereal would be 1½ servings and the second one 2½ servings.
- A medium-size fruit is usually considered to be 1 serving. A large fruit could provide as many as 2 or more servings.
- In the milk, yogurt, and cheese groups, 1 serving represents 120 calories. A cup of whole milk has about 160 calories, compared with a cup of skim milk, which contains 88 calories. A cup of whole milk, therefore, would provide 1⅓ servings in this food group.

Using Low-Fat Entrees

To be more accurate with caloric intake and to simplify meal preparation, use commercially prepared low-fat frozen entrees as the main dish for lunch and dinner meals (only one entree for the 1,200-calorie diet plan— see Activity 6.2, page 147). Look for entrees that provide about 300 calories and no more than 6 grams of fat per entree. These two entrees can be used as the meat and beans group selections and will provide most of the daily protein requirement for the body. Along with each entree, supplement the meal with some of your servings from the other food groups.

This diet plan has been used successfully in weight loss research programs.[15] If you choose not to use these low-fat entrees, prepare a similar meal using 3 ounces (cooked) of lean meat, poultry, or fish with additional beans, vegetables, rice, or pasta that will provide 300 calories with fewer than 6 grams of fat per dish.

Analyze Your Intake

As you record your food choices, be sure to write the precise amount for each serving. If you choose to do so, you then can run a computerized nutrient analysis to verify your caloric intake and food distribution pattern (percent of total calories from carbohydrate, fat, and protein).

Tips for Behavior Modification and Adherence to a Lifetime Weight Management Program

Achieving and maintaining recommended body composition is by no means impossible, but it does require desire and commitment. If weight management is to become a priority in life, people must realize that they have to transform their behavior to some extent.

Modifying old habits and developing new, positive behaviors take time. The following management techniques have been used successfully to change detrimental behavior and help adhere to a positive lifetime weight control program. In developing a retraining program, people are not expected to use all of the strategies listed, but should pick the ones that apply to them.

- Make a commitment to change. The first necessary ingredient is the desire to modify your behavior. You need to stop precontemplating and contemplating change and get going! The reasons for change must be more compelling than the reasons for continuing your present lifestyle patterns. You must accept that you have a problem and decide by yourself whether you really want to change. If you are sincerely committed, your chances for success are enhanced already.
- Set realistic goals. Most people with a weight problem would like the pounds to melt away, failing to realize that the weight problem developed over several years. A sound weight reduction and maintenance program can be accomplished only by establishing new lifetime eating and exercise habits, both of which take time to develop. In setting a realistic long-term goal, short-term objectives also should be planned. The long-term goal may be to decrease body fat to 20 percent of total body weight. The short-term objective may be a 1 percent decrease in body fat each month. Objectives such as these allow for regular evaluation and help maintain motivation and renewed commitment to attain the long-term goal.
- Incorporate exercise into the program. Choosing enjoyable activities, places, times, equipment, and people to work out with helps a person adhere to an

"Super-sized" portion sizes at restaurants in the United States contribute to the growing epidemic of obesity.

exercise program. Details on developing a complete exercise program are given in Chapter 3.
- Differentiate hunger from appetite. Hunger is the actual physical need for food. Appetite is a desire for food, usually triggered by factors such as stress, habit, boredom, depression, availability of food, or just the thought of food itself. People should eat only when they have a physical need. In this regard, developing and sticking to a regular meal pattern help control hunger.
- Eat less fat. Each gram of fat provides 9 calories, and protein and carbohydrates provide only 4 calories. In essence, you can eat more food on a low-fat diet because you consume fewer calories with each meal.
- Pay attention to calories. Some people think that because a certain food is low in fat, they can eat as much as they want. People have consumed entire boxes of fat-free cookies and bags of pretzels under this pretense. A homemade chocolate-chip cookie might have 100 calories, whereas a low-fat one might have 50. Simple math will tell you that eating one homemade cookie is better than eating a half dozen low-fat ones. When reading food labels, don't just look at the fat content. Pay attention to calories as well.
- Cut unnecessary items from your diet. Many people regularly drink a 140-calorie can of soda pop (or more) each day. Substituting a glass of water would cut 51,100 (140 × 365) calories yearly from the diet—the equivalent of 14.6 (51,000 ÷ 3,500) pounds of fat.
- Maintain daily intake of calcium-rich foods, especially low-fat or non-fat dairy products.

- Add foods to your diet that reduce cravings. Many people have a biological imbalance of insulin. Insulin helps the body use and conserve energy. Some people produce so much insulin that their bodies can't use it all. This imbalance leads to an overpowering craving for carbohydrates. As they eat more carbohydrates, even more insulin is released. Foods that reduce cravings include eggs, red meat, fish, poultry, cheese, tofu, oils, fats, and nonstarchy vegetables such as lettuce, green beans, peppers, asparagus, broccoli, mushrooms, and Brussels sprouts. If you watch your portion sizes, eating foods that reduce cravings at regular meals and for snacks helps to decrease the intense desire for carbohydrates, prevent overeating, and aid with weight loss.

- Avoid automatic eating. Many people associate certain daily activities with eating. For example, people may eat while cooking, watching television, or reading. Most of the time the foods consumed in these situations lack nutritional value or are high in sugar and fat.

- Stay busy. People tend to eat more when they sit around and do nothing. Occupying the mind and body with activities not associated with eating helps take away the desire to eat. Some options are walking; cycling; playing sports; gardening; sewing; or visiting a library, a museum, or a park. To break the routine of life, you might develop other skills and interests or try something new and exciting.

- Plan meals ahead of time. Sensible shopping is necessary to accomplish this objective. Always shop on a full stomach, because hungry shoppers tend to buy unhealthy foods impulsively—and then snack on the way home. The shopping list should include whole-grain breads and cereals, fruits and vegetables, low-fat milk and dairy products, lean meats, fish, and poultry.

- Cook wisely.
  - Use less fat and fewer refined foods in food preparation.
  - Trim all visible fat from meats and remove skin from poultry before cooking.
  - Skim the fat off gravies and soups.
  - Bake, broil, boil, or steam instead of frying.
  - Use butter, cream, mayonnaise, and salad dressings sparingly.
  - Avoid coconut oil, palm oil, and cocoa butter.
  - Prepare plenty of foods that contain fiber.
  - Include whole-grain breads and cereals, vegetables, and legumes in most meals.
  - Eat fruits for dessert.
  - Stay away from soda pop, fruit juices, and fruit flavored drinks.
  - In addition to using less sugar, cut down on other refined carbohydrates such as corn syrup, malt sugar, dextrose, and fructose.
  - Drink plenty of water—at least six glasses a day.

- Do not serve more food than you should eat. Measure the food in portions and keep serving dishes away from the table. In this way you will eat less, have a harder time getting seconds, and have less appetite because the food is not visible. People should not be forced to eat when they are satisfied (including children after they already have had a healthy, nutritious serving).

- Try "junior size" instead of "super size." Studies indicate that people who are served larger portions eat more, whether they are hungry or not. For junior size, use smaller plates, bowls, cups, and glasses. Try eating half as much food as you commonly eat. Over the years, the sizes of dishes and glasses have gotten bigger. Consequently, people serve and eat a lot more food than they need. If you use a smaller plate, it will look like more food and you'll tend to eat less. Watch for portion sizes at restaurants as well. Plate and portion sizes at restaurants now are so large that people overeat and still end up with leftovers to take home. Similarly, the original bottle of Coca-Cola contained 6.5 ounces. Machines now routinely dispense 20-ounce bottles, and convenience stores sell 64-ounce "buckets" of soda pop (about 750 calories). Supersized foods create supersized people.

- Eat out infrequently. Research indicates that the more often people of all ages eat out, the more body fat they have. People who eat out six or more times per week consume an average of about 300 extra calories per day and 30 percent more fat than those who eat out less often.

- Eat slowly and at the table only. Eating is one of the pleasures of life, and we need to take time to enjoy it. Eating on the run is not good because the body doesn't have enough time to "register" nutritive and caloric consumption, and people overeat before the body perceives the fullness signal. Eating at the table also forces people to take time out to eat, and it deters snacking between meals, primarily because of the extra time and effort required to sit down and eat. When people are done eating, they should not sit around the table but, rather, clean up and put away the food to avoid snacking.

- Avoid social binges. Social gatherings tend to entice self-defeating behavior. Visual imagery might help before attending social gatherings. Plan ahead and visualize yourself there. Don't feel pressured to eat or drink, and don't rationalize in these situations. Choose low-calorie foods and entertain yourself with other activities such as dancing and talking.

- Don't raid the refrigerator or the cookie jar. In these tempting situations, take control. Stop and think.

- Do not place unhealthy foods within easy reach. Ideally, avoid bringing high-calorie, high-sugar, or high-fat foods into the house. If they are there already, store them where they are hard to get to or see—perhaps the garage or basement.

Critical Thinking

What behavioral strategies have you used to properly manage your body weight? How do you think those strategies would work for others?

- Avoid evening food raids. Most people with weight problems do well during the day but then "lose it" at night. Excessive snacking following the evening meal is a common pitfall. Stay busy after your evening meal. Go for a short walk; floss and brush your teeth; get to bed earlier. In most cases the intense desire for food that you get during the evening hours disappears following a good night's rest.
- Practice stress-management techniques (more on stress in Chapter 7). Many people snack and increase food consumption in stressful situations. Eating is not a stress-releasing activity and, instead, can aggravate the problem if weight control is an issue.
- Get support. People who receive support from friends, relatives, and formal support groups are much more likely to lose and maintain weight loss than those without such support. The more support you receive, the better off you will be.
- Monitor changes and reward accomplishments. Feedback on fat loss and lean tissue gain is a reward in itself. Awareness of changes in body composition also helps reinforce new behaviors. Being able to exercise without interruption for 15, 20, 30, or 60 minutes; swimming a certain distance; running a mile—all

these accomplishments deserve recognition. Meeting objectives calls for rewards that are not related to eating: new clothing, a tennis racquet, a bicycle, exercise shoes, or something else that is special and you would not have acquired otherwise.
- Be prepared for slips. Most people will slip and occasionally splurge. If that happens, don't despair and give up. Reevaluate and continue with your efforts. An occasional slip will not make much difference in the long run.
- Think positive. Avoid negative thoughts about how difficult changing past behaviors might be. Instead, think of the benefits you will reap, such as feeling, looking, and functioning better, plus enjoying better health and improving your quality of life. Avoid negative environments and people who will not be supportive.

You Can Do It!

The challenge of taking off excessive body fat and keeping it off for good has no simple solution. Weight management is accomplished through lifetime commitment to physical activity and proper food selection. When taking part in a weight-reduction program, people have to decrease their caloric intake moderately and implement strategies to modify unhealthy eating behaviors.

Relapses into past negative behaviors are almost inevitable. Making mistakes is human and does not mean failure. Failure comes to those who give up and do not use previous experiences to build upon and, instead, develop skills that will prevent self-defeating behaviors in the future. Where there's a will, there's a way, and those who persist will reap the rewards.

Aetna InteliHealth. This site provides articles on Healthful Lifestyles, including weight management. The Nutrition database offers tips on weight management, exercise and assessing your diet. Interactive tools include healthful recipe, food pyramid, and a body mass index calculator.
http://www.intelihealth.com

ASSESS YOUR KNOWLEDGE

Evaluate how well you understand the concepts presented in this chapter using the Assess Your Knowledge and Practice Quizzes options on your Profile Plus CD-ROM.

1. Obesity is defined as a body mass index equal to or above
   a. 10.
   b. 25.
   c. 30.
   d. 45.
   e. 50.

2. The yearly estimated number of deaths attributed to excessive body weight and physical inactivity in the United States is
   a. 28,000.
   b. 55,000.
   c. 93,000.
   d. 112,000.
   e. 350,000.

3. Obesity increases the risk for
   a. hypertension.
   b. congestive heart failure.
   c. atherosclerosis.
   d. type 2 diabetes.
   e. all of the above.

4. Tolerable weight is a body weight
   a. that is not ideal but one that you can live with.
   b. that will tolerate the increased risk of chronic diseases.
   c. with a BMI range between 25 and 30.
   d. that meets both ideal values for percent body weight and BMI.
   e. All are correct choices.

5. When the body uses protein instead of a combination of fats and carbohydrates as a source of energy,
   a. weight loss is very slow.
   b. a large amount of weight loss is in the form of water.
   c. muscle turns into fat.
   d. fat is lost very rapidly.
   e. fat cannot be lost.

6. One pound of fat represents
   a. 1,200 calories.
   b. 1,500 calories.
   c. 3,500 calories.
   d. 5,000 calories.
   e. None of the above.

7. The mechanism that seems to regulate how much a person weighs is known as
   a. setpoint.
   b. weight factor.
   c. basal metabolic rate.
   d. metabolism.
   e. energy-balancing equation.

8. The key to successful weight management is
   a. frequent dieting.
   b. very low-calorie diets when "normal" dieting doesn't work.
   c. a lifetime physical activity program.
   d. regular low carbohydrate/high protein meals.
   e. All are correct choices.

9. The daily amount of physical activity recommended for weight loss maintenance is
   a. 15 to 20 minutes.
   b. 20 to 30 minutes.
   c. 30 to 60 minutes.
   d. 60 to 90 minutes.
   e. Any amount is sufficient as long as it is done daily.

10. A daily energy expenditure of 300 calories through physical activity is the equivalent of approximately _____ pounds of fat per year.
    a. 12
    b. 15
    c. 22
    d. 27
    e. 31

Correct answers can be found on page 261.

Daily Caloric Requirement: Computation Form

Name _____   Date _____

Course _____   Section _____

A. Current body weight   _____

B. Caloric requirement per pound of body weight (use Table 6.1, page 137)   _____

C. Typical daily caloric requirement without exercise to maintain body weight
    (A × B)   _____

D. Selected physical activity (e.g., jogging)*   _____

E. Number of exercise sessions per week   _____

F. Duration of exercise session (in minutes)   _____

G. Total weekly exercise time in minutes (E × F)   _____

H. Average daily exercise time in minutes (G ÷ 7)   _____

I. Caloric expenditure per pound per minute (cal/lb/min) of physical activity
    (use Table 6.2, page 138)   _____

J. Total calories burned per minute of exercise (A × I)   _____

K. Average daily calories burned as a result of the exercise program (H × J)   _____

L. Total daily caloric requirement with exercise to maintain body weight (C + K)   _____

M. Number of calories to subtract from daily requirement to achieve a
    negative caloric balance (multiply current body weight by 5)**   _____

N. Target caloric intake to lose weight (L − M)   _____

---

* If more than one physical activity is selected, you will need to estimate the average daily calories burned as a result of each
 additional activity (steps D through K) and add all of these figures to L above.

** This figure should never be below 1,200 calories for women or 1,500 calories for men. See Activity 6.2 for the 1,200-, 1,500-,
 1,800-, and 2,000-calorie diet plans.

1. How much effort are you willing to put into reaching your weight loss goal?

   _____

   _____

2. Indicate your feelings about participating in an exercise program.

   _____

   _____

3. Will you commit to be more physically active and to participate in a combined aerobic and strength-training program?   Yes [ ]   No [ ]

   If your answer is "Yes," proceed to the next question; if you answered "No," please review Chapters 3 and 6 again.

4. Indicate your current number of daily steps: [_____]

5. List aerobic activities you enjoy or may enjoy doing.

   _____

   _____

6. Select one or two aerobic activities in which you will participate regularly.

   [_____]   [_____]

7. List facilities available to you where you can carry out the aerobic and strength-training programs.

   _____

   _____

8. Indicate days and times you will set aside for your aerobic and strength-training program (accumulate 60 to 90 minutes of physical activity 6 to 7 days per week, including 3 to 5 weekly sessions of aerobic exercise lasting about 30 minutes each and 2 to 3 weekly strength training sessions).

   Monday: _____

   Tuesday: _____

   Wednesday: _____

   Thursday: _____

   Friday: _____

   Saturday: _____

   Sunday: _____

9. Conclusion: Briefly describe whether you think you can meet the goals of your physical activity, aerobic, and strength-training programs. What obstacles will you have to overcome and how will you overcome them?

   _____

   _____

   _____

Daily Food Intake Record: 1,200-Calorie Diet Plan

Name _____   Date _____

Course _____   Section _____

Instructions

The objective of the diet plan is to meet (not exceed) the number of servings allowed for the food groups listed. Each time you eat a particular food, record it in the space provided for each group along with the appropriate serving size. Be sure not to exceed the number of calories allowed per serving listed below. Instead of the meat and beans group, you are allowed to have a commercially available low-fat frozen entree for your meal (this entree should provide no more than 300 calories and less than 6 grams of fat). You can make additional copies of this form as needed.

Meat & Beans: 1 low-fat frozen entree
Milk: 2 servings
Fruits: 2 servings
Veggies: 3 servings
Grains: 6 servings

Bread, Cereal, Rice, Pasta Group (80 calories/serving): 6 servings

1 _____

2 _____

3 _____

4 _____

5 _____

6 _____

Vegetable Group (25 calories/serving): 3 servings

1 _____

2 _____

3 _____

Fruit Group (60 calories/serving): 2 servings

1 _____

2 _____

Milk Group (120 calories/serving, use low-fat milk and low-fat milk products): 2 servings

1 _____

2 _____

Low-fat Frozen Entree (300 calories and less than 6 grams of fat): 1 serving

1 _____

Daily Food Intake Record: 1,500-Calorie Diet Plan

Instructions

The objective of the diet plan is to meet (not exceed) the number of servings allowed for the food groups listed. Each time you eat a particular food, record it in the space provided for each group along with the appropriate serving size. Be sure not to exceed the number of calories allowed per serving listed below. Instead of the meat and beans group, you are allowed to have two commercially available low-fat frozen entree for your meal (this entree should provide no more than 300 calories and less than 6 grams of fat). You can make additional copies of this form as needed.

Meat & Beans: 2 low-fat frozen
                entrees
Milk: 2 servings
Fruits: 2 servings
Veggies: 3 servings
Grains: 6 servings

Bread, Cereal, Rice, Pasta Group (80 calories/serving): 6 servings

1 _____

2 _____

3 _____

4 _____

5 _____

6 _____

Vegetable Group (25 calories/serving): 3 servings

1 _____

2 _____

3 _____

Fruit Group (60 calories/serving): 2 servings

1 _____

2 _____

Milk Group (120 calories/serving, use low-fat milk and low-fat milk products): 2 servings

1 _____

2 _____

Two Low-fat Frozen Entrees (300 calories and less than 6 grams of fat): 2 servings

1 _____

2 _____

Daily Food Intake Record:
1,800-Calorie Diet Plan

Name

Date

Course

Section

Instructions

The objective of the diet plan is to meet (not exceed) the number of servings allowed for the food groups listed. Each time you eat a particular food, record it in the space provided for each group along with the appropriate serving size. Be sure not to exceed the number of calories allowed per serving listed below. Instead of the meat and beans group, you are allowed to have two commercially available low-fat frozen entrees for two of your meals (these entrees should provide no more than 300 calories and less than 6 grams of fat). You can make additional copies of this form as needed.

Meat & Beans: 2 low-fat frozen entrees
Milk: 2 servings
Fruits: 3 servings
Veggies: 5 servings
Grains: 8 servings

Bread, Cereal, Rice, Pasta Group (80 calories/serving): 8 servings

1 _____ 5 _____

2 _____ 6 _____

3 _____ 7 _____

4 _____ 8 _____

Vegetable Group (25 calories/serving): 5 servings

1 _____ 4 _____

2 _____ 5 _____

3 _____

Fruit Group (60 calories/serving): 3 servings

1 _____

2 _____

3 _____

Milk Group (120 calories/serving, use low-fat milk and low-fat milk products): 2 servings

1 _____

2 _____

Two Low-fat Frozen Entrees (300 calories and less than 6 grams of fat): 2 servings

1 _____

2 _____

Daily Food Intake Record: 2,000-Calorie Diet Plan

Instructions

The objective of the diet plan is to meet (not exceed) the number of servings allowed for the food groups listed. Each time you eat a particular food, record it in the space provided for each group along with the appropriate serving size. Be sure not to exceed the number of calories allowed per serving listed below. Instead of the meat and beans group, you are allowed to have two commercially available low-fat frozen entrees for two of your meals (these entrees should provide no more than 300 calories and less than 6 grams of fat). You can make additional copies of this form as needed.

Meat & Beans: 2 low-fat frozen entrees
Milk: 2 servings
Fruits: 4 servings
Veggies: 5 servings
Grains: 10 servings

Bread, Cereal, Rice, Pasta Group (80 calories/serving): 10 servings

1 _____   6 _____
2 _____   7 _____
3 _____   8 _____
4 _____   9 _____
5 _____   10 _____

Vegetable Group (25 calories/serving): 5 servings

1 _____   4 _____
2 _____   5 _____
3 _____

Fruit Group (60 calories/serving): 4 servings

1 _____
2 _____
3 _____
4 _____

Milk Group (120 calories/serving, use low-fat milk and low-fat milk products): 2 servings

1 _____
2 _____

Two Low-fat Frozen Entrees (300 calories and less than 6 grams of fat): 2 servings

1 _____
2 _____

Stress Management

CHAPTER 7

OBJECTIVES

- Define stress, eustress, and distress.
- Explain how stress affects health and optimal performance.
- Define the two major types of behavior patterns or personality types.
- Learn whether you have a hostile personality.
- Develop time management skills.
- Identify the major sources of stress in your life.
- Define the role of physical exercise in reducing stress.
- Learn to use various stress management techniques.

tress has become one of the most common problems we face. Learning to live and get ahead today is not possible without stress. To succeed in an unpredictable world that changes with every new day, working under pressure has become the rule rather than the exception for most people. Estimates indicate that the annual cost of stress and stress-related diseases in the United States exceeds $100 billion—a direct result of health-care costs, lost productivity, and absenteeism.

Stress is a fact of modern life. Every person has an optimal level of stress that is most conducive to adequate health and performance. When stress levels reach mental, emotional, and physiological limits, however, stress becomes distress and the person no longer functions effectively.

The human body's response to stress has been the same ever since our species first walked the earth. Stress prepares the organism to react to the stress-causing event, called the **stressor**. The difference is the way in which we react to stress. Many people thrive under stress; others under similar circumstances are unable to handle it. An individual's reaction to a stress-causing agent determines whether stress is positive or negative.

Chronic negative reactions to stress raise the risk for many health disorders, including coronary heart disease, hypertension, eating disorders, ulcers, diabetes, asthma, depression, migraine headaches, sleep disorders, and chronic fatigue, and may even play a role in the

How vulnerable to stress are you? Find out with the activities on your CD-ROM.

development of certain types of cancer. To maintain emotional and physiological stability, it's crucial to recognize when stress has a negative effect and to overcome the stressful condition quickly and efficiently.

The good news is that stress can be self-controlled. Most people have accepted stress as a normal part of daily life and, even though everyone has to deal with it, few seem to understand it and know how to cope effectively. People should not try to avoid stress entirely, because a certain amount is necessary for optimum health, performance, and well-being. It is difficult to succeed and have fun in life without "hits, runs, and errors."

The Body's Reaction to Stress

Dr. Hans Selye, one of the foremost authorities on stress, defined it as "the nonspecific response of the human organism to any demand that is placed upon it."[1] "Nonspecific" indicates that the body reacts in a similar way regardless of the nature of the event that leads to the stress response. In simpler terms, stress is the body's mental, emotional, and physiological response to any situation that is new, threatening, frightening, or exciting.

The body responds to stress with a rapid-fire sequence of physical changes known as **fight or flight** (see Figure 7.1). The hypothalamus activates the sympathetic nervous system, and the pituitary gland triggers the release of catecholamines (hormones) from the adrenal glands. These hormonal changes increase heart rate, blood pressure, blood flow to active muscles and the brain, glucose levels, oxygen consumption, and strength—all necessary for the body to either fight or flee. In cases of both fight and flight, the body relaxes and stress dissipates. If the person is unable to take action, however, the muscles tense and tighten instead.

Stress isn't necessarily bad. Dr. Selye further defined stress as either **eustress** or **distress**. In both cases, the nonspecific response is almost the same. In eustress, health and performance continue to improve even as stress increases. With distress, health and performance begin to deteriorate.

Critical Thinking

Can you identify sources of eustress and distress in your personal life during this past year? Explain your emotional and physical response to each stressor and how the two differ.

FIGURE **7.1** Physiological response to stress: fight or flight.

From *Lifetime Physical Fitness & Wellness*, by W. W. K. Hoeger and S. A. Hoeger (Belmont, CA: Wadsworth/Thomson Learning, 2007), p. 368.

Adaptation to Stress

Human physiology is such that the body continually strives to maintain a constant internal environment. This state of physiological balance, known as **homeostasis**, allows the body to function as effectively as possible. When a stressor triggers a nonspecific response, homeostasis is disrupted. This reaction to stressors, best explained by Dr. Selye through the **general adaptation syndrome (GAS)**, is composed of three stages: alarm reaction, resistance, and exhaustion/recovery.

Alarm Reaction

The alarm reaction is the immediate response to a stressor, whether positive or negative. During the alarm reaction, the body evokes an instant physiological reaction that involves the mobilization of systems and processes within the organism to minimize the threat

FIGURE **7.2** General Adaptation Syndrome: The body's response to stress.

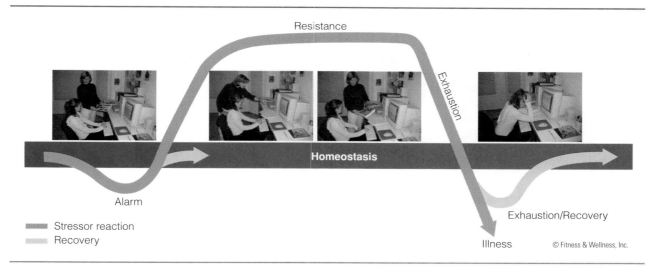

Resistance

Exhaustion

Homeostasis

Alarm

Exhaustion/Recovery

▬▬ Stressor reaction
▬▬ Recovery

Illness

© Fitness & Wellness, Inc.

to homeostasis (see "Coping with Stress," pages 158–160). If the stressor subsides, the body recovers and returns to homeostasis.

Resistance

If the stressor persists, the body calls upon its limited reserves to build up resistance as it strives to maintain homeostasis. For a short while, the body copes effectively and meets the challenge of the stressor until it can be overcome (see Figure 7.2).

Exhaustion/Recovery

If stress becomes chronic and intolerable, the body spends its limited reserves and loses its ability to cope, entering the exhaustion/recovery stage. During this stage, the body functions at a diminished capacity while it recovers from stress. In due time, following an "adequate" recovery period, the body recuperates and is able to return to homeostasis. If chronic stress persists during the exhaustion stage, however, immune function is compromised, which can damage body systems and lead to disease.

An example of the stress response through the general adaptation syndrome can be illustrated in college test performance. As you prepare to take an exam, you experience an initial alarm reaction. If you understand the material, study for the exam, and do well (eustress), the body recovers and stress is dissipated. If, however, you are not adequately prepared and fail the exam, the resistance stage is triggered. You are now concerned about your grade, and you remain in the resistance stage until the next exam. If you prepare and do well, the body

recovers. But if you fail once again and no longer can bring up your grade, exhaustion sets in, with possible physical and emotional breakdowns as a result. Exhaustion may be aggravated if you are struggling in other courses as well.

The exhaustion stage is often manifested in athletes and the most ardent fitness participants. Staleness is usually a consequence of overtraining. Peak performance can be sustained for only about 2 to 3 weeks at a time. Any attempts to continue intense training after peaking leads to exhaustion, diminished fitness, and mental and physical problems associated with overtraining. Thus, athletes and some fitness participants also need an active recovery phase following the attainment of peak fitness.

KEY TERMS

Stress The mental, emotional, and physiological response of the body to any situation that is new, threatening, frightening, or exciting.

Stressor Stress-causing agent.

Fight or flight A series of physical responses activated automatically in response to environmental stressors.

Eustress Positive stress.

Distress Negative or harmful stress under which health and performance begin to deteriorate.

Homeostasis A natural state of equilibrium. The body attempts to maintain this equilibrium by constantly reacting to external forces that attempt to disrupt this delicate balance.

General adaptation syndrome (GAS) A theoretical model that explains the body's adaptation to sustained stress, which includes three stages: alarm reaction, resistance, and exhaustion/recovery.

Taking time out during stressful life events
is vital for good health and wellness.

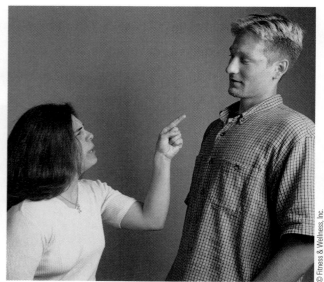

Anger and hostility can be a health risk factor.

Behavior Patterns

Common life events are not the only source of stress in
life. All too often, individuals bring on stress as a result
of their characteristic behavior patterns. The two main
types of behavior patterns are **Type A** and **Type B**. Each
type is based on several characteristics.

Type A behavior characterizes a primarily hard-
driving, overly ambitious, aggressive, at times hostile
and overly competitive person. Type A individuals often
set their own goals, are self-motivated, try to accomplish many tasks at the same time, are excessively
achievement-oriented, and have a sense of time urgency.
By contrast, Type B behavior is characteristic of calm,
casual, relaxed, easy-going individuals. Type B people
take one thing at a time, do not feel pressured or hurried,
and seldom set their own deadlines.

Over the years, experts have indicated that individuals classified as Type A have a significantly higher incidence for disease, especially cardiovascular conditions.[2]
Not all typical Type A people, however, are at higher
risk for disease. Type A individuals who are chronically
angry and hostile are at higher risk.[3] The questionnaire
provided in Figure 7.3 can help you determine whether
you have a hostile personality.

Some experts believe that emotional stress is far
more likely than physical stress to trigger a heart attack.
Especially vulnerable are people who are impatient and
are readily annoyed when they have to wait for someone or something—an employee, a traffic light, in a
restaurant line.

Research also is focusing on individuals who have
anxiety, depression, and feelings of helplessness when

Releasing Anger the Healthy Way

- Recognize the anger for what it is. Don't be afraid of
  it or try to suppress it.

- Figure out what made you so angry, then decide
  whether it's worth being so upset. Chances are that
  it's really a minor irritation or hassle.

- Stop before you act. Calm down first. Count to 10,
  take a deep breath, mentally recite the words to a
  favorite verse, or initiate some other distracting and
  relaxing activity. Then get ready to deal with the
  anger.

- If you're ticked off at somebody else, use calm tact to
  say why, without ripping into the other person. Tell
  him or her how you're feeling and try to negotiate
  some things.

- Be generous with the other person. Maybe he just
  failed an exam. Maybe she just heard bad news from
  home. Maybe he's having a rotten day. Listen carefully to her side of things and try as much as you can
  to understand.

- When all else fails, forgive the other person. Everyone makes mistakes. Carrying a grudge will hurt you
  worse than it hurts the other person.

From *Wellness: Guidelines for a Healthy Lifestyle,* by W. W. K. Hoeger, L. Turner,
and B. Q. Hafen (3d ed.) (Belmont, CA: Wadsworth/Thomson Learning, 2007).

FIGURE **7.3** Hostility and heart disease risk scale.

HOSTILITY COULD HARM YOUR HEART

Experts now conclude that feelings of hostility increase your risk of heart disease. Dr. Redford Williams, Duke University Medical Center, has designed a questionnaire to help you determine whether you have a hostile personality. Circle the answer that most closely fits how you would respond to the given situation:

1. A teenager drives by my yard blasting the car stereo:
   A. I begin to understand why teenagers can't hear.
   B. I can feel my blood pressure starting to rise.

2. A boyfriend/girlfriend calls at the last minute "too tired to go out tonight." I'm stuck with two $15 tickets:
   A. I find someone else to go with.
   B. I tell my friend how inconsiderate he/she is.

3. Waiting in the express checkout line at the supermarket where a sign says "No More Than 10 Items Please":
   A. I pick up a magazine and pass the time.
   B. I glance to see if anyone has more than 10 items.

4. Most homeless people in large cities:
   A. Are down and out because they lack ambition.
   B. Are victims of illness or some other misfortune.

5. At times when I've been very angry with someone:
   A. I was able to stop short of hitting him/her.
   B. I have, on occasion, hit or shoved him/her.

6. When I am stuck in a traffic jam:
   A. I am usually not particularly upset.
   B. I quickly start to feel irritated and annoyed.

7. When there's a really important job to be done:
   A. I prefer to do it myself.
   B. I am apt to call on my friends to help.

8. The cars ahead of me start to slow and stop as they approach a curve:
   A. I assume there is a construction site ahead.
   B. I assume someone ahead had a fender-bender.

9. An elevator stops too long above where I'm waiting:
   A. I soon start to feel irritated and annoyed.
   B. I start planning the rest of my day.

10. When a friend or co-worker disagrees with me:
    A. I try to explain my position more clearly.
    B. I am apt to get into an argument with him or her.

11. At times when I was really angry in the past:
    A. I have never thrown things or slammed a door.
    B. I've sometimes thrown things or slammed a door.

12. Someone bumps into me in a store:
    A. I pass it off as an accident.
    B. I feel irritated at their clumsiness.

13. When my spouse (significant other) is fixing a meal:
    A. I keep an eye out to make sure nothing burns.
    B. I talk about my day or read the paper.

14. Someone is hogging the conversation at a party:
    A. I look for an opportunity to put him/her down.
    B. I soon move to another group.

15. In most arguments:
    A. I am the angrier one.
    B. The other person is angrier than I am.

Score one point for each of these answers: 1. B, 2. B, 3. B, 4. A, 5. B, 6. B, 7. A, 8. B, 9. A, 10. B, 11. B, 12. B, 13. A, 14. A, 15. A. If you scored 4 or more points you may be hostile. Questions 1, 6, 9, 12, and 15 reflect anger. Questions 2, 5, 10, 11, 14, reflect aggression. Questions 3, 4, 7, 8, 13 reflect cynicism. If you scored 2 points in any category, you should work on that area of your personality.

From *Anger Kills*, by Redford B. Williams, and Virginia Williams. Copyright © 1993 by Redford B. Williams, M.D., and Virginia Williams, Ph.D. Reprinted by permission of Random House, Inc.

they encounter setbacks and failures in life. People who lose control of their lives, those who give up on their dreams in life, knowing that they could and should be doing better, may be more likely to have heart attacks than hard-driving people who enjoy their work.

Many of the Type A characteristics are learned behaviors. Consequently, if people can learn to identify the sources of stress, they can change their behavioral

K E Y   T E R M S

Type A Behavior pattern characteristic of a hard-driving, over-ambitious, aggressive, at times hostile and overly competitive person.

Type B Behavior pattern characteristic of a calm, casual, relaxed, and easy-going individual.

Changing a Type A Personality

- Make a contract with yourself to slow down and take it easy. Put it in writing. Post it in a conspicuous spot, then stick to the terms you set up. Be specific. Abstracts ("I'm going to be less uptight") don't work.

- Work on only one or two things at a time. Wait until you change one habit before you tackle the next one.

- Eat more slowly and eat only when you are relaxed and sitting down.

- If you smoke, quit.

- Cut down on your caffeine intake, because it increases the tendency to become irritated and agitated.

- Take regular breaks throughout the day, even as brief as 5 or 10 minutes, when you totally change what you're doing. Get up, stretch, get a drink of cool water, walk around for a few minutes.

- Work on fighting your impatience. If you're standing in line at the grocery store, study the interesting things people have in their carts instead of getting upset.

- Work on controlling hostility. Keep a written log. When do you flare up? What causes it? How do you feel at the time? What preceded it? Look for patterns and figure out what sets you off. Then do something about it. Either avoid the situations that cause you hostility or practice reacting to them in different ways.

- Plan some activities just for the fun of it. Load a picnic basket in the car and drive to the country with a friend. After a stressful physics class, stop at a theater and see a good comedy.

- Choose a role model, someone you know and admire who does not have a Type A personality. Observe the person carefully, then try out some techniques the person demonstrates.

- Simplify your life so you can learn to relax a little bit. Figure out which activities or commitments you can eliminate right now, then get rid of them.

- If morning is a problem time for you and you get too hurried, set your alarm clock half an hour earlier.

- Take time out during even the most hectic day to do something truly relaxing. Because you won't be used to it, you may have to work at it at first. Begin by listing things you'd really enjoy that would calm you. Include some things that take only a few minutes: Watch a sunset, lie out on the lawn at night and look at the stars, call an old friend and catch up on news, take a nap, sauté a pan of mushrooms and savor them slowly.

- If you're under a deadline, take short breaks. Stop and talk to someone for 5 minutes, take a short walk, or lie down with a cool cloth over your eyes for 10 minutes.

- Pay attention to what your own body clock is saying. You've probably noticed that every 90 minutes or so, you lose the ability to concentrate, get a little sleepy, and have a tendency to daydream. Instead of fighting the urge, put down your work and let your mind wander for a few minutes. Use the time to imagine and let your creativity run wild.

- Learn to treasure unplanned surprises: a friend dropping by unannounced, a hummingbird outside your window, a child's tightly clutched bouquet of wildflowers.

- Savor your relationships. Think about the people in your life. Relax with them and give yourself to them. Give up trying to control others and resist the urge to end relationships that don't always go as you'd like them to.

From *Wellness: Guidelines for a Healthy Lifestyle*, by W. W. K. Hoeger, L. Turner, and B. Q. Hafen (3d ed.) (Belmont, CA: Wadsworth/Thomson Learning, 2007).

responses. The main assessment tool to determine behavioral type is the structured interview, in which the interviewee is asked to reply to several questions that describe Type A and Type B behavior patterns. The interviewer notes the responses to the questions and also mental, emotional, and physical behaviors the individual exhibits as he or she replies to each question. Based on the answers and the associated behaviors, the interviewer rates the person along a continuum ranging from Type A to Type B.

Vulnerability to Stress

Researchers have identified a number of factors that can affect the way in which people handle stress. How people deal with these factors can actually increase or decrease vulnerability to stress. The questionnaire provided in Figure 7.4 lists these factors so you can determine your vulnerability rating. It will help you identify specific areas in which you can make improvements to help you cope more efficiently.

FIGURE **7.4** Stress vulnerability questionnaire.

Item	Strongly Agree	Mildly Agree	Mildly Disagree	Strongly Disagree
1. I try to incorporate as much physical activity* as possible in my daily schedule.	1	2	3	4
2. I exercise aerobically 20 minutes or more at least three times per week.	1	2	3	4
3. I regularly sleep 7 to 8 hours per night.	1	2	3	4
4. I take my time eating at least one hot, balanced meal a day.	1	2	3	4
5. I drink fewer than two cups of coffee (or equivalent) per day.	1	2	3	4
6. I am at recommended body weight.	1	2	3	4
7. I enjoy good health.	1	2	3	4
8. I do not use tobacco in any form.	1	2	3	4
9. I limit my alcohol intake to no more than one drink per day.	1	2	3	4
10. I do not use hard drugs (chemical dependency).	1	2	3	4
11. I have someone I love, trust, and can rely on for help if I have a problem or need to make an essential decision.	1	2	3	4
12. There is love in my family.	1	2	3	4
13. I routinely give and receive affection.	1	2	3	4
14. I have close personal relationships with other people who provide me with a sense of emotional security.	1	2	3	4
15. There are people close by whom I can turn to for guidance in time of stress.	1	2	3	4
16. I can speak openly about feelings, emotions, and problems with people I trust.	1	2	3	4
17. Other people rely on me for help.	1	2	3	4
18. I am able to keep my feelings of anger and hostility under control.	1	2	3	4
19. I have a network of friends who enjoy the same social activities I do.	1	2	3	4
20. I take time to do something fun at least once a week.	1	2	3	4
21. My religious beliefs provide guidance and strength to my life.	1	2	3	4
22. I often provide service to others.	1	2	3	4
23. I enjoy my job (major or school).	1	2	3	4
24. I am a competent worker.	1	2	3	4
25. I get along well with co-workers (or students).	1	2	3	4
26. My income is sufficient for my needs.	1	2	3	4
27. I manage time adequately.	1	2	3	4
28. I have learned to say "no" to additional commitments when I am already pressed for time.	1	2	3	4
29. I take daily quiet time for myself.	1	2	3	4
30. I practice stress management as needed.	1	2	3	4

Total Points: [ ]

Scoring:

0–30 points	. . . .	Excellent (great resistance to stress)
31–40 points	. . . .	Good (little vulnerability to stress)
41–50 points	. . . .	Average (somewhat vulnerable to stress)
51–60 points	. . . .	Fair (vulnerable to stress)
≥61 points	. . . .	Poor (highly vulnerable to stress)

*Walk instead of driving, avoid escalators and elevators, or walk to neighboring offices, homes, and stores.

From *Lifetime Physical Fitness & Wellness*, by W. W. K. Hoeger and S. A. Hoeger (Belmont, CA: Wadsworth/Thomson Learning, 2007), p. 365.

The benefits of physical fitness have already been discussed extensively in this book. In addition, social support, self-worth, and nurturance (the sense of being needed) are essential to cope effectively with stressful life events. These factors play a supportive and protective role in people's lives and are crucial for a person's physical, social, mental, and emotional well-being. The more integrated people are in society, the less vulnerable they are to stress and illness.

Positive correlations have been found between social support and health outcomes. People can draw upon social support to weather crises. Knowing that someone else cares, that people are there to lean on, that support is out there, is valuable for survival (or growth) in times of need.[4]

As you complete the questionnaire, you will notice that many of the items describe situations and behaviors that are within your own control. To make yourself less vulnerable to stress, you will want to improve the behaviors that make you more vulnerable to stress. You should start by modifying the behaviors that are easiest to change before undertaking some of the most difficult ones.

Sources of Stress

Before addressing techniques that you can use to cope more effectively with stress, attempt to identify your current life stressors using the stress test provided in Figure 7.5. This test will help you determine stressors that you have encountered recently in your life. Think back over this past year and circle the "stress points" listed for each event that you experienced during this time. Then total the points and determine the amount of stress in your life during the past year.

Now, to help you cope more effectively, use the stress analysis form provided in Activity 7.1, page 169. On this form, record the results of your stress questionnaires and list the stressors that affect you the most in your daily life. For each stressor, explain, in the space provided, the situation(s) under which it occurs, your response to it, the impact it is having in your life, and how you presently are handling the stressor. Based on what you have learned already, also indicate what you can do to either avoid the stressor or cope more effectively with it in the future. Common stressors in the lives of college students are depicted in Figure 7.6, page 160.

After completing the exercise in Activity 7.1, proceed to the discussion of relaxation techniques, pages 162–167. Once you have learned and mastered some of these techniques, return to your stress analysis and reevaluate your approach to cope with each stressor.

Regular leisure-time physical activity helps prevent psychological burnout.

Coping with Stress

The ways in which people perceive and cope with stress seem to be more important in the development of disease than the amount and type of stress itself. If individuals perceive stress as a definite problem in their lives, when it interferes with optimal level of health and performance, several techniques can help in coping more effectively.

First, of course, the person must recognize that a problem is present. Many people either do not want to believe they are under too much stress or fail to recognize some of the typical symptoms of distress. Noting some of the stress-related symptoms will help a person respond more objectively and initiate an adequate coping response.

When people have stress-related symptoms, they first should try to identify and remove the stressor or stress-causing agent. This is not as simple as it may seem, because eliminating the stressor may not be possible, or a person may not even know what the stressor

FIGURE **7.5** Stress test.

Take the Stress Test

To get a feel for the possible health impact of the various recent changes in your life, think back over the past year and circle the "stress points" listed for each of the events that you experienced during that time. Then add up your points. A total score of anywhere from about 250 to 500 or so would be considered a moderate amount of stress. If you score higher than that, you may face an increased risk of illness; if you score lower than that, consider yourself fortunate.

Health

An injury or illness which:	
kept you in bed a week or more, or sent you to the hospital	74
was less serious than that	44
Major dental work	26
Major change in eating habits	27
Major change in sleeping habits	26
Major change in your usual type or amount of recreation	28

Work

Change to a new type of work	51
Change in your work hours or conditions	35
Change in your responsibilities at work:	
more responsibilities	29
fewer responsibilities	21
promotion	31
demotion	42
transfer	32
Troubles at work:	
with your boss	29
with co-workers	35
with persons under your supervision	35
other work troubles	28
Major business adjustment	60
Retirement	52
Loss of job:	
laid off from work	68
fired from work	79
Correspondence course to help you in your work	18

Home and Family

Major change in living conditions	42
Change in residence:	
move within the same town or city	25
move to a different town, city, or state	47
Change in family get-togethers	25
Major change in health or behavior of family member	55
Marriage	50
Pregnancy	67
Miscarriage or abortion	85
Gain of a new family member:	
birth of a child	66
adoption of a child	65
a relative moving in with you	59
Spouse beginning or ending work	46
Child leaving home:	
to attend college	41
due to marriage	41
for other reasons	45
Change in arguments with spouse	50
In-law problems	38
Change in the marital status of your parents:	
divorce	59
remarriage	50
Separation from spouse:	
due to work	53
due to marital problems	76
Divorce	96
Birth of grandchild	43
Death of spouse	119
Death of other family member:	
child	123
brother or sister	102
parent	100

Personal and social

Change in personal habits	26
Beginning or ending school or college	38
Change of school or college	35
Change in political beliefs	24
Change in religious beliefs	29
Change in social activities	27
Vacation trip	24
New, close, personal relationship	37
Engagement to marry	45
Girlfriend or boyfriend problems	39
Sexual difficulties	44
"Falling out" of a close personal relationship	47
An accident	48
Minor violation of the law	20
Being held in jail	75
Death of a close friend	70
Major decision about your immediate future	51
Major personal achievement	36

Financial

Major change in finances:	
increased income	38
decreased income	60
investment or credit difficulties	56
Loss or damage of personal property	43
Moderate purchase	20
Major purchase	37
Foreclosure on a mortgage or loan	58

Total Score: [   ]

Source: Reprinted from the *Journal of Psychosomatic Research*, Vol. 43, Miller and Rahe, "Life Changes Scaling for the 1990's," 1997, with permission from Elserier Science.

F I G U R E **7.6** Stressors in the lives of college students.

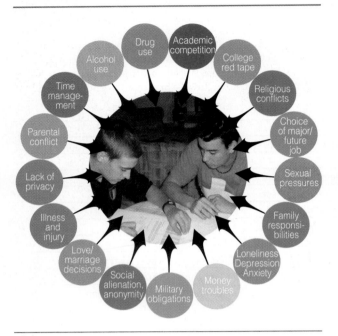

Adapted from W. W. K. Hoeger, L. W. Turner, and B. Q. Hafen. *Wellness: Guidelines for a Healthy Lifestyle* (Belmont, CA: Wadsworth/Thomson Learning, 2002).

is. If the cause is unknown, keeping a log of the time and days when the symptoms arise, as well as the events preceding and following the onset of symptoms, might be helpful.

For instance, a couple noted that every afternoon around 6 o'clock, the wife became nauseated and had abdominal pain. After seeking professional help, both were instructed to keep a log of daily events. It soon became clear that the symptoms did not appear on weekends but always started just before the husband came home from work during the week. Following some personal interviews with the couple, it was determined that the wife felt a lack of attention from her husband and responded subconsciously by becoming ill to the degree that she required personal attention and affection from her husband. Once the stressor was identified, they initiated appropriate behavior changes to correct the situation.

In many instances, however, the stressor cannot be removed. Examples of situations in which little or nothing can be done to eliminate the stress-causing agent are the death of a close family member, first year on the job, an intolerable boss, a change in work responsibility. Nevertheless, stress can be managed through time management and relaxation techniques.

Common Symptoms of Stress

- headaches
- muscular aches (mainly in neck, shoulders, and back)
- grinding teeth
- nervous tic, finger-tapping, toe-tapping
- increased sweating
- increase in or loss of appetite
- insomnia
- nightmares
- fatigue
- dry mouth
- stuttering
- high blood pressure
- tightness or pain in the chest
- impotence
- hives
- dizziness
- depression
- irritation
- anger
- hostility
- fear, panic, anxiety
- stomach pain, flutters
- nausea
- cold, clammy hands
- poor concentration
- pacing
- restlessness
- rapid heart rate
- low-grade infection
- loss of sex drive
- rash or acne

Time Management

According to Benjamin Franklin, "Time is the stuff life is made of." The current "hurry-up" style of life is not conducive to wellness. The hassles involved in getting through a typical day often lead to stress-related illnesses. People who do not manage their time properly may experience chronic stress, fatigue, despair, discouragement, and illness.

Based on various national surveys, most Americans report that time moves too fast for them and more than half of those surveyed think they have to get everything done. The younger the respondents, the more they struggled with lack of time. Almost half wished they had more time for exercise and recreation, hobbies, and family.

Healthy and successful people are good time managers, able to maintain a pace of life within their comfort zone. In a survey of 1954 Harvard graduates from the school of business, only 27 percent had reached the goals they established in college. All of these successful graduates had rated themselves superior time managers, and only 8 percent of the remaining graduates perceived themselves as superior time managers. The successful graduates attributed their success to "smart work," not necessarily "hard work."

Trying to achieve one or more goals in a limited time can create a tremendous amount of stress. Many people just don't seem to have enough hours in the day to accomplish their tasks. The greatest demands on our time, nonetheless, frequently are self-imposed—trying to do too much, too fast, too soon.

Although some time killers—such as eating, sleeping, and recreation—are necessary for health and wellness, in excess they will cause stress. To make better use of your time:

1. Find the time killers. Many people do not know how they spend each part of the day. Keep a 4- to 7-day log and record your activities at half-hour intervals. As you go through your typical day, record the activities so you will remember all of them. At the end of each day, decide when you wasted time. You might be shocked by the amount of time you spent on the phone, sleeping (more than 8 hours per night), or watching television.

2. Set long-range and short-range goals. Setting goals requires some in-depth thinking and helps put your life and daily tasks in perspective. Write down three goals that you want to accomplish: (a) in life, (b) 10 years from now, (c) this year, (d) this month, and (e) this week. You may want to file this form and review it in years to come.

3. Identify your immediate goals and prioritize them for today and this week. Each day, sit down and determine what you need to accomplish that day and that week. Rank your "today" and "this week" tasks in three categories: (a) top-priority, (b) medium-priority, and (c) "trash." Top-priority tasks are clearly the most important ones. If you were to reap most of your productivity from 30 percent

Planning and prioritizing your daily activities simplifies your days.

© Fitness & Wellness, Inc.

of your activities, which would they be? Medium-priority activities must be done but can wait a day or two. Trash activities are those that are not worth your time (for example, cruising the hallways).

4. Use a daily planner to help you organize and simplify your day. In this way you can access your priority list, appointments, notes, references, names, places, phone numbers, and addresses conveniently from your coat pocket or purse. Many individuals think that planning daily and weekly activities is a waste of time. A few minutes to schedule your time each day, however, will pay off in hours saved.

As you plan your day, be realistic and find your comfort zone. Determine what is the best way to organize your day. Which is the most productive time for work, study, errands? Are you a morning person, or are you getting most of your work done when other people are quitting for the day? Pick your best hours for top-priority activities. Be sure to schedule enough time for exercise and relaxation. Recreation is not necessarily wasted time. You need to take care of your physical and emotional well-being. Otherwise your life will be seriously imbalanced.

5. Take 10 minutes each night to figure out how well you accomplished your goals that day. Successful time managers evaluate themselves daily. This simple task will help you see the entire picture. Cross off the goals you accomplished and carry over

Common Time Killers

- watching television
- listening to radio/music
- sleeping
- eating
- daydreaming
- shopping
- socializing/parties
- recreation
- talking on the telephone
- worrying
- procrastinating
- drop-in visitors
- confusion (unclear goals)
- indecision (what to do next)
- interruptions
- perfectionism (every detail must be done)

to the next day those you did not get done. You also may realize that some goals can be moved down to low-priority or be trashed.

In addition to the above steps, the following general suggestions can help you make better use of your time:

- *Delegate.* When possible, delegate activities that someone else can do for you. Having another person type your paper while you prepare for an exam might be well worth the expense and your time.
- *Say "no."* Learn to say no to activities that keep you from getting your top priorities done. You can do only so much in a single day. Nobody has enough time to do everything he or she would like to get done. Don't overload either. Many people are afraid to say no because they feel guilty if they do. Think ahead, and think of the consequences. Are you doing it to please others? What will it do to your well-being? Can you handle one more task? At some point you have to balance your activities and look at life and time realistically.
- *Protect against boredom.* Doing nothing can be a source of stress. People need to feel that they are contributing and that they are productive members of society. It also is good for self-esteem and self-worth. Set realistic goals and work toward them each day.
- *Plan ahead for disruptions.* Even a careful plan of action can be disrupted. An unexpected phone call or

visitor can ruin your schedule. Planning your response ahead of time will help you deal with these saboteurs.

- *Get it done.* Select only one task at a time, concentrate on it, and see it through. Many people do a little here, a little there, then do something else. In the end, nothing gets done. An exception to working on just one task at a time is when you are doing a difficult task. Rather than "killing yourself," interchange with another activity that is not as hard.
- *Eliminate distractions.* If you have trouble adhering to a set plan, remove distractions and trash activities from your eyesight. Television, radio, computers, magazines, open doors, or studying in a park might distract you and become time killers.
- *Set aside "overtimes."* Regularly schedule time you did not think you would need as overtime to complete unfinished projects. Most people underschedule rather than overschedule time. The result is usually late-night burnout! If you schedule overtimes and get your tasks done, enjoy some leisure time, get ahead on another project, or work on some of your trash priorities. Plan time for you.
- *Set aside special time for yourself daily.* Life is not meant to be all work. Use your special time to walk, read, or listen to your favorite music.
- *Reward yourself.* As with any other healthy behavior, positive change or a job well done deserves a reward. We often overlook the value of rewards, even if they are self-given. People practice behaviors that are rewarded and discontinue those that are not.

Relaxation Techniques

Stress management skills are essential to cope effectively and move forward in today's fast-paced world. Although you may reap benefits immediately after engaging in any of the several relaxation techniques described in this chapter, several months of regular practice may be necessary for total mastery. The relaxation exercises that follow should not be considered cure-alls or panaceas. If they do not prove to be effective, more specialized resources and professional help are indicated. In some instances a person's symptoms may not be caused by stress but, rather, may be related to an undiagnosed medical disorder.

Physical Activity

Physical exercise is one of the simplest tools to control stress. Exercise and fitness are thought to reduce the intensity of stress and recovery from a stressful event. The value of exercise in reducing stress is related to several factors, the main one being less muscular tension.

Imagine you are distressed after a miserable day at work. The job requires 8 hours of work with an intolerable boss. To make matters worse, it is late and on the way home the car in front of you is going much slower than the speed limit. The body's fight-or-flight mechanism is activated. Your heart rate and blood pressure shoot up, your breathing quickens and deepens, your muscles tense, and all systems say "go." Under the circumstances, you can take no action, and the stress will not be dissipated because you simply cannot hit your boss or the car in front of you. Instead, you could take action by "hitting" the tennis ball, the weights, the swimming pool, or the jogging trail. By engaging in physical activity, you are able to reduce the muscular tension and eliminate the physiological changes that triggered the fight-or-flight mechanism.

Physical exercise gives people an overall boost by:

● Lessening feelings of anxiety, depression, frustration, aggression, anger, and hostility.
● Alleviating insomnia.
● Providing an opportunity to meet social needs and develop new friendships.
● Allowing people to share common interests and problems.
● Developing self-discipline.
● Providing the opportunity to do something enjoyable and constructive that will lead to better health and total well-being.

Although exercise has enhanced the health and quality of life of millions of people, exercise, for a few, can become an obsessive behavior with potentially addictive qualities. Compulsive exercisers often express feelings of guilt and discomfort when they miss a day's workout. These individuals sometimes continue to exercise even when they are injured or ill and should get proper rest for adequate recovery. Under these circumstances, exercise becomes a biological stressor that will compromise performance and health. As a biological stressor, compulsive exercise or overtraining produces both physiological and psychological symptoms. Many physical activities (for example, jogging, basketball, aerobics) performed at high-intensity levels or for unusually long periods (overtraining) can be detrimental to a person's physical and emotional well-being.

Psychological symptoms of overtraining include lower motivation, depression, sleep disturbances, increased irritability, and lack of confidence. Physiological symptoms include musculoskeletal injuries, lower performance, slower recovery time, chronic fatigue, decreased appetite, loss of weight and lean tissue, fat gain, increased muscle tension, higher resting heart rate and blood pressure, and even ECG abnormalities. If

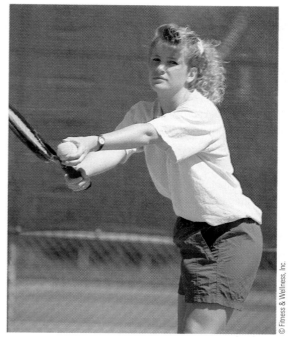

Physical activity is an excellent tool to control stress.

© Fitness & Wellness, Inc.

you experience any of these symptoms, you need to re-evaluate your exercise program and make adjustments accordingly. People who exceed the recommended guidelines for fitness development and maintenance (see Chapters 3 and 4) are exercising for reasons other than health, and some actually may be aggravating an already stressful situation.

Progressive Muscle Relaxation

One of the most popular methods used to dissipate stress is **progressive muscle relaxation**, which enables individuals to relearn the sensation of deep relaxation. Acute awareness of how it feels to progressively tighten and relax the muscles releases muscle tension and teaches the body to relax at will. Feeling the tension during the exercises also helps the person to be more alert to signs of distress, because this tension is similar to that experienced in stressful situations. In everyday life, these feelings then can cue the person to do relaxation exercises.

Relaxation exercises should be done in a quiet, warm, well-ventilated room. The exercises should

KEY TERMS

Progressive muscle relaxation A relaxation technique that involves contracting, then relaxing muscle groups in the body in succession.

Characteristics of Good Stress Managers

Good stress managers

- are physically active, eat a healthy diet, and get adequate rest every day.

- believe they have control over events in their life (have an internal locus of control, see pages 14–16).

- understand their own feelings and accept their limitations.

- recognize, anticipate, monitor, and regulate stressors within their capabilities.

- control emotional and physical responses when distressed.

- use appropriate stress management techniques when confronted with stressors.

- recognize warning signs and symptoms of excessive stress.

- schedule daily time to unwind, relax, and evaluate the day's activities.

- control stress when called upon to perform.

- enjoy life despite occasional disappointments and frustrations.

- look success and failure squarely in the face and keep moving along a predetermined course.

- move ahead with optimism and energy and do not spend time and talent worrying about failure.

- learn from previous mistakes and use them as building blocks to prevent similar setbacks in the future.

- give of themselves freely to others.

- find deep meaning in life.

encompass all muscle groups of the body. Most important is to pay attention to the sensation you feel each time you tense and relax your muscles.

The instructions can be read to the person, or memorized, or tape-recorded. You should set aside at least 20 minutes to complete the entire sequence. Doing the exercises any faster will defeat their purpose. Ideally, you should complete the sequence twice a day.

First, stretch out comfortably on the floor, face up, with a pillow under your knees, and assume a passive attitude, allowing your body to relax as much as possible. Then contract each muscle group in sequence, taking care to avoid any strain. Tighten each muscle to only about 70 percent of the total possible tension to avoid cramping or some type of injury to the muscle itself.

To produce the relaxation effects, pay attention to the sensation of tensing and relaxing. Hold each contraction about 5 seconds, then allow the muscles to go totally limp. Take enough time to contract and relax each muscle group before going on to the next. An example of a complete progressive muscle relaxation sequence is as follows:

1. Point your feet, curling your toes downward. Study the tension in the arches and top of your feet. Hold, continue to note the tension, then relax. Repeat once.

2. Flex the feet upward toward your face, and note the tension in your feet and calves. Hold and relax. Repeat once.

3. Push your heels down against the floor as if burying them in the sand. Hold and note the tension at the back of the thigh. Relax. Repeat once.

4. Contract your right thigh by straightening your leg, gently raising your leg off the floor. Hold and study the tension. Relax. Repeat with the left leg. Hold and relax. Repeat each leg once.

5. Tense your buttocks by raising your hips ever so slightly off the floor. Hold and note the tension. Relax. Repeat once.

6. Contract your abdominal muscles. Hold them tight and note the tension. Relax. Repeat once.

7. Suck in your stomach. Try to make it reach your spine. Flatten your lower back to the floor. Hold and feel the tension in the stomach and lower back. Relax. Repeat once.

8. Take a deep breath and hold it, then exhale. Repeat. Note your breathing becoming slower and more relaxed.

9. Place your arms at the side of your body and clench both fists. Hold, study the tension, and relax. Repeat once.

10. Flex the elbow by bringing both hands to your shoulders. Hold tight and study the tension in the biceps. Relax. Repeat once.

11. Place your arms flat on the floor, palms up, and push the forearms hard against the floor. Note the tension on the triceps. Hold and relax. Repeat once.

12. Shrug your shoulders, raising them as high as possible. Hold and note the tension. Relax. Repeat once.

13. Gently push your head backward. Note the tension in the back of the neck. Hold, then relax. Repeat once.

14. Gently bring the head against the chest, push forward, hold, and note the tension in the neck. Relax. Repeat once.

15. Press your tongue toward the roof of your mouth. Hold, study the tension, and relax. Repeat once.

16. Press your teeth together. Hold and study the tension. Relax. Repeat once.
17. Close your eyes tightly. Hold them closed and note the tension. Relax, leaving your eyes closed. Repeat once.
18. Wrinkle your forehead and note the tension. Hold and relax. Repeat once.

When time is a factor during the daily routine and you are not able to go through the entire sequence, you may do only the exercises specific to the area that feels most tense. Performing a partial sequence is better than not doing the exercises at all. Completing the entire sequence, of course, yields the best results.

Breathing Techniques

Breathing exercises, too, can be an antidote to stress. These exercises have been used for centuries in Asian countries to improve mental, physical, and emotional stamina. In breathing exercises the person concentrates on "breathing away" the tension and inhaling fresh air to the entire body. Breathing exercises can be learned in only a few minutes and require considerably less time than the progressive muscle relaxation exercises.

As with any other relaxation technique, these exercises should be done in a quiet, pleasant, well-ventilated room. Any of the three examples of breathing exercises presented here will help relieve tension induced by stress.

Deep Breathing

Lie with your back flat against the floor and place a pillow under your knees, feet slightly separated, with your toes pointing outward. (This exercise also may be done while sitting up in a chair or standing straight up.) Place one hand on your abdomen and the other hand on your chest. Breathe in and out slowly so the hand on your abdomen rises when you inhale and falls as you exhale. The hand on your chest should not move much at all. Repeat the exercise about 10 times. Then scan your body for tension and compare your present tension with the tension you felt at the beginning of the exercise. Repeat the entire process once or twice.

Sighing

Using the abdominal breathing technique, breathe in through your nose to a specific count (such as 4, 5, or 6). Now exhale through pursed lips to double the intake count (such as 8, 10, or 12). Repeat the exercise 8 to 10 times whenever you feel tense.

Complete Natural Breathing

Sit in an upright position or stand straight up. Breathing through your nose, fill your lungs gradually from the bottom up. Hold your breath for several seconds. Now exhale slowly by allowing your chest and abdomen to relax completely. Repeat the exercise 8 to 10 times.

Meditation

More than 700 scientific studies have verified that meditation induces relaxation and alleviates the harmful physiological effects of stress. **Meditation** is a mental exercise that can bring about psychological and physical benefits. Regular meditation has been shown to decrease blood pressure, stress, anger, anxiety, fear, negative feelings, chronic pain, and increase activity in the brain's left frontal region—an area associated with positive emotions.[5] The objective of meditation is to gain control over one's attention by clearing the mind and blocking out the stressor(s) responsible for the higher tension.

This technique can be learned rather quickly and can be used frequently during times of increased stress. Initially, choose a room that is comfortable, quiet, and free of all disturbances (including telephones). After learning the technique, you will be able to meditate just about anywhere. A time block of approximately 15 minutes, twice a day, is suggested for meditation.

1. Sit in a chair or in a quiet place in an upright position with your hands resting either in your lap or on the arms of the chair. Close your eyes and focus on your breathing. Allow your body to relax as much as possible. Do not consciously try to relax, because trying means work. Rather, assume a passive attitude and concentrate on your breathing.
2. Allow your body to breathe regularly, at its own rhythm, and repeat in your mind the word "one" every time you inhale, and the word "two" every time you exhale. Paying attention to these two words keeps distressing thoughts from entering into your mind.
3. Continue to breathe in this way about 15 minutes. Because the objective of meditation is to bring about a hypometabolic (slower metabolism) state leading to body relaxation, do not use an alarm clock to remind you that the 15 minutes have expired. The

KEY TERMS

Meditation A mental exercise in which the objective is to gain control over one's attention, clearing the mind and blocking out stressors.

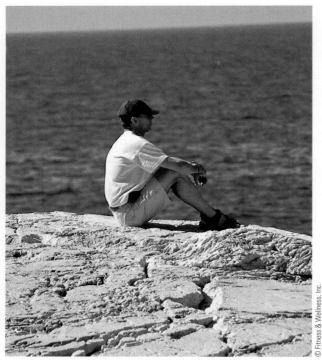

Meditation is an effective stress-coping technique.

© Fitness & Wellness, Inc.

alarm will only trigger the stress response again, defeating the purpose of the exercise. Opening your eyes once in a while to keep track of the time is fine, but do not rush or anticipate the end of the 15 minutes. This time has been set aside for meditation, and you need to relax, take your time, and enjoy the exercise.

CT Critical Thinking

List the most significant stressor that you face as a college student. What technique(s) have you used to manage this situation, and in what way has it helped you cope?

Yoga

Yoga is an excellent stress-coping technique. **Yoga** is a school of thought in the Hindu religion that seeks to help the individual attain a higher level of spirituality and peace of mind. Although its philosophical roots can be considered spiritual, yoga is based on principles of self-care.

Yoga practitioners adhere to a specific code of ethics and a system of mental and physical exercises that promote control of the mind and the body. In Western countries, many people are mainly familiar with the exercise portion of yoga. This system of exercises (postures) can be used as a relaxation technique for stress management. The exercises include a combination of postures, diaphragmatic breathing, muscle relaxation, and meditation that help buffer the biological effects of stress.

Western interest in yoga exercises gradually developed over the last century, particularly since the 1970s. People pursue yoga exercises for their potential to dispel stress by raising self-esteem, clearing the mind, slowing respiration, promoting neuromuscular relaxation, and increasing body awareness. In addition, the exercises help control involuntary body functions including heart rate, blood pressure, oxygen consumption, and metabolic rate. Doing yoga exercises can increase muscular flexibility, muscular strength and endurance, and balance, and provide a better-aligned musculoskeletal system.[6] Yoga is also used in many hospital-based programs for cardiac patients to help manage stress and decrease blood pressure.

Further, yoga exercises have been used to help treat chemical dependency and insomnia, and to prevent injury. Research on patients with coronary heart disease who practiced yoga (among other lifestyle changes) has shown that it slows or even reverses atherosclerosis.[7] These patients were compared with others who did not use yoga as one of the lifestyle changes.

There are many different styles of yoga. Classes vary according to their emphasis. Some styles of yoga are athletic, and others are passive in nature. The most popular variety in the Western world is **hatha yoga**, which incorporates a series of static-stretching postures performed in specific sequences (also known as "asanas") that help induce the relaxation response. Participants hold the postures for several seconds while concentrating on breathing patterns, meditation, and body awareness.

Most yoga classes are now variations of hatha yoga, and many of the typical stretches used in flexibility exercises today have been adapted from hatha yoga. Examples include:

1. *integral yoga* and *viny yoga*, which focus on gentle/static stretches,
2. *iyengar yoga*, which promotes muscular strength and endurance,
3. *yogalates*, incorporating Pilates exercises to increase muscular strength, and
4. *power yoga* or *yogarobics*, a high-energy form that links many postures together in a dance-like routine to promote cardiorespiratory fitness.

As with flexibility exercises, the stretches in hatha yoga should not be performed to the point of discomfort. Instructors should not push participants beyond

Yoga exercises help induce the relaxation response.

their physical limitations. Similar to other stress management techniques, yoga exercises are best performed in a quiet place for about 15 to 60 minutes per session. Many yoga participants like to perform the exercises daily.

To appreciate yoga exercise, a person has to experience it. We are only introducing yoga here. Although participants can practice yoga exercises with the instruction of a book or video, most participants take classes. Many of the postures are difficult and complex, and few individuals can master the entire sequence in the first few weeks.

Individuals who are interested in yoga exercise should initially pursue it under qualified instruction. Many colleges and universities offer yoga courses, and you also can check the phone book for a listing of yoga instructors or classes. Yoga courses are offered at many health clubs and recreation centers. Because instructors and yoga styles vary, you may want to observe a class before enrolling. You should look for an instructor whose views on wellness parallel your own. There are no national certification standards for instructors. If you are new to yoga, you are encouraged to compare a couple of instructors before you select a class.

Which Technique Is Best?

Each person reacts to stress differently. Therefore, the best strategy to alleviate stress depends mostly on the individual. Which technique you use does not matter as long as it works. You may want to experiment with all of them to find out which works best for you. Many people choose a combination of two or more.

All of the strategies discussed in this chapter help to block out stressors and promote mental and physical relaxation by diverting the attention to a different, non-threatening action. Some of the techniques are easier to learn and take less time per session. Regardless of which technique you select, the time you spend doing stress management exercises (several times a day, as needed) is well worth the effort when stress becomes a significant problem in your life.

People need to learn to relax and take time for themselves. What makes people ill is not stress itself but, instead, the way they react to the stress-causing agent. Individuals who are diligent and start taking control of themselves find that they can enjoy a better, happier, and healthier life.

KEY TERMS

Yoga A school of thought in the Hindu religion that seeks to help the individual attain a higher level of spirituality and peace of mind.

Hatha yoga A yoga style that incorporates a series of static-stretching postures performed in specific sequences.

Stress Assess. This is a three-part online educational tool developed by the National Wellness Institute at the University of Wisconsin–Steven's Point. This questionnaire is designed to increase your knowledge about stress and features separate evaluations for stress sources, distress symptoms, and stress-balancing strategies. Based on these results, you will learn healthy strategies to better manage your specific stressors.
http://wellness.uwsp.edu/other/stress

Are You Under Stress? Take the Discovery Health stress questionnaire to find out your level. The site offers 17 tips for dealing with stress and lists other online stress resources.
http://health.discovery.com/centers/stress/stress.html

ASSESS YOUR KNOWLEDGE

Evaluate how well you understand the concepts presented in this chapter using the Assess Your Knowledge and Practice Quizzes options on your Profile Plus CD-ROM.

1. Positive stress is also referred to as
   a. eustress.
   b. poststress.
   c. functional stress.
   d. distress.
   e. physiostress.

2. Which of the following is not a stage of the general adaptation syndrome?
   a. alarm reaction
   b. resistance
   c. compliance
   d. exhaustion/recovery
   e. All are stages of the general adaptation syndrome.

3. Which of the following characteristics seems to cause the greatest increase in the risk for illness among Type A individuals?
   a. hard-driven
   b. overly ambitious
   c. chronic hostility
   d. overly competitive
   e. All increase the risk equally.

4. Effective time managers
   a. delegate.
   b. learn to say "no."
   c. protect against boredom.
   d. set aside "overtimes."
   e. do all of the above.

5. Hormonal changes that occur during a stress response
   a. decrease heart rate.
   b. increase blood pressure.
   c. diminish blood flow to the muscles.
   d. induce relaxation.
   e. sap the body's strength.

6. Exercise decreases stress levels by
   a. deliberately diverting stress to various body systems.
   b. metabolizing excess catecholamines.
   c. diminishing muscular tension.
   d. stimulating alpha-wave activity in the brain.
   e. doing all of the above.

7. Which of the following exercises is included in the progressive muscle relaxation technique?
   a. pointing the feet
   b. wrinkling the forehead
   c. contracting the abdominal muscles
   d. pressing the teeth together
   e. All of the above exercises are used.

8. The technique in which a person breathes in through the nose to a specific count and then exhales through pursed lips to double the intake count is known as
   a. sighing.
   b. deep breathing.
   c. meditation.
   d. autonomic ventilation.
   e. release management.

9. Meditation
   a. induces relaxation.
   b. alleviates the harmful physiological effects of stress.
   c. can be performed just about anywhere.
   d. incorporates breathing exercises.
   e. includes all of the above statements.

10. Yoga exercises have been used successfully to
    a. stimulate ventilation.
    b. increase metabolism during stress.
    c. slow down atherosclerosis.
    d. decrease body awareness.
    e. accomplish all of the above.

Correct answers can be found on page 261.

Stress Analysis

Name _____ Date _____

Course _____ Section _____

I. Record your results and stress categories for each questionnaire given in this chapter.

	Points	**Category**

Hostility (see Figure 7.3, page 155): _____ _____ (≤ 3 = Good, ≥ 4 = High)

Anger (see Figure 7.3, page 155): _____ _____ (≤ 1 = Good, ≥ 2 = High)

Aggression (see Figure 7.3, page 155): _____ _____ (≤ 1 = Good, ≥ 2 = High)

Cynicism (see Figure 7.3, page 155): _____ _____ (≤ 1 = Good, ≥ 2 = High)

Stress Vulnerability
(see Figure 7.4, page 157): _____ _____ (0–30 = Excellent, 31–40 = Good, 41–50 = Average, 51–60 = Fair, ≥ 61 = Poor)

Stress Test (see Figure 7.5, page 159): _____ _____ (≤ 249 = low risk, ≥ 250–500 = moderate risk, >500 = high risk)

II. Life stressor. In the space provided below, list a stressor you frequently encounter in life. Explain the situation(s) under which it occurs, your response to it, the impact it has on your life, and how you presently are handling the stressor. Also indicate what you can do to either avoid the stressor or cope with it more effectively in the future.

_____

_____

_____

_____

_____

_____

_____

_____

_____

_____

_____

_____

_____

_____

III. In your own words, express how life stresses and your personality affect you in your daily life.

_____

_____

_____

_____

_____

_____

_____

_____

_____

_____

_____

IV. In the space provided below, list in order of priority, three behaviors that you would like to change to decrease your vulnerability to stress. Briefly indicate how you intend to accomplish these changes.

_____

_____

_____

_____

_____

V. Indicate how you plan to accomplish the changes listed in item IV above.

_____

_____

_____

_____

_____

_____

_____

_____

_____

VI. Number of current daily steps: [_____]

CHAPTER 8

A Healthy Lifestyle Approach

OBJECTIVES

- Understand the importance of implementing a healthy lifestyle program.
- Recognize the relationship between spirituality and wellness.
- Identify the major risk factors for coronary heart disease.
- Be able to differentiate physiological age and chronological age.
- Become acquainted with cancer-prevention guidelines.
- Learn the health consequences of chemical abuse and irresponsible sex.

Determine your risk for heart disease, plan for a smoke free future, assess your cancer risks, and test your understanding of HIV/AIDS with the activities on your CD-ROM.

mproving our health—the quality, and most likely the length, of our lives—is a matter of personal choice. The wellness approach—the combination of a fitness program and a healthy lifestyle program can help accomplish these goals.

A Wellness Lifestyle

Wellness is the constant and deliberate effort to stay healthy and achieve the highest potential for well-being. Ten simple lifestyle habits can increase longevity significantly:

1. Be physically active (including exercise).
2. Do not use tobacco.
3. Eat a healthy diet.
4. Maintain recommended body weight.
5. Sleep 7 to 8 hours each night.
6. Decrease your stress level.
7. Drink alcohol moderately or not at all.
8. Surround yourself with healthy relationships.
9. Be informed about the environment and avoid environmental risk factors.
10. Take personal safety measures.

Spiritual Well-Being

To enjoy a wellness lifestyle, a person has to practice behaviors that will lead to positive outcomes in the seven dimensions of wellness: physical, emotional, intellectual, social, environmental, occupational, and spiritual. These dimensions are interrelated; one dimension frequently affects the others. For example, a person who is "emotionally down" often has no desire to exercise, study, socialize with friends, or attend church and may be more susceptible to illness and disease. Because spirituality plays an important role and has not been discussed thus far, it merits some attention.

The definition of **spirituality** by the National Interfaith Coalition on Aging encompasses Christians and non-Christians alike. It assumes that all people are spiritual in nature. Spiritual health provides a unifying power that integrates the other dimensions of wellness (see Figure 8.1). Basic characteristics of spiritual people include a sense of meaning and direction in life, a relationship to a higher being, freedom, prayer, faith, love, closeness to others, peace, joy, fulfillment, and altruism.

Religion has been a major part of cultures since the beginning of time. Although not everyone claims an affiliation with a certain religion or denomination, various surveys indicate that more than 90 percent of the U. S. population believes in God or a universal spirit functioning as God. People, furthermore, believe to a varying extent that (a) a relationship with God is meaningful; (b) God can grant help, guidance, and assistance in daily living; and (c) mortal existence has a purpose. If we accept any or all of these statements, attaining spirituality will have a definite effect on our happiness and well-being. Although the reasons why religious affiliation enhances wellness are difficult to determine, possible reasons include the promotion of healthy lifestyle behaviors, social support, assistance in times of crisis and need, and counseling to overcome one's weaknesses.

Altruism—a key attribute of spiritual people— seems to enhance health and longevity. Altruism has been the focus of several studies. Researchers believe that doing good for others is good for oneself, especially for the immune system. In a classic study of more than 2,700 people in Michigan,[1] the investigators found that people who did regular volunteer work lived longer. People who did not volunteer regularly (at least once a week) had a 250 percent greater mortality risk during the course of the study. In this same study, the authors found that the health benefits of altruism could be so powerful that even just watching films of altruistic endeavors enhances the formation of an immune system chemical that helps fight disease.

The relationship between spirituality and wellness, therefore, is meaningful in our quest for a better quality

FIGURE **8.1** Components of spiritual well-being.

of life. As with other parameters of wellness, optimum spirituality requires development of the spiritual nature to its fullest potential.

Causes of Death

Of all deaths in the United States, more than 57 percent are caused by cardiovascular disease and cancer.[2] Close to 80 percent of these deaths could be prevented by following a healthy lifestyle. The third and fourth leading causes of death—chronic lower respiratory disease (CLRD) and accidents—also are preventable, primarily by abstaining from tobacco and other drugs, wearing seat belts, and using common sense. Eight of the nine underlying causes of death in the United States[3] (see Figure 8.2) are related to lifestyle and lack of common sense. The "big three"—tobacco use, poor diet and inactivity, and alcohol abuse—are responsible for more than 632,000 deaths annually.

Diseases of the Cardiovascular System

The most prevalent degenerative conditions in the United States are **cardiovascular diseases**. Based on 2003 vital statistics, almost 35 percent of all deaths in the United States were attributable to diseases of the heart and blood vessels.[4] Approximately 1.4 million people die of cardiovascular diseases in the United States each year.

Types of Cardiovascular Disease and Their Prevalence

Examples of cardiovascular diseases are coronary heart disease, heart attack, peripheral vascular disease, congenital heart disease, rheumatic heart disease, atherosclerosis, strokes, high blood pressure, and congestive

FIGURE **8.2** Underlying causes of death in the United States.

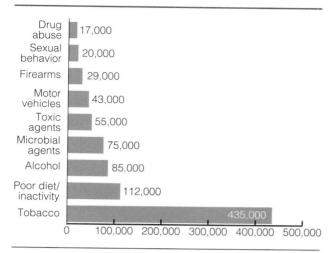

Source: Centers for Disease Control and Prevention, Atlanta.

FIGURE **8.3** Incidence of cardiovascular disease in the United States for selected years, 1900–2000.

TABLE **8.1** Estimated Prevalence and Yearly Number of Deaths from Cardiovascular Disease, 2005

	PREVALENCE	DEATHS
All forms of cardiovascular diseases*	70,100,000	1,400,000
Coronary heart disease	13,000,000**	494,382
Heart attack	1,200,000	
Stroke	5,400,000	162,672
High blood pressure	65,000,000	49,707***

  *Includes people with one or more forms of cardiovascular disease.
 **Number of deaths included under heart attack.
***Mortality figures appear to be low because many heart attacks and stroke
    deaths are caused by high blood pressure.

Source: American Heart Association, *Heart Disease and Stroke Statistics—2005
Update*, (Dallas: AHA).

heart failure. According to estimates from the Centers for Disease Control and Prevention, if all deaths from the major cardiovascular diseases were eliminated, life expectancy in the United States would increase by about 7 years. Table 8.1 provides the estimated prevalence and annual number of deaths caused by the major types of cardiovascular disease.

The American Heart Association estimated that the cost of heart and blood vessel disease in the United States exceeded $393 billion in 2005.[5] About 1.2 million people have heart attacks each year, and about a half a million of these people die as a result. More than half of these deaths occur within an hour of the onset of symptoms, before the person reaches the hospital.

Although heart and blood vessel disease is still the number-one health problem in the United States, the incidence declined by 28 percent between 1960 and 2000 (see Figure 8.3). The main reason for this dramatic decrease is health education. More people now are aware of the risk factors for cardiovascular disease and are changing their lifestyle to lower their potential risk for these diseases.

The heart and the coronary arteries are illustrated in Figure 8.4. The major form of cardiovascular disease is **coronary heart disease (CHD)**. In CHD the arteries that supply the heart muscle with oxygen and nutrients are narrowed by fatty deposits such as cholesterol and triglycerides. Narrowing of the coronary arteries diminishes the blood supply to the heart muscle, which can precipitate a heart attack.

CHD is the single leading cause of death in the United States, accounting for approximately 20 percent of all deaths and about half of all cardiovascular deaths. More than half of the people who died suddenly from

KEY TERMS

Spirituality A sense of meaning and direction in life, a relationship to a higher being; encompasses freedom, prayer, faith, love, closeness to others, peace, joy, fulfillment, and altruism.

Altruism True concern for and action on behalf of others (opposite of egoism); a sincere desire to serve others above one's personal needs.

Cardiovascular diseases The array of conditions that affect the heart and blood vessels.

Coronary heart disease (CHD) Condition in which the arteries that supply the heart muscle with oxygen and nutrients are narrowed by fatty deposits such as cholesterol and triglycerides.

FIGURE **8.4** The heart and its blood vessels.

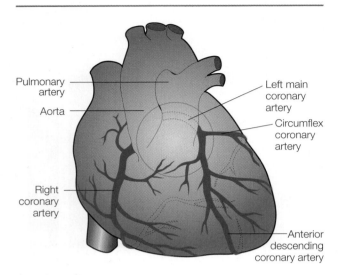

CHD had no previous symptoms of the disease. Further, the risk of death is greater in the least-educated segment of the population.

CT Critical Thinking

What are your feelings about your own risk for diseases of the cardiovascular system? Is this something that you need to concern yourself with at this point in your life? Why or why not?

Risk Factors for CHD

The leading **risk factors** for the development of CHD are:

- Physical inactivity
- High blood pressure
- Excessive body fat
- Low HDL-cholesterol
- Elevated LDL-cholesterol
- Elevated triglycerides
- Elevated homocysteine
- Inflammation
- Diabetes
- Abnormal electrocardiograms (ECG)
- Tobacco use
- Stress
- Personal and family history of cardiovascular disease
- Age
- Gender

Warning Signals of a Heart Attack and Stroke

Any or all of the following signs may occur during a heart attack or a stroke. If you experience any of these and they last longer than a few minutes, call 911 and seek medical attention immediately. Failure to do so may cause irreparable damage and even result in death.

Warning Signs of a Heart Attack

- Chest pain, discomfort, pressure, or squeezing that lasts for several minutes. These feelings may go away and return later.
- Pain that radiates to the shoulders, neck, or arms.
- Chest discomfort with shortness of breath, light-headedness, sweating, nausea, or fainting.

Warning Signs of Stroke

- Sudden weakness or numbness of the face, arm, or leg—particularly on one side of the body.
- Sudden severe headache.
- Sudden confusion, dizziness, or difficulty in speech and understanding.
- Sudden difficulty walking, loss of balance or coordination.
- Sudden visual difficulty.

An important concept in CHD risk management is that many of the risk factors are preventable and reversible. Approximately 90 percent of CHD can be prevented if people practice healthy lifestyle habits. The above risk factors are discussed in the following pages.

Physical Inactivity

Improving cardiorespiratory endurance through aerobic exercise has perhaps the greatest impact in reducing the overall risk for cardiovascular disease. In this day and age of mechanized societies, we cannot afford *not* to be physically active. Research data on the benefits of aerobic exercise in reducing cardiovascular disease are too impressive to be ignored.

Guidelines for implementing an aerobic exercise program are discussed thoroughly in Chapters 3 and 4. Following these guidelines will promote cardiorespiratory fitness, enhance health, and extend the lifespan. Even moderate amounts of aerobic exercise can reduce cardiovascular risk considerably. As shown in Figure 8.5, work conducted at the Aerobics Research Institute in Dallas showed a much higher incidence of cardiovascular deaths in low-fit people as compared to moderate- and high-fit people.[6]

FIGURE **8.5** Relationship between fitness levels and cardiovascular mortality.

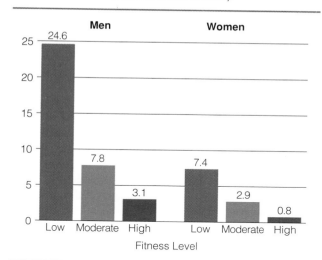

Note: Age-adjusted death rates per 10,000 person-years of follow-up, 1978–1985.

From S. N. Blair, H. W. Kohl, III, R. S. Paffenbarger, Jr., D. B. Clark, D. H. Cooper, and L. W. Gibbons, "Physical Fitness and All-Cause Mortality: A Prospective Study of Healthy Men/Women," *Journal of the American Medical Association* 262 (1989): 2395–2401.

A regular aerobic exercise program helps to control most of the major risk factors that lead to heart and blood vessel disease. Aerobic exercise will:

- increase cardiorespiratory endurance
- decrease and control blood pressure
- reduce body fat
- lower blood lipids (cholesterol and triglycerides)
- improve HDL-cholesterol (see "Abnormal Cholesterol Profile" on page 176)
- decrease low-grade (hidden) inflammation in the body
- help control or decrease the risk for diabetes
- increase and maintain good heart function, sometimes improving certain ECG abnormalities
- encourage smoking cessation
- alleviate stress
- counteract a personal history of heart disease

High Blood Pressure (Hypertension)

Blood pressure should be checked regularly, regardless of whether it is elevated or not. **Blood pressure** is measured in milliliters of mercury (mm Hg) and usually expressed in two numbers. The higher number reflects the **systolic blood pressure**, the pressure exerted during the forceful contraction of the heart. The lower value, **diastolic blood pressure**, is taken during the heart's relaxation phase, when no blood is being ejected.

Ideally, blood pressure is 120/80 or below (see Table 8.2). Most major health organizations consider all blood

TABLE **8.2** Blood Pressure Guidelines (expressed in mm Hg)

RATING	SYSTOLIC	DIASTOLIC
Normal	≤120	≤80
Prehypertension	121–139	81–89
Hypertension	≥140	≥90

Source: National Heart, Lung and Blood Institute.

pressures above 140/90 as **hypertension.** High blood pressure can be controlled with different types of medications, along with the lifestyle changes described below for people with mild hypertension. Because people respond differently to these medications, a physician may try several different medications to find out which produces the best results with the fewest side effects.

Recommended treatment for people with mild hypertension are regular aerobic exercise, weight control, a low-salt/low-fat and high potassium/high-calcium diet, lower alcohol and caffeine intake, smoking cessation, and stress management. People with high blood pressure should follow their physician's advice and stay on any prescribed medication.

Adequate potassium intake seems to regulate water retention and lower blood pressure slightly. According to the Institute of Medicine of the National Academy of Sciences, we need to consume at least 4,700 mg of potassium per day. Most Americans get only half that amount. Food items high in potassium include vegetables (especially leafy green), citrus fruit, dairy products, fish, beans, and nuts.

In terms of salt (sodium) intake, a 2004 government report indicates that, to either prevent or postpone the onset of hypertension, and to help some hypertensives control their blood pressure, we should consume less sodium than previously recommended.[7] Less than 1,500 mg of sodium are now recommended for people between 19 and 50 years of age. The current upper limit (UL) has been set at 2,300 mg per day. Among Americans

KEY TERMS

Risk factors Lifestyle and genetic variables that may lead to disease.

Blood pressure A measure of the force exerted against the walls of the vessels by the blood flowing through them.

Systolic blood pressure Pressure exerted by the blood against the walls of the arteries during the forceful contraction (systole) of the heart.

Diastolic blood pressure Pressure exerted by the blood against the walls of the arteries during the relaxation phase (diastole) of the heart.

Hypertension Chronically elevated blood pressure.

and Canadians, about 95 percent of men and 75 percent of women exceed this limit.

Comprehensive reviews on the effects of aerobic exercise on blood pressure found that, in general, an individual can expect exercise-induced reductions of approximately 4 to 5 mm Hg in resting systolic blood pressure and 3 to 4 mm Hg in resting diastolic blood pressure.[8] Although these reductions do not seem large, a decrease of about 5 mm Hg in resting diastolic blood pressure has been associated with a 40 percent decrease in the risk for stroke and a 15 percent reduction in the risk for coronary heart disease.[9]

Even in the absence of any decrease in resting blood pressure, hypertensive individuals who exercise have a lower risk of all-cause mortality compared to hypertensive/sedentary individuals.[10] Exercise, not weight loss, is the major contributor to the lower blood pressure of exercisers. If the hypertensive/sedentary individuals discontinue aerobic exercise, they do not maintain these changes.

Aerobic exercise programs for hypertensive patients should be of moderate intensity. Training at 40 to 60 percent intensity (12 to 13 on the RPE scale) seems to have the same effect in lowering blood pressure as training at 70 percent. High-intensity training (above 70 percent) in hypertensive patients may not lower the blood pressure as much as moderate-intensity exercise.

Another extensive review of research studies on the effects of at least 4 weeks of strength training on resting blood pressure yielded similar results.[11] Both systolic and diastolic blood pressures decreased by an average of 3 mm Hg. The participants in these studies, however, were primarily individuals with normal blood pressure. Of greater significance, the results showed that strength training did not cause an increase in resting blood pressure. More research remains to be done on hypertensive subjects.

Excessive Body Fat

As defined in Chapter 2, body composition refers to the fat and nonfat components of the human body. If a person has too much fat weight, he or she is overweight or obese. Obesity long has been recognized as a factor contributing to coronary heart disease. The American Heart Association lists obesity as one of the six major risk factors for this disease. The other five risk factors are tobacco smoke, high blood lipids, physical inactivity, high blood pressure, and diabetes mellitus.

Maintaining recommended body weight is essential in any cardiovascular risk-reduction program. For individuals with excessive body fat, even a modest weight reduction of 5 percent to 10 percent can reduce high blood pressure and total cholesterol levels.

The causes of obesity are complex, including an individual's combination of genetics, behavior, and lifestyle factors. Guidelines for a comprehensive weight management program are given in Chapter 6.

Abnormal Cholesterol Profile

The term **blood lipids** is used mainly with reference to cholesterol and triglycerides. Because these substances cannot float around freely in the water-based medium of the blood, they are packaged and transported in the blood by complex molecules called **lipoproteins**. If you never have had a blood lipid test, it is highly recommended. The blood test includes total **cholesterol**, **high-density lipoprotein (HDL)** cholesterol, **low-density lipoprotein (LDL)** cholesterol, and triglycerides. A significant elevation in blood lipids has been linked to heart and blood vessel disease.

A poor blood lipid profile is one of the most important predisposing factors in the development of CHD, accounting for almost half of all cases. The general recommendation by the National Cholesterol Education Program (NCEP) is to keep total cholesterol levels below 200 mg/dl (see Table 8.3). The risk for heart attack increases 2 percent for every 1 percent increase in total cholesterol.[12] Cholesterol levels between 200 and 239 mg/dl are borderline-high, and levels of 240 mg/dl and above indicate high risk for disease. Approximately 42 million American adults have total cholesterol values at or above 240 mg/dl.[13]

Although the average adult in the United States consumes between 400 and 600 mg of cholesterol daily, the body actually manufactures more than that. Saturated fats raise cholesterol levels more than anything else in the diet. The average saturated fat intake in the American diet produces approximately 1,000 mg of cholesterol per day.[14] Because of individual differences, some people can have a higher than normal intake of saturated fats and still maintain normal levels. Others, who have a lower intake, can have abnormally high levels.

As important as it is, total cholesterol is not the most accurate predictor of cardiovascular risk. Many heart attacks occur in people who have only slightly elevated total cholesterol. More significant is the way in which cholesterol is carried in the bloodstream. Cholesterol is transported primarily in the form of high-density lipoprotein (HDL) cholesterol and low-density lipoprotein (LDL) cholesterol.

In a process known as reverse cholesterol transport, HDLs act as "scavengers," removing cholesterol from the body and preventing plaque from forming in the arteries. The strength of HDL is in the protein molecules found in their coatings. When HDL comes in contact

TABLE **8.3** Standards for Blood Lipids

	AMOUNT	RATING
TOTAL CHOLESTEROL	<200 mg/dl	Desirable
	200–239 mg/dl	Borderline high
	≥240 mg/dl	High risk
LDL CHOLESTEROL	<100 mg/dl	Optimal
	100–129 mg/dl	Near or above optimal
	130–159 mg/dl	Borderline high
	160–189 mg/dl	High
	≥190 mg/dl	Very high
HDL CHOLESTEROL	<40 mg/dl	Low (high risk)
	≥60 mg/dl	High (low risk)
TRIGLYCERIDES	≤150 mg/dl	Desirable
	150–199 mg/dl	Borderline-high
	200–499 mg/gl	High
	≥500 mg/dl	High risk

Source: National Cholesterol Education Program.

with cholesterol-filled cells, these protein molecules attach to the cells and take their cholesterol. LDL-cholesterol, on the other hand, tends to release cholesterol, which then may penetrate the lining of the arteries and speed up the process of **atherosclerosis**.

Saturated fats are found mostly in meats and dairy products and seldom in foods of plant origin. Poultry and fish contain less saturated fat than beef does but should be eaten in moderation (about 3 to 6 ounces per day). Unsaturated fats are mainly of plant origin and cannot be converted to cholesterol.

The NCEP guidelines provided in Table 8.3 state that an LDL-cholesterol value below 100 mg/dl is optimal. Values above 160 mg/dl present high risk for cardiovascular disease. A genetic variation of LDL-cholesterol, known as Lp(a), is noteworthy because a high level of these particles leads to earlier development of atherosclerosis. Certain substances in the arterial wall are thought to interact with Lp(a), leading to premature formation of plaque.

The more HDL-cholesterol, the better. HDL-cholesterol, the "good cholesterol," offers some protection against heart disease. Actually, low levels of HDL-cholesterol could be the best predictor of CHD and may be more significant than the total cholesterol value. A low level of HDL-cholesterol has the strongest relationship to CHD at all levels of total cholesterol, including levels below 200 mg/dl.

The recommended HDL-cholesterol values to minimize the risk for CHD are a minimum of 40 mg/dl.

HDL-cholesterol levels above 60 mg/dl actually may reduce the risk for CHD. For the most part, HDL-cholesterol is determined genetically. Generally, women have higher levels than men. The female sex hormone estrogen tends to raise HDL, so pre-menopausal women have a much lower incidence of heart disease. African-American children and adult men have higher HDL values than whites. HDL-cholesterol also decreases with age.

INCREASING HDL-CHOLESTEROL Increasing HDL-cholesterol improves the cholesterol profile and lessens the risk for CHD. Habitual aerobic exercise, weight loss, niacin, and quitting smoking help raise HDL-cholesterol. Drug therapy (see the next page) also may promote higher HDL-cholesterol levels.

HDL-cholesterol and a regular aerobic exercise program clearly are related (high intensity or above 6 METs, for at least 20 minutes three times per week—see Chapters 3 and 4). Individual responses to aerobic exercise differ, but generally, the more you exercise, the higher your HDL-cholesterol level.

LOWERING LDL-CHOLESTEROL When more LDL-cholesterol is present than the cells can use, cholesterol seems not to cause a problem until it is oxidized by **free radicals**. When oxidized, white blood cells invade the arterial wall, take up the cholesterol, and clog the arteries. If LDL-cholesterol is higher than ideal, it can be lowered by losing body fat, manipulating the diet, taking medication, and participating in a regular aerobic exercise program.

The antioxidant effect of vitamins C and E can reduce the risk for CHD. A single unstable free radical (an oxygen compound produced during metabolism) can

KEY TERMS

Blood lipids (fat) Cholesterol and triglycerides.

Lipoproteins Complex molecules that transport cholesterol in the bloodstream.

Cholesterol A waxy substance, technically a steroid alcohol, found only in animal fats and oil; used in making cell membranes, as a building block for some hormones, in the fatty sheath around nerve fibers, and in other necessary substances.

High-density lipoprotein (HDL) Cholesterol-transporting molecules in the blood (good cholesterol).

Low-density lipoprotein (LDL) Cholesterol-transporting molecules in the blood (bad cholesterol).

Atherosclerosis Fatty/cholesterol deposits in the walls of the arteries leading to formation of plaque.

Free radicals Oxygen compounds produced in normal metabolism.

damage LDL particles. Vitamin C seems to inactivate free radicals and slow the oxidation of LDL-cholesterol. Vitamin E may protect LDL from oxidation, preventing heart disease, but studies suggest that it does not seem to be helpful in reversing damage once it has taken place.[15]

Effective medications are also available to treat elevated cholesterol and triglycerides. Most notable among them are the statins group (Lipitor, Mevacor, Pravachol, Lescol, and Zocor), which can lower cholesterol by up to 60 percent in 2 to 3 months. Statins slow down cholesterol production and increase the liver's ability to remove blood cholesterol. They also decrease triglycerides and produce a small increase in HDL levels.

Other drugs effective in reducing LDL-cholesterol are bile acid sequestrants that bind cholesterol found in bile acids. Cholesterol subsequently is excreted in the stools. These drugs are often used in combination with statin drugs.

High doses (1.5 to 3 grams per day) of nicotinic acid or niacin (a B vitamin) also help lower LDL-cholesterol and triglycerides, and increase HDL-cholesterol. (A fourth group of drugs, known as fibrates, is primarily used to lower triglycerides.)

It is better to lower LDL-cholesterol without medication, because drugs can often cause undesirable side effects. People with heart disease often must take cholesterol-lowering medication, but it is best if medication is combined with lifestyle changes to augment the cholesterol-lowering effect.

To decrease LDL-cholesterol, the diet should be low in saturated fat, cholesterol, and trans fatty acids. It should also be high in fiber. Saturated fat should be replaced by monounsaturated and polyunsaturated fats because the latter tend to decrease LDL-cholesterol. Exercise is important, as dietary manipulation by itself is not as effective in lowering LDL-cholesterol as a combination of diet plus aerobic exercise.

Foods that contain trans fatty acids, hydrogenated fat, or partially hydrogenated vegetable oil should be avoided. Studies indicate that these foods elevate cholesterol as much as saturated fats do. Hydrogen is frequently added to monounsaturated and polyunsaturated fats to increase shelf life and to solidify them so they are more spreadable. Margarine and spreads, commercially produced crackers and cookies, dairy products, meats, and fast foods often contain trans fatty acids. The label "partially hydrogenated" and "trans fat" indicates that the product carries a health risk just as high as that of saturated fat.

To have a significant effect in lowering LDL-cholesterol, total daily fiber intake must be in the range of 25 to 38 grams per day (see the discussion of fiber in Chapter 5), total fat consumption can be in the range of 30 percent of total daily caloric intake, as long as most of the fat is unsaturated fat and the average cholesterol consumption is lower than 200 mg per day.

The fiber intake of most people in the United States averages less than 15 grams per day. Fiber, in particular the soluble type, has been shown to lower cholesterol. Soluble fiber dissolves in water and forms a gel-like substance that encloses food particles. This property helps bind and excrete fats from the body. Soluble fibers are found primarily in oats, fruits, barley, legumes, and psyllium.

Psyllium, a grain that is added to some multigrain breakfast cereals, also helps lower LDL-cholesterol. As little as 3 daily grams of psyllium can lower LDL-cholesterol by 20 percent. Commercially available fiber supplements that contain psyllium (such as Metamucil) can be used to increase soluble fiber intake. Three daily tablespoons will add about 10 grams of soluble fiber to the diet.

The incidence of heart disease is low in populations in which daily fiber intake exceeds 30 grams per day. Further, a 1996 Harvard University Medical School study on 43,000 middle-aged men who were followed for more than 6 years showed that increasing fiber intake to 30 daily grams resulted in a 41 percent reduction in heart attacks.[16]

Research on the effects of a 30 percent-fat diet has shown that it has little or no effect in lowering cholesterol, and that CHD actually continues to progress in people who have the disease. Thus, some practitioners recommend a 10 percent or less fat-calorie diet combined with aerobic exercise program while trying to lower cholesterol.

A daily 10 percent-total-fat diet requires the person to limit fat intake to an absolute minimum. This type of diet is difficult to follow indefinitely. People with high cholesterol levels, however, may not have to follow that diet indefinitely but should adopt the 10 percent fat diet while attempting to lower cholesterol. Thereafter, eating a 20 percent to 30 percent fat diet may be adequate to maintain recommended cholesterol levels (current fat consumption in the United States averages 34 percent of total calories).

One drawback of very lowfat diets (less than 25 percent fat) is that they tend to lower HDL-cholesterol and increase triglycerides. If HDL-cholesterol is already low, monounsaturated and polyunsaturated fats should be added to the diet. Olive, canola, corn, and soybean oils and nuts are sample food items that are high in monounsaturated fats and polyunsaturated fats. A specialized nutrition book should be consulted to determine food items that are high in monounsaturated and polyunsaturated fats.

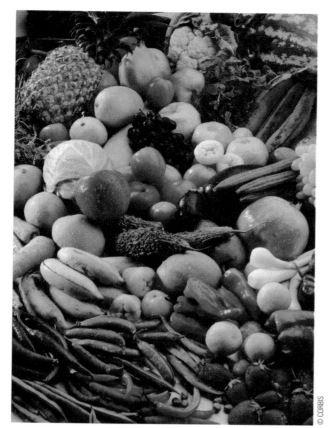

High-fiber foods are recommended
to decrease LDL-cholesterol.

Soy protein also has been recommended to lower total and LDL-cholesterol. Over the course of several weeks, a low saturated fat and cholesterol diet that includes 25 grams of soy protein a day will lower cholesterol by an additional 5 percent to 7 percent, as compared to the same diet but without the soy protein. This benefit is seen primarily in people who have total cholesterol levels above 200 mg/dl. Some people may have to consume up to 60 grams a day to see an effect.

Also, margarines and salad dressings now are available on the market that contain stanol ester, a plant derived compound that lowers cholesterol. Over time, about 3 grams of margarine or 6 tablespoons of salad dressing containing stanol ester lowers LDL-cholesterol by 14 percent.

To lower LDL-cholesterol levels, the following general dietary guidelines are recommended:

- Consume between 25 and 38 grams of fiber daily, including a minimum of 10 grams of soluble fiber (good sources are oats, fruits, barley, legumes, and psyllium).
- Do not consume more than 200 mg of dietary cholesterol a day.

- Consume red meats (3 ounces per serving) fewer than three times per week and no organ meats (such as liver and kidneys).
- Do not eat commercially baked foods.
- Avoid foods that contain trans fats, hydrogenated fat, or partially hydrogenated vegetable oil.
- Increase intake of omega-3 fatty acids by eating two or three omega-3-rich fish meals per week.
- Consume 25 grams of soy protein a day.
- Drink low-fat milk (1 percent or less fat, preferably) and use low-fat dairy products.
- Do not use coconut oil, palm oil, or cocoa butter.
- Limit egg consumption to fewer than three eggs per week (this is for people with high cholesterol only; others may consume eggs in moderation).
- Use margarines and salad dressings that contain stanol ester instead of butter and regular margarine.
- Bake, broil, grill, poach, or steam food instead of frying.
- Refrigerate cooked meat before adding to other dishes. Remove fat hardened in the refrigerator before mixing the meat with other foods.
- Avoid fatty sauces made with butter, cream, or cheese.
- Maintain recommended body weight.

Elevated Triglycerides

Triglycerides, also known as free fatty acids, in combination with cholesterol, speed up the formation of plaque. Very low-density lipoproteins (VLDLs) and **chylomicrons** carry triglycerides in the bloodstream. These fatty acids are found in poultry skin, lunch meats, and shellfish, but they are manufactured mainly in the liver from refined sugars, starches, and alcohol. High intake of alcohol and sugars (honey included) significantly raises triglyceride levels. The level can be lowered by cutting down on the previously mentioned foods along with pastries, candies, soft drinks, fruit juices, white bread, pasta, and alcohol. In addition, cutting down on overall fat consumption, quitting smoking, reducing weight (if overweight), and doing aerobic exercise are helpful. A desirable blood triglyceride level is less than 150 mg/dl (see Table 8.3, page 177).

Elevated Homocysteine

Clinical data indicating that many heart attack victims have normal cholesterol levels have led researchers to look for other risk factors that may contribute to

K E Y   T E R M S

Triglycerides Fats formed by glycerol and three fatty acids.

Chylomicrons Molecules that transport triglycerides in the blood.

atherosclerosis. Although it is not a blood lipid, a high concentration of **homocysteine** in the blood is thought to enhance the formation of plaque and subsequently lead to blockage of the arteries. The body uses homocysteine to help build proteins and carry out cellular metabolism. Homocysteine forms during an intermediate step in the creation of another amino acid. This process requires the presence of folate and vitamins B_6 and B_{12}.

Typically, homocysteine is metabolized rapidly, so it does not accumulate in the blood or damage the arteries. Many people, however, have high blood levels of homocysteine. This might be attributable to either a genetic inability to metabolize homocysteine or a deficiency in the vitamins required for its conversion.

Homocysteine is typically measured in micromoles per liter (µmol/l). A level below 9.0 µmol/l is desirable, while above 13.0 µmol/l is viewed as elevated. A 10-year follow-up study of people with high homocysteine levels showed that those individuals with a level above 14.25 µmol/l had almost twice the risk of stroke compared with individuals whose level was below 9.25 µmol/l.[17] Homocysteine accumulation is theorized to be toxic because it may:

1. Damage the inner lining of the arteries (the initial step in the process of atherosclerosis);
2. Stimulate the proliferation of cells that contribute to plaque formation; and
3. Encourage clotting that may completely obstruct an artery.

Keeping homocysteine from accumulating in the blood seems to be as simple as eating the recommended daily servings of vegetables, fruits, grains, and some meat and legumes. Increasing evidence that folate can prevent heart attacks has led to the recommendation that people consume 400 mcg per day of folate.

Unfortunately, estimates indicate that most Americans do not get 400 daily mcg of folate. Five daily servings of fruits and vegetables can provide sufficient levels of folate and vitamin B_6 to remove and clear homocysteine from the blood. People who consume these five servings are unlikely to derive extra benefits from a vitamin B-complex supplement.

Vitamin B_{12} is found primarily in animal flesh and animal products. Vitamin B_{12} deficiency is rarely a problem, as 1 cup of milk or an egg provides the daily requirement. The body also recycles most of this vitamin; therefore, it takes years to develop a deficiency.

Inflammation

For years it has been known that inflammation plays a role in CHD and that inflammation hidden deep in the body is a common trigger of heart attacks, even when

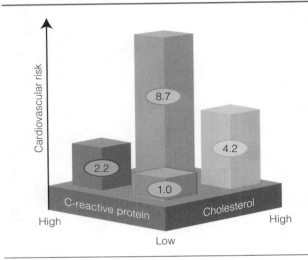

FIGURE **8.6** Relationships between C-reactive protein, cholesterol, and risk of cardiovascular disease.

Source: Adapted from P. Libby, P. M. Ridker, and A. Maseri, "Inflammation and Atherosclerosis," *Circulation* 105 (2002): 1135–1143.

cholesterol levels are normal or low and arterial plaque is minimal. Low-grade inflammation can occur in a variety of places throughout the body. To evaluate ongoing inflammation, physicians have turned to **C-reactive protein (CRP)**, a protein whose level in the blood increases with inflammation. People with elevated CRP are more prone to cardiovascular events. The evidence shows that CRP blood levels elevate years before a first heart attack or stroke and that individuals with elevated CRP have twice the risk of a heart attack. The risk of a heart attack is even higher in people with both elevated CRP and cholesterol, resulting in an almost ninefold increase in risk (see Figure 8.6).

Because high CRP levels might be a better predictor of future heart attacks than high cholesterol alone, a new test known as high-sensitivity CRP (hs-CRP), which measures inflammation in the blood vessels, has been approved by the FDA. The term "high-sensitivity" was derived from the test's capability to detect small amounts of CRP in the blood.

Hs-CRP test results provide a good measure of the probability of plaque rupturing within the arterial wall. There are two main types of plaque: soft and hard. Soft plaque is the most likely to rupture. Ruptured plaque releases clots into the bloodstream that can lead to a heart attack or stroke. A hs-CRP test is relatively inexpensive, and it is highly recommended for patients at risk for a heart attack. Guidelines for hs-CRP levels are given in Table 8.4.

CRP is increased by several factors, including obesity, excessive alcohol intake, and high-protein diets.

TABLE **8.4** High-Sensitivity CRP Guidelines	
AMOUNT	RATING
<1 mg/l	Low risk
1–3 mg/l	Average risk
>3 mg/l	High risk

Source: T. A. Pearson, et. al. "Markers of Inflammation and Cardiovascular Disease." *Circulation* 107 (2003): 499–511.

Recent evidence further indicates that high-fat, fast-food meals increase CRP levels for several hours following the meals.[18] Cooking meat and poultry at high temperatures creates damaged proteins (AGEs or advanced glycosylation end products) that trigger inflammation.

CRP levels decrease with statin drugs, which also lower cholesterol and reduce inflammation. Exercise, proper nutrition, and aspirin are also helpful. With weight loss, CRP levels decrease proportional to the amount of fat lost. Omega-3 fatty acids (found in salmon, tuna, and mackerel fish) inhibit proteins that cause inflammation, and aspirin therapy also helps by controlling inflammation.

Diabetes

In people who have **diabetes mellitus**, the pancreas totally stops producing insulin (or does not produce enough to meet the body's needs) or the cells become resistant to the effects of insulin. The role of insulin is to "unlock" the cells and escort glucose into the cell. The incidence of cardiovascular disease and death in the diabetic population is quite high. More than 75 percent of people with diabetes mellitus die from cardiovascular disease.

People with chronically elevated blood glucose levels may have problems metabolizing fats, which can make them more susceptible to atherosclerosis, coronary disease, heart attacks, high blood pressure, and strokes. Diabetics also tend to have lower HDL-cholesterol and higher triglyceride levels.

Further, chronic high blood sugar can lead to nerve damage, vision loss, kidney damage, and lower immune function (making the individual more susceptible to infections). Diabetics are four times more likely to become blind and 20 times more likely than nondiabetics to develop kidney failure. Nerve damage in the lower extremities makes the person less aware of injury and infection. A small untreated sore can lead to severe infection, gangrene, and even lead to an amputation.

An 8-hour fasting blood glucose level above 125 mg/dl on two separate tests confirms a diagnosis of diabetes. A level of 126 or higher should be brought to the attention of a physician. This guideline has changed from previous years, in which a level above 140 had been used to diagnose diabetes.

TYPES OF DIABETES Diabetes is of two types: type 1, or **insulin-dependent diabetes mellitus (IDDM)**, and type 2, or **non-insulin-dependent diabetes mellitus (NIDDM)**. Type 1 has also been known as "juvenile diabetes," because it is found mainly in young people. With type 1, the pancreas produces little or no insulin. With type 2, the pancreas either does not produce sufficient insulin or it produces adequate amounts but the cells become insulin-resistant, thereby keeping glucose from entering the cell. Type 2 accounts for 90 to 95 percent of all diabetes cases.

Although diabetes has a genetic predisposition, adult-onset (type 2) diabetes is related closely to overeating, obesity, and lack of physical activity. More than 80 percent of type 2 diabetics are overweight or have a history of excessive weight. In most cases, this condition can be corrected through a special diet, a weight loss program, and a regular exercise program.

A diet high in complex carbohydrates (unrefined whole grains) and water soluble fibers (found in fruits, vegetables, oats, and beans), low in saturated fat, and low in sugar is helpful in treating diabetes. Several research reports have shown that a habitual aerobic exercise program (walking, cycling, or swimming four or five times per week) increases the body's receptivity to insulin.

More recently, both moderate-intensity and vigorous physical activity have been associated with increased insulin sensitivity and decreased risk for diabetes. The key to increase and maintain proper insulin sensitivity

K E Y   T E R M S

Homocysteine   Intermediate amino acid in the interconversion of two other amino acids: methionine and cysteine.

C-reactive protein (CPR)   A protein whose level in the blood increases with inflammation (which may be hidden deep in the body); elevation of this protein is an indicator of potential cardiovascular events.

Diabetes mellitus   A condition in which blood glucose is unable to enter the cells because the pancreas either totally stops producing insulin or does not produce enough to meet the body's needs.

Insulin-dependent diabetes mellitus (IDDM or Type 1)   A form of diabetes in which the pancreas produces little or no insulin.

Non-insulin-dependent diabetes mellitus (NIDDM or Type 2)   A form of diabetes in which the pancreas either does not produce sufficient insulin or it produces adequate amounts but the cells become insulin-resistant, keeping glucose from entering the cell.

is regularity of the exercise program. Failure to maintain habitual physical activity voids the benefits.

Aggressive weight loss, especially if combined with increased activity, often allows Type 2 diabetic patients to normalize their blood sugar level without the use of medication. Individuals who have high blood glucose levels should consult a physician to decide on the best treatment.

METABOLIC SYNDROME As the cells resist the action of insulin, the pancreas releases even more insulin in an attempt to keep the blood glucose level from rising. A chronic rise in insulin seems to trigger a series of abnormalities referred to as **metabolic syndrome**. These abnormal conditions include low HDL-cholesterol, high triglycerides, and an increased blood-clotting mechanism. Many individuals with metabolic syndrome also have high blood pressure. All of these conditions increase the risk for CHD and other diabetic-related conditions (blindness, infection, nerve damage, and kidney failure). Approximately 70 million Americans are afflicted by metabolic syndrome.

People with metabolic syndrome have an abnormal insulin response to carbohydrates, in particular those that are absorbed rapidly (high-glycemic foods). In contrast to the American Heart Association dietary guidelines, metabolic syndrome researchers indicate that the current low-fat, high-carbohydrate diet may not be the best for prevention of CHD and actually could increase the risk for this disease in people with high insulin resistance and glucose intolerance.[19]

It might be best for these people to distribute their daily caloric intake so they derive 45 percent of their calories from carbohydrates (primarily low-glycemic), 40 percent from fat, and 15 percent from protein.[20] Of the 40 percent fat calories, 30 percent to 35 percent should come from mono- and polyunsaturated fats and only 5 percent to 10 percent should be provided by saturated fat.

Individuals with metabolic syndrome also benefit from weight loss (if overweight), exercise, and smoking cessation. Insulin resistance drops by about 40 percent in overweight people who lose 20 pounds. Forty-five minutes of daily aerobic exercise enhances insulin efficiency by 25 percent. Smoking, on the other hand, increases insulin resistance.

Abnormal Electrocardiograms (ECGs)

Electrocardiograms (ECGs or EKGs) are taken at rest, during the stress of exercise, and during recovery. An exercise or stress ECG also is known as a graded exercise stress test or a maximal exercise tolerance test. Similar to a high-speed road test on a car, a stress ECG reveals the heart's tolerance to high-intensity exercise. Based on the findings, ECGs may be interpreted as normal, equivocal, or abnormal.

A **stress electrocardiogram (stress ECG)** frequently is used to diagnose coronary heart disease. It also is administered to determine cardiorespiratory fitness levels, to screen individuals for preventive and cardiac rehabilitation programs, to detect abnormal blood pressure response during exercise, and to establish actual or functional maximal heart rate for purposes of participation in exercise.

Not every adult who wishes to start or continue in an exercise program needs a stress ECG. The following guidelines can help you determine when this type of test should be conducted:

1. Men over age 45 and women over age 55.
2. A total cholesterol level above 200 mg/dl, or an HDL-cholesterol level below 35 mg/dl.
3. Hypertensive and diabetic individuals.
4. Cigarette smokers.
5. Individuals with a family history of CHD, syncope, or sudden death before age 60.
6. People with an abnormal resting ECG.
7. All individuals with symptoms of chest discomfort, dysrhythmias, syncope, or **chronotropic incompetence**.

Tobacco Use

More than 47 million adults and 3.5 million adolescents in the United States smoke cigarettes. Each day, an additional 3,000 people under the age of 18 become smokers. Cigarette smoking is the single largest preventable cause of illness and premature death in the United States. If we include all related deaths, tobacco is responsible for more than 435,000 unnecessary deaths per year. Smoking has been linked to cardiovascular disease, cancer, bronchitis, emphysema, and peptic ulcers.

About 53,000 of those yearly deaths are nonsmokers who were exposed to secondhand smoke in their daily life. Both fatal and nonfatal cardiac events increase greatly in people who are exposed to passive smoking. Some 37,000 yearly deaths from heart disease are attributed to secondhand smoke. Even in regular smokers, adaptations to the harmful effects of smoking are slight, so the adverse effects are much greater to nonsmokers. Secondhand smoke is ranked behind active smoking and alcohol as the third leading preventable cause of death in the United States. Passive smoking is a significant risk factor for heart disease in children and adults alike.

In relation to coronary disease, smoking speeds up the process of atherosclerosis and also produces a threefold increase in the risk of sudden death following a **myocardial infarction**. Smoking increases heart rate and blood pressure and irritates the heart, which can trigger

FIGURE **8.7** Six-step smoking cessation approach.

The following six-step plan has been developed as a guide to help you quit smoking. The total program should be completed in 4 weeks or less. Steps one through four should take no longer than 2 weeks. A maximum of 2 additional weeks are allowed for the rest of the program.

Step One. Decide positively that you want to quit. Now prepare a list of the reasons why you smoke and why you want to quit.

Step Two. Initiate a personal diet and exercise program. Exercise and decreased body weight cause a greater awareness of healthy living and increase motivation for giving up cigarettes.

Step Three. Decide on the approach you will use to stop smoking. You may quit cold turkey or gradually decrease the number of cigarettes smoked daily. Many people have found that quitting cold turkey is the easiest way to do it. Although it may not work the first time, after several attempts, all of a sudden smokers are able to overcome the habit without too much difficulty. Tapering off cigarettes can be done

in several ways. You may start by eliminating cigarettes that you do not necessarily need, you can switch to a brand lower in nicotine or tar every couple of days, you can smoke less of each cigarette, or you can simply decrease the total number of cigarettes smoked each day.

Step Four. Set the target date for quitting. In setting the target date, choosing a special date may add a little extra incentive. An upcoming birthday, anniversary, vacation, graduation, family reunion—all are examples of good dates to free yourself from smoking.

Step Five. Stock up on low-calorie foods—carrots, broccoli, cauliflower, celery, popcorn (butter- and salt-free), fruits, sunflower seeds (in the shell), sugarless gum, and plenty of water. Keep such food handy on the day you stop and the first few days following cessation. Replace it for cigarettes when you want one.

Step Six. This is the day that you will quit smoking. On this day and the first few days thereafter, do not keep cigarettes handy. Stay away from friends and events that trigger your desire to smoke. Drink large

amounts of water and fruit juices and eat low-calorie foods. Replace the old behavior with new behavior. You will need to replace smoking time with new positive substitutes that will make smoking difficult or impossible. When you desire a cigarette, take a few deep breaths and then occupy yourself by doing a number of things such as talking to someone else, washing your hands, brushing your teeth, eating a healthy snack, chewing on a straw, doing dishes, playing sports, going for a walk or bike ride, going swimming, and so on.

If you have been successful and stopped smoking, a lot of events still can trigger your urge to smoke. When confronted with such events, people rationalize and think, "One won't hurt." It will not work! Before you know it, you will be back to the regular nasty habit. Be prepared to take action in those situations. Find adequate substitutes for smoking. Remind yourself of how difficult it has been and how long it has taken you to get to this point. As time goes on, it will only get easier rather than worse.

---

fatal cardiac **arrhythmias.** As far as the extra load on the heart is concerned, giving up one pack of cigarettes per day is the equivalent of smoking between 50 and 75 pounds of excess body fat! Another harmful effect is a decrease in HDL-cholesterol, the "good" type that helps control blood lipids.

The risk for cardiovascular disease starts to decrease the moment a person quits smoking. After cessation, the risk approaches that of a lifetime nonsmoker. Pipe and cigar smoking and chewing tobacco also increase the risk for heart disease. Even if no smoke is inhaled, toxic substances are absorbed through the membranes of the mouth and end up in the bloodstream.

Quitting tobacco use is not easy. The addictive properties of nicotine make quitting difficult, and physical and psychological withdrawal symptoms set in. A six-step plan to help people stop smoking is contained in Figure 8.7.

KEY TERMS

Metabolic syndrome An array of metabolic abnormalities that contribute to the development of atherosclerosis triggered by resistance to insulin; these conditions include low HDL-cholesterol, high triglycerides, high blood pressure, and an increased blood clotting mechanism.

Electrocardiogram (ECG or EKG) A recording of the electrical activity of the heart.

Stress electrocardiogram (stress ECG) An exercise test during which the workload is gradually increased (until the subject reaches maximal fatigue), with blood pressure and 12-lead electrocardiographic monitoring throughout the test.

Chronotropic incompetence A condition in which the heart rate increases slowly during exercise and never reaches maximum.

Myocardial infarction Heart attack; damage or death of an area of the heart muscle as a result of an obstructed artery to that area.

Arrhythmias Irregular heart rhythms.

Cigarette smoking is the single largest preventable cause of illness and premature death in the United States.

Physical activity is an excellent tool to control stress.

Critical Thinking

Cigarette smoking is the largest preventable cause of premature illness and death in the United States. Do you think the government should outlaw the use of tobacco in all forms? Or does the individual have the right to engage in self-destructive behavior?

The most important factor in quitting cigarette smoking is a sincere desire to do so. More than 95 percent of successful ex-smokers have been able to quit on their own, either by quitting cold turkey or by using self-help kits available from organizations such as the American Cancer Society, the American Heart Association, and the American Lung Association. Only 3 percent of ex-smokers quit as a result of formal cessation programs.

Stress

Stress has become a part of life. People have to deal daily with goals, deadlines, responsibilities, and pressures. The **stressor** itself is not what creates the health hazard but, rather, the individual's response to it.

The human body responds to stress by producing more catecholamines to prepare the body for **fight or flight**. If the person fights or flees, the body metabolizes the higher levels of catecholamines and is able to return to a normal state. If, however, a person is under constant stress and is unable to take action (as in the death of a close relative or friend, loss of a job, trouble at work, or financial insecurity), the catecholamines remain elevated in the bloodstream.

People who are not able to relax place a constant low-level strain on the cardiovascular system that could manifest itself in heart disease. In addition, when a person is in a stressful situation, the coronary arteries that feed the heart muscle constrict, reducing the oxygen supply to the heart. If the blood vessels are largely blocked by atherosclerosis, abnormal heart rhythms or even a heart attack may follow.

As outlined in Chapter 7, individuals who are under a lot of stress and do not cope well with it need to take measures to counteract the effects of stress in their lives. Identifying and learning how to cope with the sources of stress will improve health and quality of life.

Physical activity is one of the best ways to relieve stress. When a person takes part in physical activity, the body metabolizes excess catecholamines and is able to return to a normal state. Exercise also steps up muscular activity, which contributes to muscular relaxation.

Personal and Family History

Individuals who have a family history of, or already have experienced, cardiovascular problems are at higher risk than those who never have had a problem. People with this history should be encouraged strongly to keep the other risk factors as low as possible. Because most risk factors are reversible, the risk for future problems will decrease significantly.

Age and Gender

Age becomes a risk factor for men over age 45 and women over age 55. The greater incidence of heart disease may stem in part from lifestyle changes as we get older (less physical activity, poor nutrition, obesity, and so on). Earlier in life, men are at greater risk for cardiovascular disease than women are. Following menopause, the risk for women increases. Based on final mortality statistics for 2002, more women (493,623) than men (433,825) died from cardiovascular disease.[21]

Young people should not think they are immune from heart disease. The process begins early in life. Autopsies conducted in people who have died in their 20s reveal that many of them already exhibit early stages of atherosclerosis. Other studies have found elevated blood cholesterol levels in children as young as 10 years old.

Even though the aging process cannot be stopped, it certainly can be slowed. The concept of **chronological age** versus **physiological age** is important in longevity. Some individuals in their 60s or older have the body of a 30-year-old. And 30-year-olds often are in such poor condition and health that they almost seem to have the body of a 60-year-old. Managing risk factors and developing positive lifestyle habits are the best ways to slow natural aging.

Cancer

Cell growth is controlled by **deoxyribonucleic acid (DNA)** and **ribonucleic acid (RNA)**. When nuclei lose their ability to regulate and control cell growth, cell division is disrupted and mutant cells may develop. Some of these cells may grow uncontrollably and abnormally, forming a mass of tissue called a tumor, which can be either **benign** or **malignant**. Although benign tumors can interfere with normal bodily functions, they rarely cause death.

About 23 percent of all deaths in the United States come from **cancer**. Each year, close to 1.4 million new cases are reported and more than half a million people die from cancer.[22] Over 100 types of cancer can develop in the body. Cancer cells grow for no reason and multiply, destroying normal tissue. If the spread of cells is not controlled, death ensues. A cell may duplicate as many as 100 times.

Normally, the DNA molecule is duplicated perfectly during cell division. In a few cases the DNA molecule is not replicated exactly but specialized enzymes repair it quickly. Occasionally, cells with defective DNA keep dividing and ultimately form a small tumor. As more mutations occur, the altered cells continue to divide and can become malignant. A decade or more can pass between carcinogenic exposure or mutations and the time cancer is diagnosed. A critical turning point in the development of cancer is when a tumor reaches about 1 million cells. At this stage it is referred to as **carcinoma in situ**, when it has not spread. Such an undetected tumor may go for months or years without any significant growth.

While encapsulated, a tumor does not pose a serious threat to human health. To grow, the tumor requires more oxygen and nutrients. In time, a few of the cancer cells start producing chemicals that enhance **angiogenesis**. Cells break away from a malignant tumor and, through the new blood vessels, migrate to other parts of the body, in a process called **metastasis**, where they can cause new cancer.

Although the immune system and the blood turbulence destroy most cancer cells, only one abnormal cell lodging elsewhere can start a new cancer. These cells also will grow and multiply uncontrollably, destroying normal tissue. Once cancer cells metastasize, treatment becomes more difficult. Therapy can kill most cancer cells, but a few cells may become resistant to treatment. These cells then can grow into a new tumor that will not respond to the same treatment.

As with cardiovascular disease, cancer is largely preventable. As much as 80 percent of all human cancer is related to lifestyle or environmental factors (including diet, tobacco use, excessive use of alcohol, sexual and reproductive activity, and exposure to environmental hazards). Equally important is that more than 9.8 million Americans with a history of cancer were alive in 2005. Currently, 6 in 10 people diagnosed with cancer are expected to be alive 5 years from the initial diagnosis.

KEY TERMS

Stress The mental, emotional, and physiological response of the body to any situation that is new, threatening, frightening, or exciting.

Stressor Stress-causing event.

Fight or flight Physiological response of the body to stress that prepares the individual to take action by stimulating the vital defense systems.

Chronological age Calendar age.

Physiological age Age based on the individual's functional and physical capacity.

Deoxyribonucleic acid (DNA) Genetic substance of which genes are made; molecule that bears cell's genetic code.

Ribonucleic acid (RNA) Genetic material involved in the formation of cell proteins.

Benign Noncancerous.

Malignant Cancerous.

Cancer Group of diseases characterized by uncontrolled growth and spread of abnormal cells into malignant tumors.

Carcinoma in situ Encapsulated malignant tumor that is found at an early stage and has not spread.

Angiogenesis Capillary (blood vessel) formation into a tumor.

Metastasis Movement of bacteria or body cells from one part of the body to another.

Guidelines for Preventing Cancer

The biggest factor in fighting cancer today is health education. People need to be informed about the risk factors for cancer and the guidelines for early detection. The most effective way to protect against cancer is to change negative lifestyle habits and behaviors. Activity 8.1, page 197, is a questionnaire regarding the risk factors and preventive measures discussed below.

Making Dietary Changes

The American Cancer Society (ACS) estimates that one-third of all cancers in the United States are related to nutrition. A healthy diet, therefore, is crucial to decrease the risk for cancer. The diet should be predominately vegetarian—high in fiber and low in fat (particularly from animal sources). **Cruciferous vegetables**, tea, soy products, calcium, and omega-3 fats are encouraged. Protein intake should be kept within the recommended nutrient guidelines. If alcohol is consumed, it should be used in moderation. Obesity should be avoided.

Green and dark yellow vegetables, cruciferous vegetables (cauliflower, broccoli, cabbage, Brussels sprouts, and kohlrabi), and beans (legumes) seem to protect against cancer. Folate, found naturally in dark green leafy vegetables, dry beans, and orange juice, may reduce the risk of colon and cervical cancers. Brightly colored fruits and vegetables contain **carotenoids** and vitamin C. Lycopene, one of the many carotenoids (a phytochemical—see following discussion), has been linked to lowered risk of cancers of the prostate, colon, and cervix. Lycopene is especially abundant in cooked tomato products.

Researchers believe the antioxidant effect of vitamins and the mineral selenium helps protect the body from oxygen free radicals. As discussed in Chapter 5, during normal metabolism most of the oxygen in the human body is converted into stable forms of carbon dioxide and water. A small amount, however, ends up in an unstable form known as oxygen free radicals, which are thought to attack and damage the cell membrane and DNA, leading to the formation of cancers. Antioxidants absorb free radicals before they can cause damage, and they also interrupt the sequence of reactions once damage has begun.

Many studies have linked low intake of fiber to increased risk for colon cancer. Fiber binds to bile acids in the intestine for excretion from the body in the stools. The interaction of bile acids with intestinal bacteria releases cancer-causing byproducts. Bile-acid production increases with increased fat content in the small intestine.

Daily consumption of fiber (25 grams for women to 38 grams for men) is recommended. Grains are high in fiber and contain vitamins and minerals—folate,

selenium, and calcium—that seem to decrease the risk for colon cancer. Selenium also protects against prostate cancer and possibly lung cancer. Calcium may protect against colon cancer by preventing rapid growth of cells in the colon, especially in people with colon polyps.

PHYTOCHEMICALS A promising horizon in cancer prevention is the discovery of **phytochemicals.** These compounds, found in abundance in fruits and vegetables, seem to exert a powerful effect in preventing cancer by blocking the formation of cancerous tumors and disrupting the process at almost every step of the way. Experts recommend that to obtain the highest possible protection, produce should be consumed several times during the day (instead of in one meal) to maintain effective phytochemical levels throughout the day. Research indicates that phytochemical blood levels drop within 3 hours of consuming the produce.[23]

Polyphenols (phytochemicals) also are known to block the formation of **nitrosamines** (potentially cancer-causing compounds formed from chemicals in processed meats to prevent the formation of harmful bacteria) by turning up the body's natural detoxification defenses and thereby suppressing progression of the disease. Phytochemicals also are present in many grains and in regular (not herbal) teas. Green, black, and red tea all seem to provide protection. Evidence also points to certain components in tea that can block the spread of cancers to other parts of the body. Green and black tea have similar amounts of polyphenols. Herbal teas do not provide the same benefits as regular tea.

Green tea seems to be especially helpful in preventing gastrointestinal cancers, including those of the stomach, small intestines, pancreas, and colon. Consumption of green tea also has been linked to a lower incidence of lung, esophageal, and estrogen-related cancers, including most breast cancers. Other research indicates that phytochemicals in green tea induce cancer cells to self-destruct.[24] In Japan, where people drink green tea regularly but smoke twice as much as people in the United States, the incidence of lung cancer is half that of the United States. A cancer-prevention diet recommends drinking two or more cups of green tea daily.

The antioxidant effect of one of the polyphenols in green tea—epigallocatechin gallate, or EGCG—is at least 25 times more effective than vitamin E and 100 times more effective than vitamin C at protecting cells and the DNA from damage believed to cause cancer, heart disease, and other diseases associated with free radicals.[25] EGCG is also twice as strong as the red wine antioxidant resveratrol, which helps prevent heart disease.

OTHER DIETARY FACTORS High fat intake may promote cancer and excessive weight. Some experts recommend that

Phytochemicals found in abundance in fruits and vegetables seem to have a powerful effect in decreasing risk for cancer.

© 2001 PhotoDisc, Inc.

in a cancer prevention diet, total fat intake should be limited to less than 20 percent of total daily calories. Fat intake should consist of primarily monounsaturated and omega-3 fats. Omega 3-fats, found in many types of fish, flaxseeds, and flaxseed oil, seem to offer protection against colorectal, pancreatic, breast, oral, esophageal, and stomach cancers. Omega 3-fats block the synthesis of prostaglandins, bodily compounds that promote growth of tumors.

Foods high in vitamin C may deter some cancers. Salt-cured, smoked, and nitrite-cured foods have been associated with cancers of the esophagus and stomach. Processed meats should be consumed sparingly and always with orange juice or other foods rich in vitamin C. Vitamin C seems to discourage the formation of nitrosamines.

Some research suggests that grilling protein (fat or lean) at high temperatures for a long time increases the formation of carcinogenic substances on the skin or surface of the meat. Microwaving the meat for a couple of minutes before barbecuing decreases the risk, as long as the fluid released by the meat is discarded. Most of the potential **carcinogens** collect in this solution. Removing the skin before serving and cooking at lower heat to a medium stage rather than well done also seem to lower the risk.

Mixing soy protein in powder form with meats also seems to decrease the formation of carcinogens when cooking meats. Soy foods may help because soy contains chemicals that prevent cancer. Although further research is merited, isoflavones (phytochemicals) found in soy are structurally similar to estrogen and may prevent breast, prostate, lung, and colon cancers. These isoflavones are frequently referred to as phytoestrogens or plant estrogens. Isoflavones also block angiogenesis. Presently, it is not known if the health benefits of soy are related to isoflavones by themselves or in combination with other nutrients found in soy.

In animal studies, when animals with tumors were given large amounts of soy, the estrogen activity of soy isoflavones actually led to the growth of estrogen-dependent tumors. Experts, therefore, caution women with breast cancer or a history of this disease to limit soy intake because it may stimulate cancer cells by closely imitating the actions of estrogen.

No specific recommendations are presently available as to the amount of daily soy protein intake for cancer prevention. The FDA allows the health claim that 25 grams per day in conjunction with a diet low in saturated fat and cholesterol lowers the risk for cardio-vascular disease. Based on the traditional diets of people in China and Japan, including children, who regularly consume soy foods, there doesn't seem to be an unsafe level of consumption. Soy protein powder supplementation, however, may not be safe, because this may elevate soy protein intake to an unnaturally high level.

People who consume alcohol should do so in moderation, because too much alcohol raises the risk for developing certain cancers, especially when it is combined with tobacco smoking or smokeless tobacco. In combination, these substances significantly increase the risk for cancers of the mouth, larynx, throat, esophagus, and liver. According to the ACS, approximately 17,000 deaths from cancer yearly are attributed to excessive use of alcohol, often in combination with smoking. The

KEY TERMS

Cruciferous vegetables Plants that produce cross-shaped leaves (cauliflower, broccoli, cabbage, Brussels sprouts, kohlrabi); these seem to have a protective effect against cancer.

Carotenoids Pigment substances (more than 600) in plants, about 50 of which are precursors to vitamin A; the most potent carotenoid is beta-carotene.

Phytochemicals Compounds found in fruits and vegetables that block formation of cancerous tumors and disrupt the process of cancer.

Nitrosamines Potentially cancer-causing compounds formed when nitrites and nitrates—which are used to prevent the growth of harmful bacteria in processed meats—combine with other chemicals in the stomach.

Carcinogens Substances that contribute to the formation of cancers.

combined action of heavy use of alcohol and tobacco can increase cancer of the oral cavity fifteenfold.

Maintaining recommended body weight also is encouraged. Obesity may be associated with cancers of the colon, rectum, breast, prostate, endometrium, and kidney.

Abstaining From Tobacco

Cigarette smoking by itself is a major health hazard. As stated earlier in this chapter, if we include all related deaths, smoking is responsible for more than 440,000 unnecessary deaths in the United States each year. The World Health Organization estimates that smoking causes 3 million deaths worldwide annually. The average life expectancy for a chronic smoker is about 15 years less than for a nonsmoker. The most prevalent carcinogenic exposure in the workplace is cigarette smoke. At least 28 percent of all cancer is tied to smoking, and 87 percent of lung cancer is tied to smoking. Use of smokeless tobacco can lead to nicotine addiction and dependence as well as increased risk for mouth, larynx, throat, and esophageal cancers.

Avoiding Excessive Sun Exposure

Too much exposure to ultraviolet radiation (both UVB and UVA rays) is a major contributor to skin cancer. The most common sites of skin cancer are those exposed to the sun most often (face, neck, and back of the hands). The three types of skin cancer are:

1. Basal cell carcinoma
2. Squamous cell carcinoma
3. Malignant melanoma.

Nearly 90 percent of the almost 1 million cases of basal cell or squamous cell skin cancers reported yearly in the United States could have been prevented by protecting the skin from the sun's rays. ACS data indicates that **melanoma** is the most deadly, causing approximately 7,700 deaths in 2005. One in every six Americans will develop some type of skin cancer eventually.

Nothing is healthy about a "healthy tan." Tanning of the skin is the body's natural reaction to permanent and irreversible damage from too much exposure to the sun. Even brief exposures to sunlight add up to a greater risk for skin cancer and premature aging. The tan fades at the end of the summer season, but the underlying skin damage does not disappear. People with sensitive skin in particular should avoid sun exposure between 10:00 AM and 4:00 PM.

The stinging sunburn comes from ultraviolet B (UVB) rays, which also are thought to be the main cause of premature wrinkling and skin aging, roughened/

Sunburns and tanning pose a risk for skin cancer from overexposure to the sun's ultraviolet rays.

© Fitness & Wellness, Inc.

leathery/sagging skin, and skin cancer. Unfortunately, the damage may not become evident until up to 20 years later. In contrast, skin that has not been overexposed to the sun remains smooth and unblemished, and, over time, shows less evidence of aging.

Sun lamps and tanning parlors provide mainly ultraviolet A (UVA) rays. Once thought to be safe, they are now known to damage skin and have been linked to melanoma, the most serious form of skin cancer. As little as 15 to 30 minutes of exposure to UVA can be as dangerous as a day spent in the sun.

Sunscreen lotion should be applied about 30 minutes before lengthy exposure to the sun, because the skin takes that long to absorb the protective ingredients. A **sun protection factor (SPF)** of at least 15 is recommended. SPF 15 means that the skin takes 15 times longer to burn than with no lotion. If you ordinarily get a mild sunburn after 20 minutes of noonday sun, an SPF 15 allows you to remain in the sun about 300 minutes before burning. The higher the number, the longer the protection. When swimming or sweating, you should reapply waterproof sunscreens more often, because all sunscreens lose strength when they are diluted.

Critical Thinking

You have learned about many of the risk factors for major cancer sites. How will this information affect your health choices in the future? Will it be valuable to you, or will you quickly forget all you have learned and remain in a contemplation stage at the end of this course?

Monitoring Estrogen, Radiation Exposure, and Potential Occupational Hazards

Estrogen use has been linked to endometrial cancer in some studies, although other evidence contradicts those findings. And, even though exposure to radiation increases the risk for cancer, the benefits of x-rays may outweigh the risk involved, and most medical facilities use the lowest dose possible to keep the risk to a minimum. Occupational hazards, such as asbestos fibers, nickel and uranium dusts, chromium compounds, vinyl chloride, and bischlormethyl ether, increase the risk for cancer. Cigarette smoking magnifies the risk from occupational hazards.

Physical Activity

An active lifestyle seems to have a protective effect against cancer. Although the mechanism is not clear, physical fitness and cancer mortality in men and women may have a graded and consistent inverse relationship.

A daily 30-minute moderate-intensity exercise program lowers the risk for colon cancer and may lower the risk for cancers of the breast and reproductive system. Research has shown that regular exercise lowers the risk for breast cancer in women by 20 percent to 30 percent. In addition, growing evidence suggests that the body's autoimmune system may play a role in preventing cancer. Moderate exercise improves the autoimmune system.[26]

Early Detection

Fortunately, many cancers can be controlled or cured through early detection. The real problem comes when cancerous cells spread, because they are difficult to wipe out then. Therefore, effective prevention, and early detection, is crucial. Herein lies the importance of periodic screening. Table 8.5 summarizes the ACS recommendations for early detection of cancer. At home, once a month, women should practice breast self-examination (BSE), and men, testicular self-examination (TSE). Men should pick a regular day each month (for example, the first day of the month) to practice TSE, and women should perform BSE 2 or 3 days after the menstrual period is over.

Other Risk Factors for Cancer

Contributions to cancer of many of the other much publicized factors are not as significant as those just pointed out. Intentional food additives, saccharin, processing agents, pesticides, and packaging materials

---

Warning Signals for Cancer

Everyone should become familiar with the following warning signs of cancer and bring them to a physician's attention if any are present:

1. Change in bowel or bladder habits.
2. Sore that does not heal.
3. Unusual bleeding or discharge.
4. Thickening or lump in breast or elsewhere.
5. Indigestion or difficulty in swallowing.
6. Obvious change in wart or mole.
7. Nagging cough or hoarseness.

---

currently used in the United States and other developed countries seem to have minimal consequences. High levels of stress and poor coping may affect the autoimmune system negatively and thereby render the body less effective in dealing with the various cancers.

Genetics plays a role in susceptibility in about 10 percent of all cancers. Most of the effect is seen in the early childhood years. Some cancers result from a combination of genetic and environmental liability. Genetics may add to the environmental risk of certain types of cancers. The biggest carcinogenic exposure in the workplace is cigarette smoke.

Environmental factors are more than pollution and smoke. These factors incorporate diet, lifestyle-related events, viruses, and physical agents such as x-rays and exposure to the sun.

Scientific evidence and testing procedures for prevention and early detection of cancer do change. Studies continue to provide new information. The intent of cancer prevention programs is to educate and guide individuals toward a lifestyle that will help prevent cancer and enable early detection of malignancy. The Recommendations for Early Detection of Cancer in Asymptomatic People by the ACS (Table 8.5) should be heeded in regular physical examinations as part of a cancer-prevention program.

Treatment of cancer always should be left to specialized physicians and cancer clinics. Current treatment modalities include surgery, radiation, radioactive substances, chemotherapy, hormones, and immunotherapy.

KEY TERMS

Melanoma The most virulent, rapidly spreading form of skin cancer.

Sun protection factor (SPF) Degree of protection offered by ingredients in sunscreen lotion; at least SPF 15 is recommended.

TABLE **8.5** Summary of Recommendations for Early Detection of Cancer in Asymptomatic People

SITE	RECOMMENDATION
BREAST	• Yearly mammograms are recommended starting at age 40. The age at which screening should be stopped should be individualized by considering the potential risks and benefits of screening in the context of overall health status and longevity.
	• Clinical breast exam should be part of a perodic health exam, about every three years for women in their 20s and 30s, and every year for women 40 and older.
	• Women should know how their breasts normally feel and report any breast change promptly to their health care providers. Breast self-exam is an option for women starting in their 20s.
	• Women at increased risk (e.g., family history, genetic tendency, past breast cancer) should talk with their doctors about the benefits and limitations of starting mammography screening earlier, having additional tests (i.e., breast ultrasound and MRI), or having more frequent exams.
COLON & RECTUM	Beginning at age 50, men and women should follow one of the examination schedules below: • A fecal occult blood test (FOBT) or fecal immunochemical test (FIT) every year • A flexible sigmoidoscopy (FSIG) every five years • Annual FOBT or FIT and flexible sigmoidoscopy every five years* • A double-contrast barium enema every five years • A colonoscopy every 10 years * Combined testing is preferred over either annual FOBT or FIT, or FSIG every five years, alone. People who are at moderate or high risk for colorectal cancer should talk with a doctor about a different testing schedule.
PROSTATE	The PSA test and the digital rectal exam should be offered annually, beginning at age 50, to men who have a life expectancy of at least 10 years. Men at high risk (African-American men and men with a strong family history of one or more first-degree relatives diagnosed with prostate cancer at an early age) should begin testing at age 45. For both men at average risk and high risk, information should be provided about what is known and what is uncertain about the benefits and limitations of early detection and treatment of prostate cancer so that they can make an informed decision about testing.
UTERUS	**Cervix:** Screening should begin approximately three years after a woman begins having vaginal intercourse, but no later than 21 years of age. Screening should be done every year with regular Pap tests or every two years using liquid-based tests. At or after age 30, women who have had three normal test results in a row may get screened every two to three years. Alternatively, cervical cancer screening with HPV DNA testing and conventional or liquid-based cytology could be performed every three years. However, doctors may suggest a woman get screened more often if she has certain risk factors, such as HIV infection or a weak immune system. Women 70 years and older who have had three or more consecutive normal Pap tests in the last 10 years may choose to stop cervical cancer screening. Screening after total hysterectomy (with removal of the cervix) is not necessary unless the surgery was done as a treatment for cervical cancer. **Endometrium:** The American Cancer Society recommends that at the time of menopause all women should be informed about the risks and symptoms of endometrial cancer, and strongly encouraged to report any unexpected bleeding or spotting to their physicians. Annual screening for endometrial cancer with endometrial biopsy beginning at age 35 should be offered to women with or at risk for hereditary nonpolyposis colon cancer (HNPCC).
CANCER-RELATED CHECKUP	For individuals undergoing periodic health examinations, a cancer-related checkup should include health counseling and, depending on a person's age and gender, might include examinations for cancers of the thyroid, oral cavity, skin, lymph nodes, testes, and ovaries, as well as for some nonmalignant diseases.

From *Cancer Facts and Figures.* © 2004, American Cancer Society, Inc.

Chronic Lower Respiratory Disease

Chronic lower respiratory disease (CLRD) encompasses diseases that limit air flow, such as chronic obstructive pulmonary disease, emphysema, and chronic bronchitis (all diseases of the respiratory system). The incidence of CLRD increases proportionately with cigarette smoking (and other forms of smoked tobacco) and exposure to certain types of industrial pollution. In the case of emphysema, genetic factors also may play a role.

Accidents

Even though most people do not consider accidents to be a health problem, accidents rank as the fourth leading cause of death in the United States, affecting the total well-being of millions of Americans each year. Accident prevention and personal safety also are part of a health enhancement program aimed at achieving a higher quality of life. Proper nutrition, exercise, abstinence from cigarette smoking, and stress management are of little help if the person is involved in a disabling or fatal accident caused by distraction, a single reckless decision, or not wearing safety belts properly.

Accidents do not always just happen. We sometimes cause accidents. Other times we are victims of accidents. Although some factors in life—earthquakes, tornadoes, and airplane crashes, for example—are completely beyond our control, more often than not personal safety and accident prevention are a matter of common sense. Many accidents result from poor judgment and a confused mental state. Frequently accidents happen when we are upset, not paying attention to the task with which we are involved, or abusing alcohol and other drugs.

Alcohol abuse is the number-one cause of all accidents. Alcohol intoxication is the leading cause of fatal automobile accidents. Other drugs commonly abused in society alter feelings and perceptions, cause mental confusion, and impair judgment and coordination, greatly increasing the risk for accidental morbidity and mortality.

Substance Abuse

Chemical dependencies presently encompass some of the most self-destructive behaviors in society. Abused substances include alcohol, hard drugs, and cigarettes (the latter has been discussed already in this chapter). Problems associated with substance abuse include drunken or impaired driving, mixing drug prescriptions, family difficulties, and drugs to improve athletic performance (anabolic steroids). Although all forms of substance abuse are recognized to be unhealthy, the following information focuses on alcohol and on the illegal drugs marijuana, cocaine, methamphetamine, heroin, and MDMA (Ecstasy).

Alcohol

Alcohol use represents one of the most significant health-related drug problems in the United States today. Estimates indicate that 7 in 10 adults, or more than 100 million Americans 18 years and older, are drinkers.

Approximately 18 million of them abuse alcohol or are alcohol dependent and will struggle with **alcoholism** throughout life. Among younger people, about 7.2 million between the ages of 12 and 20 are binge drinkers.

Alcohol intake impedes peripheral vision, impairs the ability to see and hear, decreases reaction time, hinders concentration and motor performance (including increased swaying), and causes impaired judgment of distance and speed of moving objects. Further, it lessens fear, increases risk-taking behaviors, stimulates urination, and induces sleep.

A single large dose of alcohol also may decrease sexual function. One of the most unpleasant, dangerous, and life-threatening effects of drinking is the **synergistic action** of alcohol when combined with other drugs, particularly central nervous system depressants. Long-term manifestations of alcohol abuse can be serious and life threatening. These conditions include **cirrhosis** of the liver (often fatal); greater risk for oral, esophageal, and liver cancer; **cardiomyopathy**; high blood pressure; greater risk for strokes; inflammation of the esophagus, stomach, small intestine, and pancreas; stomach ulcers; sexual impotence; malnutrition; brain cell damage and consequent loss of memory; depression, psychosis, and hallucinations. Additional information on the physiological effects of alcohol is given in Chapter 9.

Illegal Drugs

Approximately 60 percent of the world's production of illegal drugs is consumed in the United States. An estimated 35 million people in the United States use an illegal drug. Each year we spend more than $65 billion on illegal drugs.

According to the U. S. Department of Education, today's drugs are stronger and more addictive, posing a greater risk than ever before. Drugs lead to physical and psychological dependence. If used regularly, they integrate into the body's chemistry, raising drug tolerance

---

K E Y   T E R M S

Chronic lower respiratory disease (CLRD) A group of diseases that limit air flow, such as chronic obstructive pulmonary disease, emphysema, and chronic bronchitis (all diseases of the respiratory system).

Alcoholism Disease in which an individual loses control over drinking alcoholic beverages.

Synergistic action The effect of mixing two or more drugs, the effects of which can be much greater than the sum of two or more drugs acting by themselves.

Cirrhosis A disease characterized by scarring of the liver.

Cardiomyopathy A disease affecting the heart muscle.

and forcing the person to increase the dosage constantly for similar results. In addition to the serious health problems caused by drug abuse, more than half of all adolescent suicides are drug-related.

Marijuana

Marijuana (pot or grass) is the most widely used illegal drug in the United States. Approximately 31 million people in the country use marijuana regularly. Earlier studies in the 1960s indicated that the potential effects of marijuana were exaggerated and that the drug was relatively harmless. The drug as it is used today, however, is as much as 10 times stronger than it was when the initial studies were conducted. Long-term harmful effects of marijuana use include atrophy of the brain leading to irreversible brain damage, as well as decreased resistance to infectious diseases, chronic bronchitis, lung cancer, and possible sterility and impotence.

Cocaine

Similar to marijuana, for many years cocaine was thought to be a relatively harmless drug. This misconception came to an abrupt halt in the 1980s when two well-known athletes, Len Bias (basketball) and Don Rogers (football), died suddenly following cocaine overdose. Approximately 6 million people in the United States use cocaine, 96 percent of whom had used marijuana previously.

Sustained cocaine snorting can lead to a constant runny nose, nasal congestion and inflammation, and perforation of the nasal septum. Long-term consequences of cocaine use in general include loss of appetite, digestive disorders, weight loss, malnutrition, insomnia, confusion, anxiety, and cocaine psychosis (characterized by paranoia and hallucinations). Large overdoses of cocaine can end in sudden death from respiratory paralysis, cardiac arrhythmias, and severe convulsions. For individuals who lack an enzyme used in metabolizing cocaine, as few as two to three lines of cocaine may be fatal.

Methamphetamine

Methamphetamine or "meth" is a more potent form of amphetamine and has become the fastest-growing drug threat in the United States. More than 12 million Americans have tried this powerfully addictive drug. Typically it comes as a white, odorless, bitter-tasting powder that dissolves readily in water or alcohol. The drug is a potent central nervous system stimulant that produces a general feeling of well-being, decreases appetite, increases motor activity, and decreases fatigue and the need for sleep.

Methamphetamine is easily manufactured with over-the-counter ingredients in clandestine "meth labs." The risk of injury in a meth lab is high because potentially explosive environmental contaminants are discarded during production of the drug. Users of methamphetamine experience increases in body temperature, blood pressure, heart rate, and breathing rate; a decrease in appetite; hyperactivity; tremors; and violent behavior. High doses produce irritability, paranoia, irreversible damage to blood vessels in the brain (causing strokes), and risk of sudden death from hyperthermia and convulsions if not treated at once.

Chronic abusers experience insomnia, confusion, hallucinations, inflammation of the heart lining, schizophrenia-like mental disorder, and brain-cell damage similar to that caused by strokes. Physical changes to the brain may last months or perhaps permanently. Over time, methamphetamine use may reduce brain levels of dopamine, which can lead to symptoms of Parkinson's disease. In addition, users frequently are involved in violent crime, homicide, and suicide. Using methamphetamines during pregnancy may cause prenatal complications, premature delivery, and abnormal physical and emotional development of the child.

Heroin

For the first time in decades, heroin use is on the increase. Approximately 3.1 million Americans ages 12 and older reported trying heroin at least once. Common nicknames for heroin include Diesel, Dope, Dynamite, White Death, Nasty Boy, China White, H. Harry, Gumball, Junk, Brown Sugar, Smack, Tootsie Roll, Black Tar, and Chasing the Dragon. The most serious health threat to heroin users today is that they have no way of determining the strength of the drug purchased on the street, thus placing them at a constant risk for overdose and death. An estimated 15 percent of all drug-related hospital emergency room cases involve heroin use.

Heroin use induces a state of euphoria that comes within seconds of intravenous injection or within 5 to 15 minutes when other methods of administration are used. The drug is a sedative, so during the initial rush the person has a sense of relaxation and does not feel any pain. In users who inhale the drug, the rush may be accompanied by nausea, vomiting, intense itching, and at times severe asthma attacks. As the rush wears off, users become drowsy and confused and have reduced cardiac function and breathing rate.

A heroin overdose can cause convulsions, coma, and death. During an overdose, heart rate, breathing, blood pressure, and body temperature drop dramatically. These physiological responses can induce vomiting, tighten the muscles, and cause breathing to stop. Death is often the result of lack of oxygen or choking to death on vomit.

Within 4 to 5 hours after the drug is taken, withdrawal sets in. Heroin withdrawal is painful and may last up to 2 weeks but could go on several months. Symptoms of withdrawal for long-term users include red/raw nostrils, bone and muscle pains, muscle spasms and cramps, sweating, hot and cold flashes, runny nose and eyes, drowsiness, sluggishness, slurred speech, loss of appetite, nausea, diarrhea, restlessness, and violent yawning. Heroin use also can kill a developing fetus or cause a spontaneous abortion.

Symptoms of long-term use of heroin include hallucinations, nightmares, constipation, sexual difficulties, impaired vision, reduced fertility, boils, collapsed veins, and significantly elevated risk for lung, liver, and cardiovascular diseases, including bacterial infections in blood vessels and heart valves. Additives in street heroin can clog vital blood vessels because they do not dissolve in the body and therefore can lead to infections and death of cells in vital organs. Sudden infant death syndrome (SIDS) is seen more frequently in children born to addicted mothers.

MDMA (Ecstasy)

MDMA, also known as "ecstasy," became popular among teenagers and young adults in the United States in the mid-1980s. Prior to 1985, few Americans abused this drug. MDMA is named for its chemical structure: 3,4-methylenedioxymethamphetamine. Besides ecstasy, other street names for the drug are X-TC, E, Adam, and love drug. More than 10 million persons aged 12 and older have reported using Ecstasy at least once.

Although MDMA usually is swallowed in the form of one or two pills in doses of 50–240 mg, it also can be smoked, snorted, or occasionally injected. Because the drug is often prepared with other substances, users have no way of knowing the exact potency of the drug or additional substances found in each pill.

MDMA has a reputation among young people for being fun and harmless as long as it is used sensibly. MDMA, however, is not a harmless drug. Users may experience rapid eye movement, faintness, blurred vision, chills, sweating, nausea, muscle tension, and teeth-grinding. Individuals with heart, liver, or kidney disease or high blood pressure are especially at risk because MDMA increases blood pressure, heart rate, and body temperature; thus, it may lead to kidney failure, a heart attack, a stroke, and seizures.

Other evidence suggests that a pregnant woman using MDMA may find long-term learning and memory difficulties in her child. Other long-term side effects, lasting for weeks after use, include confusion, depression, sleep disorders, anxiety, aggression, paranoia, and impulsive behavior. Verbal and visual memory may be significantly impaired for years after prolonged use.

Treatment for Chemical Dependency

Recognizing the hazards of chemical use, families, teams, and communities can assist each other in preventing problems, as well as help those who already have problems with chemical use. Treating chemical dependency (including alcohol) seldom is accomplished without professional guidance and support. To secure the best available assistance, people in need should contact a physician or obtain a referral from a local mental health clinic (see Yellow Pages in the phone book).

Sexually Transmitted Infections

As the name implies, **sexually transmitted infections (STIs)** are infections spread through sexual contact. STIs have reached epidemic proportions in the United States. Of the more than 25 known STIs, some are still incurable. The American Social Health Association projected that 25 percent of all Americans will acquire at least one STI during their lifetime. Each year, more than 19 million people in the United States are newly infected with STIs, and almost half of them are seen in young people between the ages of 15 and 24.[27]

HIV/AIDS

AIDS (acquired immunodeficiency syndrome) is the most frightening of all STIs because it has no cure and in most cases is fatal. It is the end result of **human immunodeficiency virus (HIV)**, which spreads among individuals who engage in risky behavior such as having unprotected sex or sharing hypodermic needles. When a person becomes infected with HIV, the virus multiplies and attacks and destroys white blood cells. These cells are part of the immune system, whose function is to fight off infections and diseases in the body. As the number of white blood cells killed increases, the body's immune system breaks down gradually or may be destroyed totally. Without a functioning immune system,

---

KEY TERMS

Sexually transmitted infections (STIs) Communicable infections spread through sexual contact.

Acquired immunodeficiency syndrome (AIDS) End stage of HIV infection, manifested by any of a number of diseases that arise when the body's immune system is compromised by HIV.

Human immunodeficiency virus (HIV) Virus that leads to acquired immunodeficiency syndrome (AIDS).

a person becomes susceptible to **opportunistic infections** or cancers ordinarily not seen in healthy people.

HIV is a progressive infection. At first, people who contract the virus may not know they are infected. An incubation period of weeks, months, or years may go by during which time they have no symptoms. The virus may live in the body 10 years or longer before any symptoms emerge.

As the infection progresses to the point at which certain diseases develop, the person is said to have AIDS. HIV itself doesn't kill. Nor do people die from AIDS. AIDS is the term used to define the final stage of HIV infection. Death is caused by a weakened immune system that is unable to fight off opportunistic diseases. The virus has been known to live in the body 10 years or longer before symptoms emerge. Once the individual develops the symptoms that fit the case definition of AIDS, the person may live another 3 years or so.

No one has to become infected with HIV. At present, once infected with the virus, a person never will become uninfected. The only answer is to protect oneself against this infection. No one should be so ignorant as to believe that it can never happen to him or her!

HIV is transmitted by the exchange of cellular body fluids—blood, semen, vaginal secretions, and maternal milk. These fluids may be exchanged during sexual intercourse, by using hypodermic needles that infected individuals have used previously, between a pregnant woman and her developing fetus, in babies from infected mothers during childbirth, less frequently during breast feeding, and, rarely, from a blood transfusion or an organ transplant.

AIDS is an "equal opportunity epidemic." People do not get HIV because of who they are but, rather, because of what they do. HIV and AIDS threaten anyone, anywhere: men, women, children, teenagers, young people, older adults, Whites, Blacks, Hispanics, homosexuals, heterosexuals, bisexuals, druggies, Americans, Africans, Asians, Europeans. Nobody is immune to HIV.

You cannot tell if people are infected with HIV or have AIDS simply by looking at them or taking their word. Not you, not a nurse, not even a doctor can tell, without an HIV antibody test. Therefore, every time you engage in risky behavior, you run the risk of contracting HIV. The two most basic risky behaviors are (a) having unprotected vaginal, anal, or oral sex with an HIV-infected person, and (b) sharing hypodermic needles or other drug paraphernalia with someone who is infected.

Estimates by the Centers for Disease Control and Prevention indicate that, through the end of 2003, a cumulative total of 902,223 AIDS cases had been diagnosed in the United States, and 505,801 people had died from the diseases caused by HIV. One in every 300

Americans is infected at present, and about 27 percent of the diagnosed HIV/AIDs cases are women.

Although more than half of all AIDS cases in the United States initially occurred in homosexual or bisexual men, HIV infection now is spreading at a faster rate in heterosexuals. About 40,000 new infections are reported each year. Of these new infections, 45 percent of cases are reported in men who have sex with men, 30 percent in men and women through heterosexual sex, and 24 percent by injection drug use. Many heterosexuals practice unprotected sex because they don't believe it can happen to their segment of the population. But HIV is an epidemic that does not discriminate by sexual orientation. Worldwide, up to 80 percent of the AIDS cases have been reported in heterosexuals.

As with any other serious illness, AIDS patients deserve respect, understanding, and support. Rejection and discrimination are traits of immature, hateful, and ignorant people. Education, knowledge, and responsible behaviors are the best ways to minimize fear and discrimination.

Guidelines for Preventing STIs

With all the grim news about STIs, the good news is that you can do things to prevent their spread and take precautions to keep yourself from becoming a victim. The facts are in: The best preventive technique is a mutually monogamous sexual relationship—sex with only one person who has sexual relations only with you. That one behavior will remove you almost completely from any risk for developing an STI.

Unfortunately, in today's society, trust is an elusive concept. You may be led to believe you are in a monogamous relationship when your partner actually (a) may be cheating on you and gets infected, (b) ends up having a one-night stand with someone who is infected, (c) got the virus several years ago before the present relationship and still isn't aware of the infection, (d) may not be honest with you and chooses not to tell you about the infection, or (e) is shooting up drugs and becomes infected. In any of these cases, HIV can be passed on to you.

Because your future and your life are at stake and because you may never know if your partner is infected, you should give serious and careful consideration to postponing sex until you believe you have found a lifetime monogamous relationship. In doing so, you will not have to live with the fear of catching HIV or other STIs or deal with an unplanned pregnancy.

As strange as this may seem to some, many people postpone sexual activity until they are married. This is the best guarantee against HIV. Young people should understand that married life will provide plenty of time for fulfilling and rewarding sex. If you choose to delay sex, do not let peers pressure you into having sex. Some people would have you believe you are not a real man or woman if you don't have sex. Manhood and womanhood are not proven during sexual intercourse but, instead, through mature, responsible, and healthy choices. Other people lead you to believe that love doesn't exist without sex. Sex in the early stages of a relationship is not the product of love but is simply the fulfillment of a physical, and often selfish, drive. A loving relationship develops over a long time with mutual respect for each other.

Teenagers are especially susceptible to peer pressure leading to premature sexual intercourse. As a result, more than a million teens become pregnant each year, with a 43 percent pregnancy rate for all girls at least once as a teenager. Too many young people wish they had postponed sex and silently admire those who do. Sex lasts only a few minutes. The consequences of irresponsible sex may last a lifetime. In some cases they are fatal. Then there are those who enjoy bragging about their sexual conquests and mock people who choose to wait. In essence, many of these conquests are only fantasies expounded in an attempt to gain popularity with peers.

Sexual promiscuity never leads to a trusting, loving, and lasting relationship. Mature people respect others' choices. If someone does not respect your choice to wait, he or she certainly does not deserve your friendship or, for that matter, anything else. There is no greater sex than that between two loving and responsible individuals who mutually trust and admire each other. Contrary to many beliefs, these relationships are possible. They are built upon unselfish attitudes and behaviors.

As you look around, you will find people who have these values. Seek them out and build your friendships and future around people who respect you for who you are and what you believe. You don't have to compromise your choices or values. In the end, you will reap the greater rewards of a fulfilling and lasting relationship, free of AIDS and other STIs.

Also, be prepared so that you will know your course of action before you get into an intimate situation. Look for common interests and work together toward them. Express your feelings openly: "I'm not ready for sex; I just want to have fun and kissing is fine

with me." If your friend does not accept your answer and is not willing to stop the advances, be prepared with a strong response. Statements such as "Please stop" or "Don't!" are for the most part ineffective. Use a firm statement such as, "No, I'm not willing to do it" or "I've already thought about this, and I'm not going to have sex." If this still doesn't work, label the behavior rape: "This is rape, and I'm going to call the police."

What about those who do not have—or do not desire —a monogamous relationship? Risky behaviors that significantly increase the chances of contracting an STI, including HIV infection, are:

1. Multiple or anonymous sexual partners such as a pick-up or prostitute.
2. Anal sex with or without a condom.
3. Vaginal or oral sex with someone who shoots drugs or engages in anal sex.
4. Sex with someone you know who has several sex partners.
5. Unprotected sex (without a condom) with an infected person.
6. Sexual contact of any kind with anyone who has symptoms of AIDS or who is a member of a group at high risk for AIDS.
7. Sharing toothbrushes, razors, or other implements that could become contaminated with blood with anyone who is, or might be, infected with the HIV virus.

Avoiding risky behaviors that destroy quality of life and life itself is a critical component of a healthy lifestyle. Learning the facts so you can make responsible choices can protect you and those around you from startling and unexpected conditions. Using alcohol moderately (or not at all), refraining from substance abuse, and preventing sexually transmitted infections are keys to averting both physical and psychological damage.

K E Y   T E R M S

Opportunistic infections Diseases that arise in the absence of a healthy immune system that would fight them off in healthy people.

Create a Diet to Lower your Cholesterol. This interactive site will provide personalized guidelines on how to eat healthy and decrease your risk of heart disease, based on your height, weight, age, gender, and activity level.
http://www.nhlbisupport.com/chd1/create.htm

Cancer Quiz: Test Your Prevention Smarts. Take this seven-question quiz to assess your knowledge regarding cancer prevention.
http://mayoclinic.com/health/cancer-prevention/QZ00021

ASSESS YOUR KNOWLEDGE

Evaluate how well you understand the concepts presented in this chapter using the Assess Your Knowledge and Practice Quizzes options on your Profile Plus CD-ROM.

1. Coronary heart disease
   a. is the single leading cause of death in the United States.
   b. is the leading cause of sudden cardiac deaths.
   c. is a condition in which the arteries that supply the heart muscle with oxygen and nutrients are narrowed by fatty deposits.
   d. accounts for approximately 20 percent of all deaths.
   e. All of the above are correct choices.

2. The risk of heart disease increases with
   a. high LDL-cholesterol.
   b. high HDL-cholesterol.
   c. lack of homocysteine.
   d. low levels of hs-CRP.
   e. all of the above factors.

3. Type 2 diabetes is related closely to
   a. low BMI.
   b. obesity and lack of physical activity.
   c. genetically low homocysteine.
   d. increased insulin sensitivity.
   e. all of the above factors.

4. Metabolic syndrome is related to
   a. low HDL-cholesterol.
   b. high triglycerides.
   c. increased blood-clotting mechanism.
   d. an abnormal insulin response to carbohydrates.
   e. all of the above.

5. Cancer can be defined as
   a. a process whereby some cells invade and destroy the immune system.
   b. an uncontrolled growth and spread of abnormal cells.
   c. the spread of benign tumors throughout the body.
   d. the interference of normal body functions through blood flow disruption caused by angiogenesis.
   e. All are correct choices.

6. Cancer
   a. is primarily a preventable disease.
   b. is often related to tobacco use.
   c. has been linked to dietary habits.
   d. risk increases with obesity.
   e. All are correct choices.

7. A cancer prevention diet should include
   a. ample amounts of fruit and vegetables.
   b. cruciferous vegetables.
   c. phytochemicals.
   d. soy products.
   e. all of the above.

8. The biggest carcinogenic exposure in the workplace is
   a. asbestos fibers.
   b. cigarette smoke.
   c. biological agents.
   d. nitrosamines.
   e. pesticides.

9. Treatment of chemical dependency is
   a. primarily accomplished by the individual alone.
   b. most successful when there is peer pressure to stop.
   c. best achieved with the help of family members.
   d. seldom accomplished without professional guidance.
   e. usually done with the help of friends.

10. The best way to protect yourself against sexually transmitted infections is
   a. through the use of condoms with a spermicide.
   b. by knowing about the people who have previously had sex with your partner.
   c. through a mutually monogamous sexual relationship.
   d. by having sex only with an individual who has no symptoms of STIs.
   e. All of the above choices provide equal protection against STIs.

Correct answers can be found on page 261.

Managing Cardiovascular Disease and Cancer Risks

Name _____   Date _____

Course _____   Section _____

I. Cardiovascular Disease

	Yes	**No**
1. I accumulate between 30 and 60 minutes of physical activity on most days of the week.	☐	☐
2. I exercise aerobically a minimum of three times a week in the appropriate target zone for at least 20 minutes per session.	☐	☐
3. I am at or slightly below the health fitness recommended percent body fat (see Table 2.12, page 44, or a BMI below 25).	☐	☐
4. My blood lipids are within normal range..	☐	☐
5. I get 25 (women) to 38 (men) grams of fiber in my daily diet.	☐	☐
6. I eat more than five servings of fruits and vegetables every day.	☐	☐
7. I limit saturated fat, and cholesterol in my daily diet.	☐	☐
8. I am not a diabetic.	☐	☐
9. My blood pressure is normal.	☐	☐
10. I do not smoke cigarettes or use tobacco in any other form.	☐	☐
11. I manage stress adequately in daily life.	☐	☐
12. I do not have a personal or family history of heart disease.	☐	☐

Evaluation

A "no" answer to any of the above items increases your risk for cardiovascular disease. The greater the number of "no" responses, the higher the risk for developing cardiovascular disease.

Please indicate lifestyle changes you will implement or maintain to decrease your personal risk for cardiovascular disease.

_____

_____

_____

_____

_____

_____

II. Cancer Prevention Questionnaire: Cancer Risk: Are You Taking Control?

Today, scientists think most cancers may be related to lifestyle and environment—what you eat and drink, whether you smoke, and where you work and play. The good news, then, is that you can help reduce your own cancer risk by taking control of things in your daily life.

15 Steps to a Healthier Life and Reduced Cancer Risk

	Yes	No
1. Are you eating more cruciferous vegetables? They include broccoli, cauliflower, Brussels sprouts, all cabbages, and kohlrabi.	☐	☐
2. Are high-fiber foods included in your diet? Fiber is present in whole grains, fruits and vegetables (including peaches, strawberries, potatoes, spinach, and tomatoes), wheat and bran cereals, rice, popcorn, and whole-wheat bread.	☐	☐
3. Do you choose foods with vitamin A? Fresh foods with beta-carotene—including carrots, peaches, apricots, squash, and broccoli—are the best source, not vitamin pills.	☐	☐
4. Is vitamin C included in your diet? You'll find it naturally in lots of fresh fruits and vegetables including grapefruit, cantaloupe, oranges, strawberries, red and green peppers, broccoli, and tomatoes.	☐	☐
5. Do you eat sufficient selenium-bearing foods (fish, Brazil nuts, whole grains) so you obtain at least 100 mcg of selenium per day?	☐	☐
6. Do you exercise and monitor calorie intake to avoid weight gain? Walking is ideal exercise for many people.	☐	☐
7. Are you cutting overall fat intake? This is done by eating lean meat, fish, skinned poultry, and low-fat dairy products.	☐	☐
8. Do you limit salt-cured, smoked, and nitrite-cured foods? Choose bacon, ham, hot dogs, or salt-cured fish only occasionally if you like them a lot.	☐	☐
9. Are you a non-smoker?	☐	☐
10. If you smoke, have you tried quitting?	☐	☐
11. Do you abstain from all other forms of tobacco?	☐	☐
12. If you drink alcohol, are you moderate in your intake?	☐	☐
13. Do you respect the sun's rays? Protect yourself with sunscreen (at least SPF 15), and wear long sleeves and a hat, especially during midday hours (10 AM to 4 PM).	☐	☐
14. Do you have a family history of any type of cancer? (If so, you should bring this to the attention of your personal physician.)	☐	☐
15. Are you familiar with the seven warning signals for cancer?	☐	☐

Evaluation

If you answered yes to most of these questions, congratulations. You are taking control of simple lifestyle factors that will help you feel better and reduce your risk for cancer.

Please indicate lifestyle changes you will implement or maintain to decrease your personal risk for cancer:

_____

_____

_____

Adapted from the American Cancer Society, Texas Division.

© Ariel Skelley/CORBIS

CHAPTER 9 — Relevant Fitness and Wellness Issues

OBJECTIVES

- Dispel common misconceptions related to physical fitness and wellness.
- Give practical advice and tips regarding safety.
- Address some concerns specific to women.
- Clarify additional concepts regarding nutrition and weight control.
- Answer some questions regarding wellness and aging.
- Provide guidelines related to fitness/wellness consumer issues.

For this chapter the activities on your Profile Plus CD-ROM will help you determine your risk for heart disease and cancer, help you plan for a smoke-free future, and help you evaluate your knowledge of HIV/AIDS.

This chapter addresses some of the most frequently asked questions about various facets of physical fitness and wellness. The answers will further clarify concepts discussed throughout the book, as well as put to rest several myths that misinform fitness and wellness participants. "Q" denotes the question, and "A" designates the answer.

Safety of Exercise Participation and Injury Prevention

Q Can aerobic exercise make a person immune to heart and blood vessel disease?

A Scientific evidence clearly indicates that aerobically fit individuals have a much lower incidence of cardiovascular disease. A regular aerobic exercise program by itself, however, is not an absolute guarantee against diseases of the heart and blood vessels. Several factors increase a person's risk for cardiovascular disease.

Though physical inactivity is one of the most significant risk factors, studies have documented that these risk factors have multiple interrelations. Physical inactivity, for instance, often contributes to an increase in (a) body fat, (b) LDL-cholesterol, (c) triglycerides, (d) inflammation, (e) stress, (f) blood pressure, and (g) risk for diabetes (see Figure 9.1). As discussed in Chapter 8, most risk factors for cardiovascular

FIGURE 9.1 Interrelationships among leading cardiovascular risk factors.

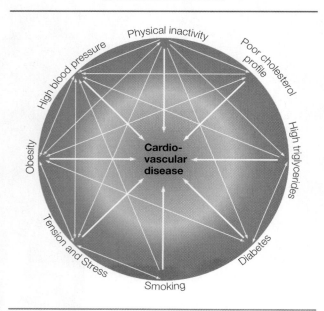

TABLE 9.1 Minimum Amount of Walking (Aerobic Activity) Required for Moderate Fitness in Adults

PROGRAM 1	DAYS/ WEEK	DISTANCE (MILES)	TIME (MIN)
Women	≥3	2	≤30
Men	≥3	2	≤27
PROGRAM 2			
Women	5–6	2	30–40
Men	6–7	2	30–40

From S. N. Blair, *Fitness and Mortality* (Dallas: Aerobics Research Center, 1991).

disease are preventable and reversible. Overall management of the risk factors is the best way to minimize the risk for cardiovascular disease. Research also indicates that the odds of surviving a heart attack are much higher for people who engage in a regular aerobic exercise program.

Q What amount of aerobic exercise is optimal to significantly decrease the risk for cardiovascular disease?

A The amount of exercise required to maintain cardiorespiratory fitness calls for a training session approximately every 48 hours for 20 to 30 minutes in the appropriate target training zone (see Chapter 3). People who accumulate 30 minutes of moderate-intensity physical activity on most days of the week, however, can expect to reap many of the health benefits provided by a regular exercise program. The amount of exercise required to offset the risk cannot be pinpointed specifically because of the many individual differences (genetic and lifestyle) between people. Research, however, has shed some light on this subject.

One of the earlier studies indicated that about 300 calories should be expended daily through aerobic exercise to obtain a certain degree of protection against cardiovascular disease.[1] A study among Harvard alumni (see Figure 1.7, page 9) found that expending 2,000 calories per week as a result of physical activity yielded the lowest risk for cardiovascular disease in this group of

almost 17,000 people. The 2,000 calories per week represents about 300 calories per daily exercise session.

The work alluded to in Chapter 8 (see Figure 8.5, page 175), conducted at the Aerobics Research Institute in Dallas, indicated that even moderate fitness levels can reduce the incidence of cardiovascular problems substantially.[2] The minimum dose for moderate fitness requires an expenditure of about 200 calories five to seven times per week (see Table 9.1). Slightly greater protection is achieved at higher fitness levels.

Clinical data on individuals with or at risk for coronary heart disease suggest that more than 1,400 calories per week may have to be expended to improve cardiorespiratory fitness, more than 1,500 weekly calories to stop the progression of atherosclerotic lesions, and more than 2,200 calories per week, or the equivalent of 5 to 6 hours of weekly exercise, for regression of lesions.[3] As noted in the previous question, neither physical activity nor exercise by itself provides an absolutely risk-free guarantee against cardiovascular disease.

Q At what age should I start concerning myself with cardiovascular disease?

A The disease process for cardiovascular disease, as well as cancer, starts early in life as a result of poor lifestyle habits. Studies have shown beginning stages of atherosclerosis and elevated blood lipids in children as young as 10 years old.

Many positive habits can be established early in life within the walls of one's own home. If people are taught at a young age that they should avoid excessive calories, sweets, salt, and alcohol; not use tobacco; and participate in physical activity, their chances of leading a healthier life are much greater than is true with the present generation. When it comes to teaching, some of the best advice that can be given is, "Come and follow me." If you cultivate positive health habits in your own life, your children will be more likely to follow.

Regular physical activity during youth enhances the likelihood of lifetime participation in an exercise program.

© Fitness & Wellness, Inc.

Q Does alcohol protect against cardiovascular disease?

A The health benefits of moderate alcohol consumption have been extensively reported by the media, but also widely exaggerated. The media love to discuss this topic because it appears to be "a vice that's good for you." The research supports the consumption of no more than two alcoholic beverages a day for men and one a day for women as providing modest benefits in decreasing the risk for cardiovascular disease. Not reported in the media, however, is that these modest health benefits do not always apply to African Americans.

The benefits of modest alcohol use can be equated to benefits obtained through a small daily dose of aspirin (about 81 mg per day, or the equivalent of a baby aspirin), or eating a small amount of nuts each day. And aspirin or a few nuts do not lead to impaired judgment or actions that you may later regret or have to live with the rest of your life.

Alcohol is not for everyone. Alcoholism seems to have both a genetic and an environmental component. The reasons why some people can drink for years without becoming addicted, whereas others follow the downward spiral of alcoholism are not understood. The addiction develops slowly. Most people think they are in control of their drinking habits and do not realize they have a problem until they become alcoholics, when they find themselves physically and emotionally dependent on alcohol.

Short- and long-term detrimental consequences of alcohol abuse are discussed in Chapter 8 (page191). If

you don't drink alcohol, don't start. Better ways to take care of your heart are to engage in regular physical activity and adhere to a healthy diet.

Q Can too much exercise be detrimental to health?

A Moderate exercise training provides many health benefits and strengthens immune function. Prolonged and intense exercise, however, can negatively affect immune function and result in increased susceptibility to upper respiratory tract infections (common cold and influenza) and viral infections. The primary concern in this area is with endurance athletes who are more susceptible to infections during intense training and competition.

Q Will exercise help me feel better?

A Yes. Many studies have found that exercise helps people feel better, improves self-esteem and self-confidence, relieves stress, and even alleviates depression. As with the physiological benefits of exercise, regular participation in exercise yields psychological benefits. Hence, a lifetime of physical activity is just as important for mental wellness.

CT Critical Thinking

What role do physical activity and exercise play in your life? What impact do these have on your emotional well-being?

Q How can I tell if I'm exceeding the safe limits for exercising?

A The best way to determine whether you are exercising too strenuously is to check your heart rate and make sure it doesn't exceed the limits of your target zone. Exercising above this target zone may not be safe for unconditioned or high-risk individuals. You do not need to exercise beyond your target zone to gain the desired benefits for the cardiorespiratory system. Also, if your heart rate has not returned to under 120 beats per minute 5 minutes after you stopped exercise, you have overexerted yourself. If elevated recovery heart rates persist after you decrease exercise intensity and duration, you may have a medical condition that should be investigated.

In addition, several physical signs will tell you when you are exceeding functional limitations: rapid or irregular heart rate, difficult breathing, nausea, vomiting, lightheadedness, headaches, dizziness, pale skin, flushness, extreme weakness, lack of energy, shakiness, sore muscles, cramps, and tightness in the chest. These are all signs of exercise intolerance—the physical aversion to exercise conducted at intensity levels beyond a person's functional capacity. Learn to listen to your body. If you notice any of these symptoms, seek medical attention before continuing your exercise program.

◖ Should I exercise when I have a cold or the flu?

◖ The most important consideration is to use common sense and pay attention to your symptoms. Usually you may continue exercise if your symptoms are a runny nose, sneezing, or a scratchy throat. But if you have a fever or achy muscles; if you are vomiting, have diarrhea, or have a hacking cough, you should avoid exercise. Following an illness, be sure to ease back gradually into your program. Do not attempt to return at the same intensity and duration that you were used to prior to your illness.

◖ How fast does a person lose the benefits of exercise after stopping an exercise program?

◖ How quickly the benefits of exercise are lost differs among the various components of physical fitness and also depends on the condition the person achieves before discontinuing the exercise. Specifically with regard to cardiorespiratory endurance, it has been estimated that 4 weeks of aerobic training are completely reversed in 2 consecutive weeks of physical inactivity.

If you have been exercising regularly for months or years, 2 weeks of inactivity will not hurt you as much as it will someone who has exercised only a few weeks. Generally speaking, within 2 to 3 days of aerobic inactivity, the cardiorespiratory system starts to lose some of its capacity. Flexibility can be maintained with two or three stretching sessions per week, and strength is maintained with just one maximal training session per week. If you have to interrupt the program for reasons beyond your control, do not attempt to resume your training at the same level you left off but, instead, build up gradually again.

You should maintain a regular fitness program even during traveling and vacation periods. When traveling, plan ahead and examine your options before you leave home. Many hotels provide in-house fitness facilities. Although the equipment often is limited, it's generally sufficient for an adequate cardiorespiratory and strength workout. Frequent travelers would benefit from joining a nationally franchised health club, a YMCA, or a YWCA. In this manner, you can continue the same exercise program while visiting different cities.

Activities that require a minimum of equipment and no facilities, such as walking, jogging, and rope jumping, are excellent alternatives for the road. If you are going to venture out in a new city, always ask for safe places to jog. Nearby parks or a high school track are usually safe and help you stay away from traffic and stop lights. The strength-training (without equipment) and flexibility exercises provided in Appendixes A and B, pages 227–238, can be used to maintain your strength and flexibility. If you are visiting a resort area, fitness rental equipment, such as bikes and roller blades, is often available.

◖ What type of clothing should I wear when I exercise?

◖ The type of clothing you wear during exercise is important. In general, clothing should fit comfortably and allow free movement of the various body parts. Select clothing according to expected air temperature, humidity, and exercise intensity. Avoid nylon and rubberized materials and tight clothes that interfere with the body's cooling mechanism or obstruct normal blood flow. Fabrics made from polypropylene, Capilene, Thermax, and synthetics are best. These types of fabrics wick (draw) moisture away from the skin, enhancing evaporation and cooling the body. Exercise intensity also is important because the harder you exercise, the more heat your body produces.

When exercising in the heat, avoid the hottest time of the day, between 11:00 AM and 5:00 PM. Avoid surfaces such as asphalt, concrete, and artificial turfs because they absorb heat, which then radiates to the body. (Also see the discussion on exercise in hot and humid conditions on pages 205–206).

Only minimal clothing is necessary during exercise in the heat, to allow for maximal evaporation. Clothing should be lightweight, light-colored, loose-fitting, airy, and absorbent. Examples of commercially available products that can be used during exercise in the heat are Asci's Perma Plus, Cool-max, and Nike's Dri-F.I.T. Double-layer acrylic socks are more absorbent than cotton and help to prevent blistering and chafing of the feet. A straw-type hat can be worn to protect the eyes and head from the sun. Clothing for exercise in the cold is discussed on page 207.

A good pair of shoes is vital to prevent lower-limb injuries. You should wear shoes manufactured specifically for your choice of activity. Other considerations for proper footwear include body type, tendency toward pronation or supination, and exercise surfaces. Shoes should have good stability, motion control, and comfortable fit. It's best to purchase shoes in the middle of the day when the feet have expanded and might be one-half size larger. For increased breatheability, choose shoes with nylon or mesh uppers. Generally, salespeople

Activity-specific shoes are recommended to prevent injury to the lower extremities.

at reputable athletic shoe stores are knowledgeable and can help you select a good shoe that fits your needs. Examine your shoes after 500 miles or 6 months and obtain a new pair if they are worn out. Old shoes frequently are responsible for lower-limb injuries.

◻ What time of the day is best for exercise?

◺ A person can exercise at almost any time of the day except about 2 hours following a large meal, or the noon and early afternoon hours on hot and humid days. Many people enjoy exercising early in the morning because it gives them a good boost to start the day. If you have a difficult time sticking to an exercise program, early morning exercise is best because the chances of some other activity or conflict interfering with your exercise time are minimal. Some people prefer the lunch hour for weight-control reasons. By exercising at noon, they do not eat as big a lunch, which helps keep down daily caloric intake. Highly stressed people seem to like the evening hours because of the relaxing effects of exercise.

◻ How long should a person wait after a meal before engaging in strenuous physical exercise?

◺ The length of time to wait before exercising after a meal depends on the amount of food eaten. On the average, after a regular meal a person should wait about 2 hours before participating in strenuous physical activity. Light physical activity, such as a walk, is fine. If anything, it helps burn extra calories and may help the body metabolize fats more efficiently.

◻ How should acute sports injuries be treated?

◺ The best treatment always has been prevention. If an activity causes unusual discomfort or chronic irritation, you need to treat the cause by decreasing the intensity, switching activities, substituting equipment, or upgrading clothing, such as buying properly fitted shoes.

In cases of acute injury, the standard treatment is rest, cold application, compression or splinting (or both), and elevation of the affected body part. The applicable acronym is RICE:

R = rest
I = ice application
C = compression
E = elevation.

Cold should be applied three to five times a day for 15 to 20 minutes at a time during the first 36 to 48 hours, by submerging the injured area in cold water, using an ice bag, or applying ice massage to the affected part. An elastic bandage or wrap can be used for compression. Elevating the body part decreases blood flow to it. The purpose of these treatment modalities is to minimize swelling in the area, which hastens recovery time.

After the first 36 to 48 hours, heat can be used if the injury shows no further swelling or inflammation. If you have doubts regarding the nature or seriousness of the injury (such as suspected fracture), you should seek a medical evaluation.

Obvious deformities (such as in fractures, dislocations, or partial dislocations) call for splinting, cold application with an ice bag, and medical attention. Never try to reset any of these conditions by yourself, as muscles, ligaments, and nerves could be damaged further. These injuries should be treated by specialized medical personnel. A quick reference guide for the signs or symptoms and treatment of exercise-related problems is provided in Table 9.2.

◻ What causes muscle soreness and stiffness?

◺ Muscle soreness and stiffness are common in individuals who (a) begin an exercise program or participate after a long layoff from exercise, (b) exercise beyond their customary intensity and duration, and (c) perform eccentric training. The acute soreness that sets in during the first few hours after exercise is related to general fatigue caused by chemical waste products that build up in the exercised muscles.

The delayed-onset muscle soreness (DOMS) that appears several hours after exercise (usually 12 hours or so later) and lasts 2 to 4 days may be related to

TABLE 9.2 Reference Guide for Exercise-Related Problems

INJURY	SIGNS/SYMPTOMS	TREATMENT*
Bruise (contusion)	Pain, swelling, discoloration	Cold application, compression, rest
Dislocations/Fractures	Pain, swelling, deformity	Splinting, cold application, seek medical attention
Heat cramps	Cramps, spasms and muscle twitching in the legs, arms, and abdomen	Stop activity, get out of the heat, stretch, massage the painful area, drink plenty of fluids
Heat exhaustion	Fainting, profuse sweating, cold/clammy skin, weak/rapid pulse, weakness, headache	Stop activity, rest in a cool place, loosen clothing, rub body with cool/wet towel, drink plenty of fluids, stay out of heat for 2–3 days
Heat stroke	Hot/dry skin, no sweating, serious disorientation, rapid/full pulse, vomiting, diarrhea, unconsciousness, high body temperature	Seek immediate medical attention, request help and get out of the sun, bathe in cold water/spray with cold water/rub body with cold towels, drink plenty of cold fluids
Joint sprains	Pain, tenderness, swelling, loss of use, discoloration	Cold application, compression, elevation, rest, heat after 36 to 48 hours (if no further swelling)
Muscle cramps	Pain, spasm	Stretch muscle(s), use mild exercises for involved area
Muscle soreness and stiffness	Tenderness, pain	Mild stretching, low-intensity exercise, warm bath
Muscle strains	Pain, tenderness, swelling, loss of use	Cold application, compression, elevation, rest, heat after 36 to 48 hours (if no further swelling)
Shin splints	Pain, tenderness	Cold application prior to and following any physical activity, rest, heat (if no activity is carried out)
Side stitch	Pain on the side of the abdomen below the rib cage	Decrease level of physical activity or stop altogether, gradually increase level of fitness
Tendinitis	Pain, tenderness, loss of use	Rest, cold application, heat after 48 hours

*Cold should be applied 3 to 4 times a day for 15 minutes. Heat can be applied 3 times a day for 15 to 20 minutes.

microscopic tears in muscle tissue, muscle spasms that increase fluid retention and thereby stimulate the pain nerve endings, and overstretching or tearing of connective tissue in and around muscles and joints.

Two types of contraction accompany muscular activity with movement (also see the Chapter 3 discussion on mode of training—concentric muscle contraction and eccentric muscle contraction—pages 60–62). **Concentric muscle contraction** is a dynamic contraction in which the muscle shortens as it develops tension. **Eccentric muscle contraction** is a dynamic contraction in which the muscle fibers lengthen while developing tension.

For example, during the arm-curl exercise, the elbow flexor muscles (biceps, brachioradialis, and brachialis) shorten as the weight is brought toward the shoulder (concentric contraction). On the way down, the muscles contract eccentrically as they lengthen while the person lowers the weight slowly to the starting position.

As you place your foot on the ground when running, the muscles contract eccentrically to absorb the weight of the body as you strike the ground. This eccentric contraction is followed by a concentric contraction of the leg as you push off the ground to propel the body forward.

Unlike running, cycling requires only concentric contractions of the leg muscles as you pedal the bicycle. Pushing down on the pedal produces a concentric contraction of the quadriceps muscles. If you use toe clips, pulling the pedal back up to the top of the circle produces a concentric contraction of the hamstring muscles.

Eccentric training has been shown to produce more muscle soreness than concentric training does. A hard running workout, therefore, produces greater muscle soreness than a hard cycling workout of similar intensity and duration.

To prevent soreness and stiffness, the recommended approach is to warm up gradually before physical activity and to stretch adequately after exercise. Do not attempt to do too much too quickly. If you become sore and stiff, you have overdone your workout. In these cases, mild stretching, low-intensity exercise to stimulate blood flow, and a warm bath can bring relief.

Stretching may be of greatest significance following exercise. Tired muscles tend to contract to a length that is shorter than normal. Byproducts of exercise metabolism also may cause muscle spasms. Post-exercise stretching thus can help return a muscle to its normal length.

How should I care for shin splints?

The **shin splint**, one of the most common injuries to the lower limbs, usually results from one or more of the following: (a) lack of proper and gradual conditioning, (b) doing physical activities on hard surfaces (wooden floors, hard tracks, cement, and asphalt), (c) fallen arches in the feet, (d) chronic overuse, (e) muscle fatigue, (f) faulty posture, (g) improper shoes, and (h) participating in weight-bearing activities when excessively overweight.

To manage shin splints:

1. Remove or reduce the cause (exercise on softer surfaces, wear better shoes or arch supports, or completely stop exercise until the shin splints heal).
2. Do stretching exercises before and after physical activity.
3. Use ice massage for 10 to 20 minutes before and after physical exercise.
4. Apply active heat (whirlpool and hot baths) for 15 minutes, two or three times a day.
5. Use supportive taping during physical activity (the proper taping technique can be learned readily from a qualified athletic trainer).

What causes muscle cramps, and what should be done when they occur?

Muscle cramps are caused by the body's depletion of essential electrolytes or a breakdown in coordination between opposing muscle groups. If you have a muscle cramp, first attempt to stretch the muscle(s) involved. In the case of the calf muscle, for example, pull your toes up toward the knees. After stretching the affected muscles, rub them down gently, and finally do some mild exercises requiring the use of those specific muscles.

In pregnant and lactating women and people who get very little calcium in the diet, muscle cramps often are caused by a lack of this nutrient. Calcium supplements are recommended in these cases and usually relieve the problem. Tight clothing also can cause cramps because it restricts blood flow to active muscle tissue.

Why is exercising in hot and humid conditions unsafe?

When a person exercises, only 30 percent to 40 percent of the energy the body produces is used for mechanical work or movement. The rest of the energy (60 percent to 70 percent) is converted into heat. If this heat cannot be dissipated properly because the weather is too hot or the relative humidity is too high, body temperature increases and, in extreme cases, can result in death.

The specific heat of body tissue (the heat required to raise the temperature of the body by 1°C) is .38 calories per pound of body weight per 1°C (.38 cal/lb/°C). This indicates that if no body heat is dissipated, a 150-pound person has to burn only 57 calories ($150 \times .38$) to increase total body temperature by 1°C. If this person were to engage in an exercise session requiring 300 calories (about 3 miles running) without dissipating any heat, the inner body temperature would increase by 5.3°C, the equivalent of going from 98.6 to 108.1°F.

This example clearly illustrates the need for caution when exercising in hot or humid weather. If the weather is too hot or the relative humidity is too high, body heat cannot be lost through evaporation because the atmosphere already is saturated with water vapor. In one instance, a football casualty occurred when the outdoor temperature was only 64°F, but the relative humidity was 100 percent. As a general rule, a person must take care when air temperature is above 90°F and relative humidity is above 60 percent.

The American College of Sports Medicine has recommended that individuals should not engage in strenuous physical activity when the readings of a wet bulb globe thermometer exceed 82.4°F. With this type of thermometer, the wet bulb is cooled by evaporation, and on dry days it shows a lower temperature than the regular (dry) thermometer. On humid days, the cooling effect is less because of less evaporation; hence, the difference between the wet and dry readings is not as great.

KEY TERMS

Concentric muscle contraction A dynamic contraction in which the muscle shortens as it develops tension.

Eccentric muscle contraction A dynamic contraction in which the muscle lengthens as it develops tension.

Shin splint Injury to the lower leg characterized by pain and irritation at the front of the leg.

Following are symptoms of and first-aid measures for the three major signs of trouble when exercising in the heat:

1. Heat cramps. Symptoms include cramps and spasms and muscle twitching in the legs, arms, and abdomen. To relieve heat cramps, stop exercising, get out of the heat, stretch slowly, massage the painful area, and drink plenty of fluids (water, fruit drinks, or electrolyte beverages).

2. Heat exhaustion. Symptoms include fainting, dizziness, profuse sweating, cold, clammy skin, weakness, headache, and a rapid, weak pulse. If you develop any of these symptoms, stop and find a cool place to rest. Drink cool water only if conscious. Loosen or remove clothing, and rub your body with a cool/wet towel or ice packs. Place yourself in a supine position with legs elevated 8 to 12 inches. If you are not fully recovered in 30 minutes, seek immediate medical attention.

3. Heat stroke. Symptoms include serious disorientation; warm, dry skin; no sweating; rapid, full pulse; vomiting; diarrhea; unconsciousness; and high body temperature. As the body temperature climbs, unexplained anxiety sets in. When the body temperature reaches 104°F to 105°F, the individual may feel a cold sensation in the trunk of the body, goose bumps, nausea, throbbing in the temples, and numbness in the extremities. Most people become incoherent after this stage. When body temperature reaches 105°F to 106°F, disorientation, loss of fine motor control, and muscular weakness set in. If the temperature exceeds 106°F, serious neurologic injury and death may be imminent.

Heat stroke requires immediate emergency medical attention. Request help and get out of the sun and into a cool, humidity-controlled environment. While you're waiting to be taken to the hospital's emergency room, you should be placed in a semi-seated position, and your body should be sprayed with cool water and rubbed with cool towels. If possible, cold packs should be placed in areas with abundant blood supply, such as the head, neck, armpits, and groin. Fluids should not be given if you are unconscious.

In any case of heat-related illness, if the person refuses water, vomits, or starts to lose consciousness, call for an ambulance immediately. Proper initial treatment of heat stroke is critical.

Q What are the recommended guidelines for fluid replacement during prolonged aerobic exercise?

A The main objective of fluid replacement during prolonged aerobic exercise is to maintain the blood

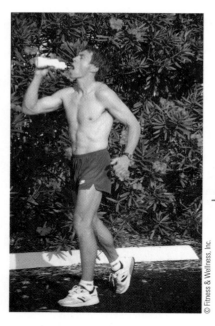

Fluid and carbohydrate replacement is essential during prolonged exercise.

© Fitness & Wellness, Inc.

volume so circulation and sweating can continue at normal levels. Adequate water replacement is the most important factor in preventing heat disorders. Drinking about 6 to 8 ounces of cool water every 15 to 20 minutes during exercise seems to be ideal to prevent dehydration. Cold fluids are absorbed more rapidly from the stomach.

Commercial fluid-replacement solutions (e.g., Powerade®, All-Sport®, Gatorade®) contain about 6 percent to 8 percent glucose, which seems to be optimal for fluid absorption and performance in most cases. Commercially prepared sports drinks are recommended especially when exercise will be strenuous and carried out for more than an hour. For exercise lasting less than an hour, water is sufficient to replace fluid loss. The sports drinks you select should be based on your personal preference. Try different drinks at 6 percent to 8 percent glucose concentration to see which drink you tolerate best and suits your taste as well. The sugar in these products does not become available to the muscles until about 30 minutes after drinking a glucose solution.

Drinks high in fructose or with a glucose concentration above 8 percent will actually slow water absorption when you exercise in the heat. Most soft drinks (cola, noncola) contain between 10 percent and 12 percent glucose, an amount that is too high for proper rehydration in these circumstances.

For long-distance events, researchers recommend that 30 to 60 grams of carbohydrate (120 to 240 calories) be consumed every hour. This is best accomplished by drinking 8 ounces of a 6 percent to 8 percent carbohydrate sports drink every 15 minutes. The percentage of the carbohydrate drink is determined by dividing the amount of carbohydrate (in grams) by the amount of fluid (in ml) and multiplying by 100. For example, 18 grams of carbohydrate in 240 ml (8 oz) of fluid yields a drink at 7.5 percent (18 ÷ 240 = 100).

Q What precautions must a person take when exercising in the cold?

A The two factors to consider when you exercise in the cold are frostbite and hypothermia. In contrast to hot and humid conditions, exercising in the cold usually is not health-threatening because clothing for heat conservation can be selected and exercise itself increases the production of body heat.

Most people actually overdress for exercise in the cold. Because exercise increases body temperature, a moderate workout on a cold day makes you feel that it is 20° to 30° warmer than the actual temperature. Overdressing for exercise can make the clothes damp from excessive perspiration. The risk for **hypothermia** increases when a person is wet or not moving around sufficiently to increase body heat. Initial warning signs of hypothermia include shivering, loss of coordination, and difficulty in speaking. With a continued drop in body temperature, shivering stops, the muscles weaken and stiffen, and the person feels elated or intoxicated and eventually loses consciousness. To prevent hypothermia, use common sense, dress properly, and be aware of environmental conditions.

The popular belief that exercising in cold temperatures (32°F and lower) freezes the lungs is false because the air is warmed properly in the air passages before it reaches the lungs. The threat is not the cold; it's the wind velocity—which affects the chill factor greatly.

For example, exercising at a temperature of 25°F with adequate clothing is not too cold, but if the wind is blowing at 25 miles per hour, the chill factor lowers the actual temperature to 15°F. This effect is even worse if a person is wet and exhausted. On windy days, exercise (jog, cycle) against the wind on the way out and with the wind when you return.

Even though the lungs are not at risk when you exercise in the cold, your face, head, hands, and feet should be protected, because they are subject to frostbite. Watch for numbness and discoloration—signs of frostbite. In cold temperatures, as much as 50 percent of the body's heat can be lost through an unprotected head and neck. A wool or synthetic cap, hood, or hat will help to hold in body heat. Mittens are better than gloves because they keep the fingers together so the surface area from which to lose heat is less. Inner linings of synthetic material are recommended because they wick moisture away from the skin. Avoid cotton next to the skin because, once it gets wet—whether from perspiration, rain, or snow—cotton loses its insulating properties.

Wearing several layers of lightweight clothing is preferable to wearing one single, thick layer because warm air is trapped between layers of clothes, enabling greater heat conservation. As body temperature increases, you can remove layers as necessary. For prolonged or long-distance workouts (cross-country skiing or long runs), take a small backpack to carry any clothing you remove. You also can carry extra warm and dry clothes in case you stop exercising away from shelter. If you remain outdoors following exercise, added clothing and continuous body movement are essential.

The first layer of clothes should wick moisture away from the skin. Polypropylene, Capilene, and Thermax are recommended. Next, a layer of wool, dacron, or polyester fleece insulates well even when wet. Lycra tights or sweatpants help to protect the legs. The outer layer should be waterproof, wind-resistant, and breatheable. A synthetic material such as Gore-Tex is best so moisture still can escape from the body. A ski mask or face mask helps to protect the face. In extremely cold conditions, petroleum jelly can be used to protect exposed skin such as the nose, cheeks, or around the eyes.

Special Considerations for Women

Q What are the physiological differences between men and women as related to exercise?

A Men and women have several basic differences that affect their physical performance. On the average, men are about 3 to 4 inches taller and 25 to 30 pounds heavier than women. The average body fat in college males is about 12 percent to 16 percent, whereas in college females it is 22 percent to 26 percent.

Maximal oxygen uptake (aerobic capacity) is about 15 percent to 30 percent greater in men, caused primarily by their lower body fat content (essential fat), higher **hemoglobin** concentration, and larger heart size. The higher hemoglobin concentration allows men to carry more oxygen during exercise, which is advantageous during aerobic events. A larger heart pumps more blood with each stroke, thereby increasing the amount of oxygenated blood available to the working muscles.

KEY TERMS

Hypothermia A breakdown in the body's ability to generate heat, resulting in body temperature below 95°F.

Hemoglobin Protein-iron compound in red blood cells that transports oxygen in the blood.

The quality of muscle in men and women is the same. Men, however, are stronger because they have more muscle mass and a greater capacity for muscle hypertrophy, the muscle's ability to increase in size. The larger capacity for muscle hypertrophy is related to sex-specific hormones. Strength differences are significantly less, though, when taking into consideration body size and composition.

Men also have wider shoulders, longer extremities, and a 10 percent greater bone width, except for pelvic width. Notwithstanding all these gender differences in physiological characteristics, the two sexes respond to training in a similar way.

Q If the potential for muscle hypertrophy in women is not as great, why do so many women body builders develop such heavy musculature?

A The idea that strength training allows women to develop muscle hypertrophy to the same extent as men do is as false as the notion that playing basketball will turn women into giants. Masculinity and femininity are established by genetic inheritance, not by the amount of physical activity. Variations in the extent of masculinity and femininity are determined by individual differences in hormonal secretions of androgen, testosterone, estrogen, and progesterone.

Women with a bigger-than-average build often are inclined to participate in sports because of their natural physical advantage. As a result, many women have associated participation in sports and strength training with large muscle size.

As the number of women who participate in sports has increased steadily during the last few years, the misconception that strength training in women leads to large increases in muscle size has abated somewhat. For example, per pound of body weight, women gymnasts are considered to be among the strongest athletes in the world. These athletes engage regularly in intense strength-training programs. Yet, of all women, female gymnasts have some of the most well-toned and graceful figures.

In recent years, improved body appearance has become the rule rather than the exception for women who participate in strength-training programs. Some of the most attractive female movie stars and participants in beauty pageants train with weights to improve their personal image.

At the same time, you may ask, "If weight training doesn't masculinize women, why do so many women body builders develop such heavy musculature?" In the sport of body building, the athletes follow intense training routines consisting of 2 or more hours of constant weight lifting with short rest intervals between sets.

Contrary to some beliefs, high levels of strength do not lead to large muscle size in women.

© Nautilus Sports/Medical Industries, Inc.

Many times, body-building training routines call for back-to-back exercises using the same muscle groups. The objective of this type of training is to pump extra blood into the muscles, which makes the muscles appear much bigger than they really are in a resting condition. Based on the intensity and the length of the training session, the muscles can remain filled with blood and appear measurably larger for several hours after completing the training session. Therefore, in real life, these women are not as muscular as they seem when they are "pumped up" for a contest.

In the sport of body building, a big point of controversy is the use of **anabolic steroids** and human growth hormones, by women as well as men. These hormones produce detrimental and undesirable side effects, which some women deem tolerable (for example, hypertension, fluid retention, smaller breasts, deepening of the voice, facial whiskers, and growth of body hair). Use of anabolic steroids in general, except for medical reasons and when monitored carefully by a physician, can have serious health consequences.

Use of anabolic steroids by women body builders is widespread. According to several sports medicine physicians and women body builders, a very high percentage of women body builders have used steroids. Furthermore, according to several women's track-and-field coaches, many women athletes in this sport around the world have used anabolic steroids and other performance-enhancing drugs to be competitive at the international level.

Undoubtedly, women who take steroids will build heavy musculature and, if they take the steroids long enough, will show masculinizing effects. As a result, the International Federation of Body Building has a mandatory steroid-testing program for women participating in the Miss Olympia contest. When drugs are not used to promote development, improved body image is the rule rather than the exception in women who participate in body building, strength training, and sports in general.

Does participation in exercise hinder menstruation?

In some instances highly trained athletes develop **oligomenorrhea** or **amenorrhea** during training and competition. These conditions are often seen in extremely lean women with disordered eating behaviors who engage in strenuous physical training over a sustained time. Amenorrhea is often associated with lower estrogen levels. Lack of estrogen leads to bone loss and a subsequent increase in risk for osteoporosis (also see question on osteoporosis on pages 211–213).

Primary amenorrhea exists when a girl has reached the age of 16 without menstruating or she has gone 2 years following the development of secondary sex characteristics without the onset of menses. Secondary amenorrhea is defined as cessation of menses following normal menstrual cycles.

At present we do not know whether the disorders are caused by physical stress or emotional stress related to high-intensity training, excessively low body fat, or other factors. Intense training and decreased caloric intake (often seen in athletes in an attempt to improve performance) appears to hinder the release of hormones needed for normal menses.

The combination of disordered eating, secondary amenorrhea, and bone mineral disorders is known as the **female athlete triad** (see Figure 9.2). The triad is seen most often in highly trained young women who participate in sports. It is also referred to as the female triad because it is seen in some non-athlete women who are very lean and extremely active. A woman can have one, two, or all three parts of the triad.

The American College of Sports Medicine has issued a position statement on the female athlete triad indicating that these disorders can lead to decreased physical capacity, illness, and premature death.[4] These conditions are by no means irreversible. Women who stop menstruating because of heavy exercise training should seek the advice of a physician. A gradual increase in daily caloric intake, slight weight gain, decreased exercise training, maintenance of adequate calcium intake, and possible estrogen replacement therapy are all recommended to treat the female athlete triad.

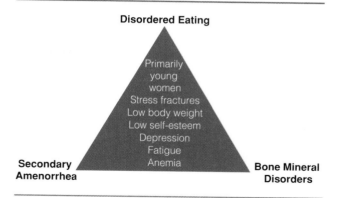

FIGURE **9.2** The female athlete triad.

Disordered Eating

Primarily young women
Stress fractures
Low body weight
Low self-esteem
Depression
Fatigue
Anemia

Secondary Amenorrhea

Bone Mineral Disorders

Does menstruation affect exercise?

Although on the average women have a lower physical capacity during menstruation, women have broken Olympic and world records at all stages of the menstrual cycle. Menstruation should not keep a woman from participating in physical activity, and it will not necessarily have a negative impact on performance.

Does exercise help relieve dysmenorrhea?

Although exercise has not been shown to either cure or aggravate **dysmenorrhea**, it has been shown to help relieve menstrual cramps because it improves circulation to the uterus. Particularly, stretching exercises of the muscles in the pelvic region seem to reduce and prevent painful menstruation that is not the result of a disease.

Is exercising safe during pregnancy?

Exercise is beneficial during pregnancy. According to the American College of Obstetricians and Gynecologists (ACOG), in the absence of contraindications,

KEY TERMS

Anabolic steroids A synthetic version of the male sex hormone testosterone, which promotes muscle development and hypertrophy.

Oligomenorrhea Irregular menstrual cycles.

Amenorrhea Absence (primary amenorrhea) or cessation (secondary amenorrhea) of normal menstrual function.

Female athlete triad Three interrelated disorders—disordered eating, amenorrhea, and bone mineral disorders—seen in some highly trained female athletes.

Dysmenorrhea Painful menstruation.

healthy pregnant women are encouraged to participate in regular moderate-intensity physical activities to continue to derive health benefits during pregnancy.[5] Pregnant women, however, should consult with their respective physicians to ensure that there are no contra-indications to exercise during pregnancy (see box).

As a general rule, healthy pregnant women can also accumulate 30 minutes of moderate-intensity physical activity on most, if not all, days of the week. Physical activity strengthens the body and helps prepare for the challenges of labor and childbirth.

The average labor and delivery lasts 10–12 hours. In most cases, labor and delivery are highly intense, with repeated muscular contractions interspersed with short rest periods. Proper conditioning will better prepare the body for childbirth. Moderate exercise during pregnancy also helps to prevent back pain and excessive weight gain, and it speeds up recovery following childbirth.

The most common recommendations for exercise during pregnancy for healthy pregnant women with no additional risk factors are as follows

1. Do not start a new or more rigorous exercise pro-gram without proper medical clearance.
2. Accumulate 30 minutes of moderate-intensity physical activities on most days of the week.
3. Instead of using heart rate to monitor intensity, ex-ercise at an intensity level that is perceived between "fairly light" and "somewhat hard." An exertion above "somewhat hard" is not recommended during pregnancy.
4. Gradually switch from weight-bearing and high-impact activities such as jogging and aerobics, to nonweight-bearing/lower-impact activities such as walking, stationary cycling, swimming, and water aerobics. The latter activities minimize the risk of injury and may allow exercise to continue through-out pregnancy.
5. Avoid exercising at an altitude above 6,000 feet (1,800 meters) or scuba diving, because these may compromise availability of oxygen to the fetus.
6. Women who are accustomed to strenuous exercise may continue in the early stages of pregnancy but should gradually decrease the amount, intensity, and exercise mode as pregnancy advances (most healthy pregnant women, however, slow down during the first few weeks of pregnancy because of morning sickness and fatigue).
7. Pay attention to the body's signals of discomfort and distress and never exercise to exhaustion. When fatigued, slow down or take a day off. Do not stop exercising altogether unless you experience any of the contraindications for exercise listed in the box at the top of this page.

Contraindications to Exercise During Pregnancy

Stop exercise and seek medical advice if you experience any of the following symptoms:

- Unusual pain or discomfort, especially in the chest or abdominal area
- Cramping, primarily in the pelvic or lower back areas
- Muscle weakness, excessive fatigue, or shortness of breath
- Abnormally high heart rate or a pounding (palpita-tions) heart rate
- Decreased fetal movement
- Insufficient weight gain
- Amniotic fluid leakage
- Nausea, dizziness, or headaches
- Persistent uterine contractions
- Vaginal bleeding or rupture of the membranes
- Swelling of ankles, calves, hands, or face

8. To prevent fetal injury, avoid activities that involve potential contact, loss of balance, or cause even mild trauma to the abdomen. Examples of these activities are basketball, soccer, volleyball, Nordic or water skiing, ice skating, road cycling, horseback riding, and motorcycle riding.
9. Do not exercise for weight-loss purposes during pregnancy.
10. Get proper nourishment (pregnancy requires be-tween 150 and 300 extra calories per day) and eat a small snack or drink some juice 20 to 30 minutes prior to exercise.
11. Prevent dehydration by drinking a cup of fluids 20 to 30 minutes before exercise and drink 1 cup of liquid every 15 to 20 minutes during exercise.
12. During the first 3 months in particular, do not exercise in the heat. Wear clothing that allows for proper dissipation of heat. A body temperature above 102.6°F (39.2°C) can harm the fetus.
13. After the first trimester, avoid exercises that require lying on the back. This position can block blood flow to the uterus and the baby.
14. Perform stretching exercises gently because hor-monal changes during pregnancy increase the laxity of muscles and connective tissue. Although these changes facilitate delivery, they also make women more susceptible to injuries during exercise.

What is **osteoporosis**, and how can it be prevented?

Osteoporosis, literally meaning "porous bones," is a condition in which bones lack the minerals required to keep them strong. In osteoporosis, bones—primarily of the hip, wrist, and spine—become so weak and brittle that they fracture readily. The process begins slowly in the third and fourth decades of life. Women are especially susceptible after menopause because of the accompanying loss of **estrogen**, which increases the rate at which bone mass is broken down.

Approximately 22 million U. S. women have osteoporosis, and 16 million don't know that they have this disease. About 30 percent of post-menopausal women have osteoporosis, but only about 2 percent are actually diagnosed and treated for this condition.[6]

Osteoporosis is the leading cause of serious morbidity and functional loss in the elderly population. One of every two women and one in eight men over age 50 will have an osteoporotic-related fracture at some point in their lives. The chances of a postmenopausal woman developing osteoporosis are much greater than her chances of developing breast cancer or incurring a heart attack or a stroke.

According to Stanford University researchers, an estimated 3.6 million Americans in 2003 had been diagnosed with osteoporosis. Up to 20 percent of people who have a hip fracture die within a year because of complications related to the fracture. As alarming as these figures are, they do not convey the pain and loss of quality of life in people who suffer the crippling effects of osteoporotic fractures.

Although osteoporosis is viewed primarily as a women's disease, more than 30 percent of all men will be affected by age 75. About 100,000 of the yearly 300,000 hip fractures in the United States occur in men.

The genetic component is strong, but osteoporosis is preventable. Maximizing bone density at a young age and subsequently decreasing the rate of bone loss later in life are critical to preventing osteoporosis.

Normal hormone levels prior to menopause and adequate calcium intake and physical activity throughout life cannot be overemphasized. These factors are all crucial to prevent osteoporosis. The absence of any one of these three factors leads to bone loss for which the other two factors never completely compensate. Smoking, excessive use of alcohol, and corticosteroid drugs also accelerate the rate of bone loss in women and men alike. Osteoporosis is also more common in whites, Asians, and small-frame people. Figure 9.3 depicts these variables.

Bone health begins at a young age. Some experts have called osteoporosis a "pediatric disease." Bone

FIGURE **9.3** Factors that diminish bone health (osteoporosis).

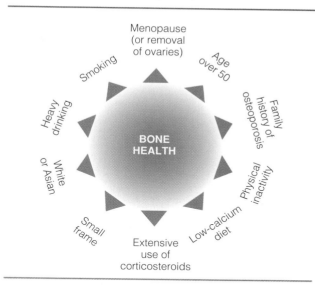

density can be promoted early in life by making sure the diet has sufficient calcium and participating in weight-bearing activities. Adequate calcium intake in both women and men is also associated with a reduced risk for colon cancer.[7] The RDA for calcium is between 1,000 and 1,300 mg per day, but leading researchers in this area recommend higher intakes (see Table 9.3). Although the recommended daily intakes can be met easily through diet alone, some experts recommend calcium supplements even for children before puberty.

To obtain your daily calcium requirement, get as much calcium as possible from calcium-rich foods, including calcium-fortified foods. If you don't get enough (most people don't), take calcium supplements.

Supplemental calcium can be obtained in the form of calcium citrate and calcium carbonate. Calcium citrate seems to be equally well absorbed with or without food, whereas calcium carbonate is not well absorbed without food. Thus if your supplement contains calcium carbonate, always take the supplement with meals. Do not take more than 500 mg at a time, because larger amounts are not well absorbed. And don't forget vitamin D, which is vital for calcium absorption.

Avoid taking calcium supplements with an iron-rich meal or in conjunction with an iron-containing

K E Y   T E R M S

Osteoporosis Softening, deterioration, or loss of bone.

Estrogen Female sex hormone; essential for bone formation and conservation of bone density.

TABLE 9.3 Recommended Daily Calcium Intake

AGE	AMOUNT (GR)
1–5	800
6–10	800–1,200
11–24	1,200–1,500
25–50 Women	1,000
25–64 Men	1,000
PMW* on HRT**	1,000
PMW not on HRT	1,500
>65	1,200–1,500

*PMW = Post-menopausal women

**HRT = Hormone replacement therapy

TABLE 9.4 Calcium-Rich Foods

FOOD	AMOUNT	CALCIUM (mg)	CALORIES
Beans, red kidney, cooked	1 cup	70	218
Beet, greens, cooked	½ cup	82	19
Bok choy (Chinese cabbage)	1 cup	158	20
Broccoli, cooked, drained	1 cup	72	44
Burrito, bean (no cheese)	1	57	225
Cottage cheese, 2% low-fat	½ cup	78	103
Ice milk (vanilla)	½ cup	102	100
Instant breakfast, nonfat milk	1 cup	407	216
Kale, cooked, drained	1 cup	94	36
Milk, nonfat, powdered	1 tbs	52	15
Milk, skim	1 cup	296	88
Oatmeal, instant, fortified, plain	½ cup	109	70
Okra, cooked, drained	½ cup	74	23
Orange juice, fortified	1 cup	300	110
Soy milk, fortified, fat free	1 cup	400	110
Spinach, raw	1 cup	56	12
Turnip greens, cooked	1 cup	197	29
Tofu (some types)	½ cup	138	76
Yogurt, fruit	1 cup	372	250
Yogurt, low-fat, plain	1 cup	448	155

multivitamin. Unfortunately, calcium interferes with iron absorption; thus, it is best to separate the intake of these two minerals. The benefit of taking your calcium supplement without food (calcium citrate) is that, in a young menstruating woman who needs iron, calcium won't interfere with the absorption of iron.

Table 9.4 provides a list of selected foods and their calcium content. Along with adequate calcium intake, taking 400 to 800 IU of vitamin D daily is the recommendation for optimal calcium absorption. People over age 50 may require 800 to 1,000 IU. About 40 percent of these adults are deficient in vitamin D.

Excessive protein intake could also affect the body's absorption of calcium. The more protein that is eaten, the higher is the calcium content in the urine (that is, the more calcium excreted). This might be the reason that countries with a high protein intake, including the United States, also have the highest rates of osteoporosis. Nonetheless, you should aim to achieve the RDA for protein, because people who consume too little protein (under 35 grams per day), lose more bone mass than those who eat too much (more than 100 grams per day). The RDA for protein is about 50 grams per day for women and 63 for men.

Soft drinks, coffee, and alcoholic beverages can also contribute to a loss in bone density if consumed in large quantities. The damage may not be caused directly by these food items but, rather, because they take the place of dairy products in the diet.

Exercise plays a key role in preventing osteoporosis by decreasing the rate of bone loss following menopause. Active people are able to maintain bone density much more effectively than their inactive counterparts. A combination of weight-bearing exercises, such as walking or jogging and weight training, is especially helpful. The benefits of exercise go beyond maintaining bone density. Exercise strengthens muscles, ligaments, and tendons—all of which provide support to the bones

(skeleton). Exercise also improves balance and coordination, which can help prevent falls and injuries.

Current studies indicate that, on the average, people who are active have denser bone mineral than inactive people do. Similar to other benefits of participating in exercise, there is no such thing as "bone in the bank." To have good bone health, people need to participate in a regular lifetime exercise program.

Prevailing research also tells us that estrogen is the most important factor in preventing bone loss. Lumbar bone density in women who have always had regular menstrual cycles exceeds that of women with a history of oligomenorrhea and amenorrhea interspersed with regular cycles. Furthermore, the lumbar density of these two groups of women is higher than that of women who have never had regular menstrual cycles.

For instance, athletes with amenorrhea (who have lower estrogen levels) have lower bone mineral density than even nonathletes with normal estrogen levels. Studies have shown that amenorrheic athletes at age 25 have the bones of women older than age 50. Over the last few years, it has become clear that sedentary women with normal estrogen levels have better bone mineral density than active amenorrheic athletes. Many experts believe the best predictor of bone mineral content is the history of menstrual regularity.

As a baseline, women age 65 and older should have a bone density test to establish the risk for osteoporosis. Younger women who are at risk for osteoporosis should discuss a bone density test with their physician at menopause. The test can also be used to monitor changes in bone mass over time and to predict the risk of future fractures. Bone density tests are painless scans requiring only small amounts of radiation to determine bone mass of the spine, hip, wrist, heel, or fingers. The amount of radiation is so low that technicians administering the test can sit right next to the person receiving it. The procedure often takes less than 10 minutes.

Following menopause, every woman should consider some type of therapy to prevent bone loss. The various therapy modalities available should be discussed with a physician.

Hormone Replacement Therapy

For decades, hormone-replacement therapy (HRT) was the most common treatment modality to prevent bone loss following menopause. A large study (16,000 healthy women, ages 50 to 79) was terminated 3 years early because the results showed that taking estrogen and progestin, a common form of HRT, actually increased the risk for disease.[8] The study was the first major long-term (8-year) clinical trial investigating the association between HRT and age-related diseases that included cardiovascular disease, cancer, and osteoporosis. Although the risk for hip fractures and colorectal cancer decreased, the risk of developing breast cancer, blood clots, strokes, and heart attacks increased.

HRT may still be the most effective treatment for the relief of acute (short-term) symptoms of menopause, such as hot flashes, mood swings, sleep difficulties, and vaginal dryness. Researchers and physicians, however, must now determine how long women can remain on HRT, how to best taper off treatment to provide maximal physical and emotional relief, and how to protect women from osteoporosis and other age-related diseases. Women who believed that HRT would help them strengthen their bones and ward off age-related diseases must now seek other treatments.

New alternative treatments to prevent bone loss are being developed. Miacalcin, a synthetic form of the hormone calcitonin, is FDA-approved for women who have osteoporosis and are at least 5-years post-menopausal. Calcitonin is a thyroid hormone that helps maintain the body's delicate balance of calcium by taking calcium from the blood and depositing it in the bones. Though it is effective in preventing bone loss, it does not help much in rebuilding bone. The drug seems to have no side effects. It is available in injectable and nasal spray forms.

Two promising nonhormonal drugs, alendronate (Fosamax) and risedronate (Actonel), prevent bone loss and even actually help to increase bone mass. Alendronate is recommended for women who already have osteoporosis. Alendronate is used primarily for bone health and does not provide benefits to the cardiovascular system. Although the research is limited, this drug seems to be safe and effective.

Selective estrogen receptor modulators (SERMs) are also used to prevent bone loss. These compounds have a positive effect on blood lipids and pose no risk to breast and uterine tissue. SERMs, however, do not help increase bone density. One SERM currently used to prevent osteoporosis is raloxifene (Evista).

Do women have special needs for iron?

Iron is a key element of hemoglobin in blood. The RDA of iron for adult women is between 15 and 18 mg per day (8 to 11 mg for men). Inadequate iron intake is often seen in children, teenagers, women of childbearing age, and endurance athletes. If iron absorption does not compensate for losses or dietary intake is low, iron deficiency develops.

As many as 50 percent of American women have a deficiency of iron. Over time, excessive depletion of iron stores in the body leads to iron-deficiency anemia, a condition in which the concentration of hemoglobin in the red blood cells is lower than it should be; this leads to fatigue and headaches, among other symptoms.

Physically active individuals, women in particular, have a greater-than-average need for iron. Heavy training creates a demand for iron that is higher than the recommended intake because small amounts of iron are lost through sweat, urine, and stools. Mechanical trauma, caused by the pounding of the feet on the pavement during extensive jogging, may also lead to destruction of iron-containing red blood cells.

A large percentage of female endurance athletes are reported to have iron deficiency. The blood **ferritin** levels of women who participate in intense physical training should be checked frequently.

The rates of iron absorption and iron loss vary from person to person. In most cases, though, people can get enough iron by eating more iron-rich foods such as beans,

KEY TERMS

Ferritin Iron stored in the body.

TABLE **9.5** Iron-Rich Foods

FOOD	AMOUNT	IRON (mg)	CALORIES	CHOLESTEROL	CALORIES FROM FAT
Beans, red kidney, cooked	1 cup	4.4	218	0	4%
Beef, ground lean	3 oz	3.0	186	81	48%
Beef, sirloin	3 oz	2.5	329	77	74%
Beef, liver, fried	3 oz	7.5	195	345	42%
Beet greens, cooked	½ cup	1.4	13	0	—
Broccoli, cooked, drained	1 sm stalk	1.1	36	0	—
Burrito, bean	1	2.4	307	14	28%
Egg, hard-cooked	1	1.0	72	250	63%
Farina (Cream of Wheat), cooked	½ cup	6.0	51	0	—
Instant breakfast, whole milk	1 cup	8.0	280	33	26%
Peas, frozen, cooked, drained	½ cup	1.5	55	0	—
Shrimp, boiled	3 oz	2.7	99	128	9%
Spinach, raw	1 cup	1.7	14	0	—
Vegetables, mixed, cooked	1 cup	2.4	116	0	—

peas, green leafy vegetables, enriched grain products, egg yolk, fish, and lean meats. Although organ meats, such as liver, are especially good sources, they also are high in cholesterol. A list of foods high in iron is given in Table 9.5.

Nutrition and Weight Control

What is the difference between a calorie and a kilo-calorie (kcal)?

A calorie is the unit of measure indicating the energy value of food to the person who consumes it. It is also used to express the amount of energy a person expends in physical activity. Technically, a kilocalorie (kcal), or large calorie, is the amount of heat necessary to raise the temperature of 1 kilogram of water 1 degree Centigrade. For simplicity, people call it a calorie rather than a kcal. For example, if the caloric value of a food is 100 calories (that is, 100 kcal), the energy in this food would raise the temperature of 100 kilograms of water 1 degree Centigrade. Similarly, walking 1 mile would burn about 100 calories (again, 100 kcal).

Are fruits and vegetables less nutritious today?

The notion that the soil is depleted of nutrients is one of those myths that has been hard to rectify. The following are comments from Dr. Gary Banuelos, a soil scientist with the USDA Research Service in Fresno, California:[9]

Fruits, vegetables, and grains will not grow, cannot be sold, and will not be bought if they contain insufficient

nutrition. If there's an inadequate amount of nutrients in the soil, plants may die because of insect infestation or disease, or cannot be sold because of poor appearance.

Many other scientists have echoed these words. Promoters of this myth are either misinformed or are not telling you the truth. Most of the time they are trying to promote supplements for personal financial gain.

In many instances, why don't the different fats listed on food labels add up to the total amount of fat listed on the labels?

Trans fatty acids have been listed on the label separately as "Trans Fat." They constitute only a small part of the total fat in most foods. As of 2006, however, food labels have to include the trans fat content. Glycerol is also included in the total amount of fat because it is used as a building block for fatty acids (triglycerides).

Hydrogen is often added to monounsaturated and polyunsaturated fats to increase shelf life and to solidify them so they are more spreadable. During this process, called "partial hydrogenation," the position of hydrogen atoms may be changed along the carbon chain, transforming the fat into a **trans fatty acid**.

Margarine and spreads, crackers, cookies, dairy products, meats, and fast foods often contain trans fatty acids. Trans fatty acids are not essential and provide no known health benefit. Health-conscious people minimize intake of these types of fats, because diets high in trans fatty acids create an inflammatory response that contributes to heart disease and cancer. Paying attention to food labels is important, because the words "partially hydrogenated" and "Trans Fat" indicate that the product carries a health risk just as high as that of saturated fat.

Ⓠ Does heavy perspiration during exercise help a person lose weight?

Ⓐ Intense exercise, especially in warm or hot conditions, greatly enhances water loss (perspiration) from the body. You sweat off water, not fat. Without fluid replacement, a person can lose between 3 and 8 pounds of weight (water) per hour, depending on body size and ambient temperature. Once fluid is replaced after exercise, the weight is regained quickly. Fluids, however, should be replaced regularly during exercise. As pointed out earlier, fluid replacement is crucial for optimal performance and proper heat balance.

Ⓠ Are rubberized sweatsuits and steam baths effective in losing weight?

Ⓐ The answer to this question is simply no! When a person wears a sweatsuit or steps into a sauna, the weight lost is not fat but is merely a significant amount of water. Sure, it looks nice when you step on the scale immediately afterward, but this represents a false loss of weight. As soon as you replace body fluids, you quickly gain back the weight.

In addition to hastening the rate of body fluid lost—fluid that is vital during prolonged exercise—wearing rubberized sweatsuits raises the body's core temperature. This combined effect puts a person in danger of dehydration, which impairs cellular function and in extreme cases even can cause death.

Ⓠ Are "natural" supplements to boost metabolism safe?

Ⓐ Supplements to boost metabolism contain stimulants that are harmful to individuals sensitive to such substances. These stimulants can also cause damage to people with metabolic disorders, heart disease, and high blood pressure. A physician or registered dietitian should be consulted prior to taking such supplements.

Ⓠ Do athletes or individuals who train for long periods need a special diet?

Ⓐ In general, athletes do not require special supplementation or any other special type of diet. Unless the diet is deficient in basic nutrients, no special, secret, or magic diet will help people perform better or develop faster as a result of what they eat. As long as the diet is balanced, based on a large variety of nutrients from the basic food groups, athletes do not require additional supplements. Even in strength training and body building, protein in excess of 20 percent of total daily caloric intake is not necessary.

The main difference between a sedentary person and a highly active individual is in the total number of calories required daily and the amount of carbohydrate intake during bouts of prolonged physical activity. During training, people consume more calories because of the greater energy expenditure required as a result of intense physical training.

A regular diet should be altered to include about 70 percent carbohydrates (carbohydrate loading) during several days of heavy aerobic training or when a person is going to participate in a long-distance event of more than 90 minutes (marathons, triathlons, road cycling races). For events shorter than 90 minutes, carbohydrate loading does not seem to enhance performance.

Exercise and Aging

Ⓠ What is the relationship between aging and physical work capacity?

Ⓐ The elderly population constitutes the fastest growing segment of the U. S. population. The number of Americans 65 and older increased from 3.1 million in 1900 (4.1 percent of the population) to more than 34 million (12.8 percent) in 1996. By the year 2030, more than 70 million people, or 22 percent of the population in the United States, are expected to be older than age 65.

The main objective of fitness programs for older adults is to help them improve their **functional fitness** and contribute to healthy aging. This implies the ability to maintain **functional independence** and to avoid disability. Older adults are encouraged to participate in programs that will help develop cardiorespiratory endurance, muscular strength and endurance, muscular flexibility, agility and balance, and motor coordination.

Data on individuals who have taken part in systematic physical activity throughout life indicate that these groups of people maintain a higher level of functional capacity and do not experience the typical declines in later years. From a functional point of view, typical sedentary Americans are about 25 years older than their chronological age indicates. Thus, an active 60-year-old person can have a work capacity similar to that of a sedentary 35-year-old.

KEY TERMS

Trans fatty acid Solidified fat formed by adding hydrogen to monounsaturated and polyunsaturated fats to increase shelf life.

Functional fitness The physical capacity of the individual to meet ordinary and unexpected demands of daily life safely and effectively.

Functional independence Ability to carry out activities of daily living without assistance from other individuals.

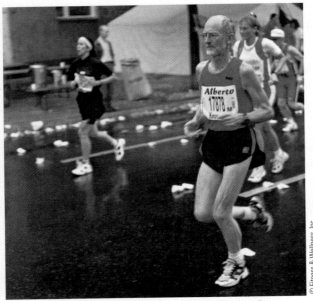

Exercise enhances quality of life and longevity.

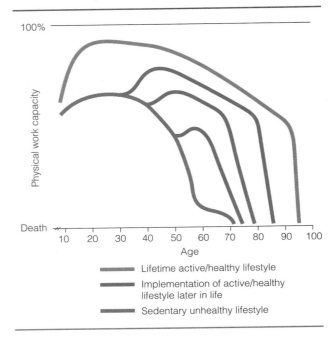

FIGURE **9.4** Relationships among physical work capacity, aging, and lifestyle habits.

Physical work capacity

100%

Death

Age

10 20 30 40 50 60 70 80 90 100

Lifetime active/healthy lifestyle

Implementation of active/healthy lifestyle later in life

Sedentary unhealthy lifestyle

Unhealthy behaviors precipitate premature aging. For sedentary people, productive life ends at about age 60. Most of these people hope to live to be 65 or 70 and often must cope with serious physical ailments. These people stop living at age 60 but choose to be buried at age 70! (See the theoretical model in Figure 9.4.)

A healthy lifestyle allows people to live a vibrant life—a physically, intellectually, emotionally, socially active, and functionally independent existence—to age 95. When death comes to active people, it usually is rather quick and not as a result of prolonged illness (see Figure 9.4). Such are the rewards of a wellness way of life.

Regular participation in physical activity provides both physiological and physical benefits to older adults.[10] Cardiorespiratory endurance training helps to increase functional capacity, decrease the risk for disease, improve health status, and increase life expectancy. Strength training decreases the rate of strength and muscle mass loss commonly associated with aging. Among the psychological benefits are preserved cognitive function, reduced symptoms and behaviors related to depression, and improved self-confidence and self-esteem.

Critical Thinking

Have you ever considered how you would like to feel and what type of activities you would like to carry on after age 65? What will it take for you to accomplish your goals?

Do older adults respond to physical training?

The trainability of older men and women alike and the effectiveness of physical activity in enhancing health have been demonstrated in prior research. Older adults who increase their physical activity experience significant changes in cardiorespiratory endurance, strength, and flexibility. The extent of the changes depends on their initial fitness level and the types of activities they select for their training (walking, cycling, strength training, and so on).

Improvements in maximal oxygen uptake in older adults are similar to those of younger people, although older people seem to require a longer training period to achieve these changes. Declines in maximal oxygen uptake average about 1 percent per year between ages 25 and 75. A slower rate of decline is seen in people who maintain a lifetime aerobic exercise program.

Results of research on the effects of aging on the cardiorespiratory system of male exercisers versus nonexercisers showed that the maximal oxygen uptake of regular exercisers was almost twice that of the nonexercisers.[11] The study revealed a decline in maximal oxygen uptake, between ages 50 and 68, of only 13 percent in the active group compared to 41 percent in the inactive group. These changes indicate that about one-third of the loss in maximal oxygen uptake results from aging and two-thirds of the loss comes from inactivity.

Blood pressure, heart rate, and body weight also were remarkably better in the exercising group. Furthermore, aerobic training seems to decrease high blood pressure in the older participants at the same rate as in young, hypertensive people.

Muscle strength declines by 10 percent to 20 percent between the ages of 20 and 50, but between ages 50 and 70 it drops by another 25 percent to 30 percent. Through strength training, frail adults in their 80s or 90s can double or triple their strength in just a few months. The amount of muscle hypertrophy achieved, however, decreases with age. Strength gains close to 200 percent have been found in previously inactive adults older than 90. In fact, research has shown that regular strength training improves balance, gait, speed, functional independence, morale, depression symptoms, and energy intake.[12]

Although muscle flexibility drops by about 5 percent per decade of life, 10 minutes of stretching every other day can prevent most of this loss as a person ages. Improved flexibility enhances mobility skills. The latter promotes independence because it helps older adults successfully perform **activities of daily living**.

In terms of body composition, inactive adults continue to gain body fat after age 60 despite the tendency toward lower body weight. The increase in body fatness is most likely caused by a decrease in basal metabolic rate and physical activity along with increased caloric intake above that required to maintain daily energy requirements.

Older adults who wish to initiate or continue an exercise program are strongly encouraged to have a complete medical exam, including a stress electrocardiogram test (see Chapter 8). Recommended activities for older adults include calisthenics, walking, jogging, swimming, cycling, and water aerobics.

Older people should avoid isometric and very high intensity strength-training exercises. Activities that require all-out effort or require participants to hold their breath (Valsalva maneuver) tend to lessen blood flow to the heart and cause a significant increase in blood pressure and the load placed on the heart. Older adults should participate in activities that require continuous and rhythmic muscular activity (about 40 percent to 60 percent of functional capacity). These activities do not cause large increases in blood pressure or place an intense overload on the heart.

Fitness/Wellness Consumer Issues

Q How do I protect myself from quackery and fraud in the fitness/wellness industry?

A The rapid growth in fitness and wellness programs during the last three decades has spurred **quackery** and **fraud**. The promotion of fraudulent products has deceived consumers into adopting "miraculous," quick, and easy ways toward total well-being.

Today's market is saturated with "special" foods, diets, supplements, pills, cures, equipment, books, and videos that promise quick, dramatic results. Advertisements for these products often are based on testimonials, unproven claims, secret research, half-truths, and quick-fix statements that the uneducated consumer wants to hear. In the meantime, the organization or enterprise making the claims stands to reap a large profit from consumers' willingness to pay for astonishing and spectacular solutions to problems related to their unhealthy lifestyle.

Television, magazine, and newspaper advertisements are not necessarily reliable. For instance, one piece of equipment sold through television and newspaper advertisements promised to "bust the gut" through 5 minutes of daily exercise that appeared to target the abdominal muscle group. This piece of equipment consisted of a metal spring attached to the feet on one end and held in the hands on the other end. According to handling and shipping distributors, the equipment was "selling like hotcakes," and companies could barely keep up with consumers' demands.

Three problems became apparent to the educated consumer. First, there is no such thing as spot-reducing; therefore, the claims could not be true. Second, 5 minutes of daily exercise burn hardly any calories and, therefore, have no effect on weight loss. Third, the intended abdominal (gut) muscles were not really involved during the exercise. The exercise engaged mostly the gluteal and lower-back muscles. This piece of equipment now can be found at garage sales for about a tenth of its original cost!

Although people in the United States tend to be firm believers in the benefits of physical activity and positive lifestyle habits as a means to promote better health, most do not reap these benefits because they simply do not know how to put into practice a sound fitness and wellness program that will give them the results they want. Unfortunately, many uneducated wellness consumers are targets of deception by organizations making fraudulent claims for their products.

Deception is not limited to advertisements. Deceit is found all around us. One can find it in newspaper and magazine articles, trade books, radio, and television

K E Y   T E R M S

Activities of daily living Everyday behaviors that people normally do to function in life (cross the street, carry groceries, lift objects, do laundry, sweep floors).

Quackery/fraud The conscious promotion of unproven claims for profit.

shows. To make a profit, popular magazines occasionally exaggerate health claims or leave out pertinent information to avoid offending advertisers. Some publishers print books on diets or self-treatment approaches that have no scientific foundation. Consumers should even be cautious about news reports of the latest medical breakthroughs. Reporters have been known to overlook important information or give certain findings greater credence than they deserve.

Precautions must also be taken when seeking health advice on the Internet. The Internet is full of both credible and dubious information. The following tips can help as you conduct a search on the Internet:

- Look for credentials of the person or organization sponsoring the site.
- Check when the site was last updated. Credible sites are updated often.
- Check the appearance of the information on the site. It should be presented in a professional manner. If every sentence ends with an exclamation point, you have good cause for suspicion.
- Be cautious if the site's sponsor is trying to sell a product. If so, be leery of opinions posted on the site. They could be biased, given that the company's main objective is to sell a product. Credible companies trying to sell a product on the Internet usually reference their sources of health information and provide additional links that support their product.
- Compare the content of a site to other credible sources. The content should compare favorably to that of other reputable sites or publications.
- Note the address and contact information for the company. A reliable company will list more than a PO box, an 800 number, and the company's e-mail address. When only the latter information is provided, consumers may never be able to locate the company for questions, concerns, or refunds.
- Be on the alert for companies that claim to be innovators while criticizing competitors or the government for being close-minded or trying to keep them from doing business.
- Watch for advertisers that use valid medical terminology in an irrelevant context or use vague pseudo-medical jargon to sell their product.

Not all people who promote fraudulent products know they are doing so. Some may be convinced that the product is effective. If you have questions or concerns about a health product, you may write to the National Council Against Health Fraud (NCAHF), PO Box 141, Fort Lee, NJ 07021. The purpose of this organization is to provide consumers with responsible, reliable, evidence-driven health information. The organization also monitors deceitful advertising, investigates complaints, and

offers public information regarding fraudulent health claims. You may also report any type of quackery to the NCAHF on its Web site at http://www.ncahf.org/. The site contains an updated list of reliable and unreliable health Web sites for the consumer.

Other consumer protection organizations offer to follow up on complaints about quackery and fraud. The existence of these organizations, however, should not give the consumer a false sense of security. The overwhelming number of complaints made each year to these organizations makes it impossible for them to follow up on each case individually.

The FDA's Center for Drug Evaluation Research, for example, has developed a priority system to determine which health fraud product it should regulate first. Products are rated on how great a risk they pose to the consumer. With this in mind, you can use the following list of organizations to make an educated decision before you spend your money. You can also report consumer fraud to these organizations:

- Better Business Bureau (BBB). The BBB can tell you whether other customers have lodged complaints about a product, a company, or a salesperson. You can find a listing for the local office in the business section of the phone book, or you can check its Web site at http://www.betterbusinessbureau.com/.
- Consumer Product Safety Commission (CPS). This independent federal regulatory agency targets products that threaten the safety of American families. Unsafe products can be researched and reported on its Web site at http://www.cpsc.gov/.
- U. S. Food and Drug Administration (FDA). The FDA regulates safety and labeling of health products and cosmetics. You can search for the office closest to you in the federal government listings (blue pages) of the phone book.

Another way to get informed before you make your purchase is to seek the advice of a reputable professional. Ask someone who understands the product but does not stand to profit from the transaction. As examples, a physical educator or an exercise physiologist can advise you regarding exercise equipment; a registered dietitian can provide information on nutrition and weight control programs; a physician can offer advice on nutritive supplements. Also, be alert to those who bill themselves as "experts." Look for qualifications, degrees, professional experience, certifications, and reputation.

Keep in mind that if it sounds too good to be true, it probably is. Fraudulent promotions often rely on testimonials or scare tactics and promise that their products will cure a long list of unrelated ailments. They use words such as quick-fix, time-tested, newfound, miraculous, special, secret, all natural, mail-order only, and money-back guarantee. Deceptive companies move often enough that customers have no way of contacting the company to ask for a reimbursement.

When claims are made, ask where the claims are published. Refereed scientific journals are the most reliable sources of information. When a researcher submits information for publication in a refereed journal, at least two qualified and reputable professionals in the field conduct blind reviews of the manuscript. A blind review means that the author does not know who will review the manuscript and the reviewers do not know who submitted the manuscript. Acceptance for publication is based on this input and relevant changes.

Q What guidelines should I follow when looking for a reputable health/fitness facility?

A As you follow a lifetime wellness program, you may want to consider joining a health/fitness facility. Or, if you have mastered the contents of this book and your choice of fitness activity is one you can pursue on your own (walking, jogging, cycling), you may not need to join a health club. Barring injuries, you may continue your exercise program outside the walls of a health club for the rest of your life. You also can conduct strength-training and stretching programs in your own home (see Chapters 3 and 4 and Appendices A, B, and C).

To stay up-to-date on fitness and wellness developments, you probably should buy a reputable and updated fitness/wellness book every 4 or 5 years. You also might subscribe to a credible health, fitness, nutrition, or wellness newsletter to stay current. You can also surf the Web—but be sure that the sites you are searching are from credible and reliable organizations.

Joining a health-fitness facility provides the opportunity to exercise in a safe environment under qualified supervision. Most likely you will have state-of-the-art equipment available for exercise and other beneficial health and wellness activities. The social component of exercising at a health/fitness center can enhance exercise compliance. If you are contemplating membership in a fitness facility:

- Make sure that the facility complies with the standards established by the American College of Sports Medicine (ACSM) for health and fitness facilities. These standards are given in Figure 9.5.
- Examine all exercise options in your community— health clubs/spas, YMCAs, gyms, colleges, schools, community centers, senior centers, and the like.
- Check to see if the facility's atmosphere is pleasurable and nonthreatening to you. Will you feel comfortable with the instructors and other people who go there? Is it clean and well kept up? If the answer is no, this may not be the right place for you.

FIGURE 9.5 American College of Sports Medicine standards for health and fitness facilities.

1. A facility must have an appropriate emergency plan.
2. A facility must offer each adult member a pre-activity screening that is relevant to the activities that will be performed by the member.
3. Each person who has supervisory responsibility must be professionally competent.
4. A facility must post appropriate signs in those areas of a facility that present potential increased risk.
5. A facility that offers services or programs to youth must provide appropriate supervision.
6. A facility must conform to all relevant laws, regulations, and published standards.

Adapted from *ACSM's Health/Fitness Facility Standards and Guidelines.* (Champaign, IL: Human Kinetics, 1997).

- Analyze costs versus facilities, equipment, and programs. Take a look at your personal budget. Will you really use the facility? Will you exercise there regularly? Many people obtain memberships and permit dues to be withdrawn automatically from a local bank account, yet seldom attend the fitness center.
- Find out what types of facilities are available: walking/running track, basketball/tennis/racquetball courts, aerobic exercise room, strength-training room, pool, locker rooms, saunas, hot tubs, handicapped access, and so on.
- Check the aerobic and strength-training equipment available. Does the facility have treadmills, bicycle ergometers, stair climbers, cross-country skiing simulators, free weights, strength-training machines? Make sure the facilities and equipment meet your activity interests.
- Consider the location. Is the facility close, or do you have to travel several miles to get there? Distance often discourages participation.
- Check on times the facility is accessible. Is it open during your preferred exercise time (for example, early morning or late evening)?
- Work out at the facility several times before becoming a member. Are people standing in line to use the equipment, or is it readily available during your exercise time?
- Inquire about the instructors' qualifications. Do the fitness instructors have college degrees or professional certifications from organizations such as the American College of Sports Medicine (ACSM) or the International Dance Exercise Association (IDEA)? These organizations have rigorous standards to ensure professional preparation and quality of instruction.
- Consider the approach to fitness (including all health-related components of fitness). Is it well rounded?

Do the instructors spend time with members, or do members have to seek them out constantly for help and instruction?

- Ask about supplementary services. Does the facility provide or contract out for regular health and fitness assessments (cardiovascular endurance, body composition, blood pressure, blood chemistry analysis)? Are wellness seminars (nutrition, weight control, stress management) offered? Do these have hidden costs?

Q What should one look for when selecting a personal trainer?

A In recent years, **personal trainers** have been in high demand by health and fitness participants. A personal trainer is an exercise specialist who works one-on-one with an individual and is typically paid by the hour or exercise session. Exercise sessions are usually conducted at a health/fitness facility or at the client's own home. A qualified personal trainer can help you start and maintain a safe exercise program, provide motivation and encouragement, design a time-effective exercise program, and provide objective health-fitness information.

Currently, anyone who prescribes exercise can call himself/herself a personal trainer without proof of education, experience, or certification. Although good trainers strive to maximize their own health and fitness, a good physique and previous athletic experience do not certify a person as a personal trainer.

Because of the high demand for personal trainers, more than 200 organizations now provide some type of certification to fitness specialists. This has led to great confusion by clients on how to evaluate the credentials of personal trainers. There is also a clear distinction between "certification" and a "certificate." Certification implies that the individual has met educational and professional standards of performance and competence. A certificate is typically awarded to individuals who attend a conference or workshop but are not required to meet any professional standards.

Presently, no licensing body oversees personal trainers. As a minimum, personal trainers should have an undergraduate degree and certification from a reputable organization such as ACSM, IDEA, or the National Strength and Conditioning Association (NSCA). Undergraduate (and graduate) degrees should be in a fitness-related area such as exercise science, exercise physiology, kinesiology, sports medicine, or physical education.

ACSM offers three certification levels: group exercise leader, health/fitness instructor, and health/fitness director. IDEA offers four levels: professional, advanced, elite, and master. For both ACSM and IDEA, each level of certification is progressively more difficult to obtain.

Before selecting a trainer, you need to establish your program goals. Below are sample questions you need to ask yourself and consider when interviewing potential trainers prior to selecting one.

- How long has the personal trainer been in practice and what education and level of certification does he or she possess?
- What type of clients does the trainer work with? Do these clients have similar needs and goals to yours?
- Can you obtain references from previous employers and past and current clients?
- Can the personal trainer provide you with a current resumé and professional certification(s)? Are you able to verify the certification with the respective professional organization?
- Is the trainer certified in CPR and does he or she have current professional liability insurance?
- What are the fees? Are several sessions cheaper than one single session? Can individuals be trained in groups? Are there discount rates for company trainers? Are there cancellation fees if you are unable to attend a given session?
- How long will the services of the personal trainer be needed: one session, several times a week, periodically, or indefinitely?
- Do you need a personal trainer to help you achieve certain fitness levels (cardiorespiratory, strength, flexibility), improve health, or is your primary concern weight loss?
- Do you prefer a male or female trainer?
- What type of personality are you looking for in the trainer: a motivator, a hard-diving trainer, a gentle approach, or just guidance without much pressure?

As a final word of caution when seeking fitness advice from a health/fitness trainer via the Internet: Be aware that certain services cannot be provided over the Internet. An Internet trainer is not able to directly administer fitness tests, motivate, observe exercise limitations, or respond effectively in an emergency situation (spotting, administering first-aid or CPR), and thus, is not able to design the most safe and effective exercise program for you.

Q What factors should I consider before purchasing exercise equipment?

A The first question you need to ask yourself is: Do I really need this piece of equipment? Most people buy on impulse because of television advertisements or because a salesperson convinced them it is a great piece of equipment that will do wonders for their health and fitness. With some creativity, you can implement an excellent and comprehensive exercise program with little, if any, equipment (see Chapters 3 and 4).

Many people buy expensive equipment only to find that they really do not enjoy that mode of activity. They do not remain regular users. Stationary bicycles (lower body only) and rowing ergometers were among the most popular pieces of equipment in the 1980s. Most of them now are seldom used and have become "fitness furniture" somewhere in the basement.

Exercise equipment does have its value for people who prefer to exercise indoors, especially during the winter months. It supports some people's motivation and adherence to exercise. The convenience of having equipment at home also allows for flexible scheduling. You can exercise before or after work or while you watch your favorite television show.

If you are going to purchase equipment, the best recommendation is to actually try it out several times before buying it. Ask yourself several questions: Did you enjoy the workout? Is the unit comfortable? Are you too short, tall, or heavy for it? Is it stable, sturdy, and strong? Do you have to assemble the machine? If so, how difficult is it to put together? How durable is it? Ask for references—people or clubs that have used the equipment extensively. Are they satisfied? Have they enjoyed using the equipment? Talk with professionals at colleges, sports medicine clinics, or health clubs.

Another consideration is to look at used units for signs of wear and tear. Quality is important. Cheaper brands may not be durable, so your investment would be wasted.

Finally, watch out for expensive gadgets. Monitors that provide exercise heart rate, work output, caloric expenditure, speed, grade, and distance may help motivate you, but they are expensive, need repairs, and do not enhance the actual fitness benefits of the workout. Look at maintenance costs and check for service personnel in your community.

healthy lifestyle program. Your activities over the last few weeks or months may have helped you develop positive habits that you should try to carry on throughout life.

Now that you are about to finish this course, the real challenge will be a lifetime commitment to fitness and wellness. Adhering to the program in a structured setting is a lot easier. Fitness and wellness is a continual process. As you proceed with the program, keep in mind that the greatest benefit is a higher quality of life.

Most people who adopt a wellness way of life recognize this new quality after only a few weeks into the program. For some people—especially individuals who have led a poor lifestyle for a long time—establishing positive habits and gaining feelings of well-being might take a few months. In the end, however, everyone who applies the principles of fitness and wellness will reap the desired benefits.

Critical Thinking

What impact has this course had on your personal fitness and healthy lifestyle program? Have you implemented changes that are improving your quality of life?

Being diligent and taking control of yourself will provide you a better, happier, healthier, and more productive life. Be sure to maintain a program based on your needs and what you enjoy doing most. This will make the journey easier, and you'll have more fun along the way. Once you reach the top, you will know there is no looking back. Improving your longevity and quality of life now is in your hands. It will require persistence and commitment, but only you can take control of your lifestyle and thereby reap the benefits of wellness.

What's Next?

The objective of this book is to provide you with the basic information necessary to implement your personal

KEY TERMS

Personal trainer An exercise specialist who works one-on-one with an individual and is typically paid by the hour or exercise session.

Lifescan Health Risk Appraisal. This site was created by Bill Hettler, M.D., of the National Wellness Institute and features a series of questions to help you identify what specific lifestyle factors can impair your health and longevity.
http://wellness.uwsp.edu/other/lifescan/index.htm

Select Your Health Quiz. Test your general health and medical knowledge; select Health and choose from the over twenty health conditions.
http://www.ivillage.com/quiz

ASSESS YOUR KNOWLEDGE

Evaluate how well you understand the concepts presented in this chapter using the Assess Your Knowledge and Practice Quizzes options on your Profile Plus CD-ROM.

1. A regular aerobic exercise program
   a. makes a person immune to heart disease.
   b. significantly decreases the risk for cardiovascular disease.
   c. decreases HDL-cholesterol.
   d. increases triglycerides.
   e. All are correct choices.

2. Which of the following is *not* a sign that you have exceeded your functional limitations during exercise?
   a. dizziness
   b. difficult breathing
   c. tightness in the chest
   d. irregular heart rate
   e. All of the above are signs of overexertion.

3. The standard treatment for an acute injury is
   a. rest.
   b. cold application.
   c. compression.
   d. elevation.
   e. All choices apply.

4. Which of the following recommendations is false regarding exercise during pregnancy?
   a. Women who are accustomed to strenuous exercise may continue to do so in the early stages of pregnancy.
   b. After the first trimester, women should avoid exercises that require lying on the back.
   c. Exercise above 6,000 feet of altitude is not recommended.
   d. Women are encouraged to exercise above a "somewhat hard" exertion level.
   e. Women may accumulate 30 minutes of moderate-intensity physical activities on most days of the week.

5. From a functional point of view, typical sedentary people in the United States are about _____ years older than their chronological age indicates.
   a. 2
   b. 8
   c. 15
   d. 25
   e. 50

6. A person suffering from heat stroke
   a. requires immediate medical attention.
   b. should be placed in a cool, humidity-controlled environment.
   c. should be sprayed with cool water and rubbed with cool towels.
   d. should not be given fluids if unconscious.
   e. All of the above are correct choices.

7. Drinking about a cup of cool water every _____ minutes seems to be ideal to prevent dehydration during exercise in the heat.
   a. 5
   b. 15 to 20
   c. 30
   d. 30 to 45
   e. 60

8. Improvements in maximal oxygen uptake in older adults (compared with younger adults) as a result of cardiorespiratory endurance training are
   a. similar.
   b. higher.
   c. lower.
   d. difficult to determine.
   e. non-existent.

9. Osteoporosis is
   a. a crippling disease.
   b. more prevalent in women.
   c. higher in people who were calcium-deficient at a young age.
   d. linked to heavy drinking and smoking.
   e. All are correct choices.

10. To protect yourself from consumer fraud when buying a new product,
    a. get as much information as you can from the salesperson.
    b. obtain details about the product from another salesperson.
    c. ask someone who understands the product but does not stand to profit from the transaction.
    d. obtain all the research information from the manufacturer.
    e. All choices are correct.

Correct answers can be found on page 261.

Fitness and Wellness Lifestyle Self-Evaluation

Name _____   Date _____

Course _____   Section _____

I. Explain the exercise program that you implemented in this course. Express your feelings about the outcomes of this program and how well you accomplished your fitness goals.

_____

_____

_____

_____

_____

_____

_____

_____

_____

_____

II. List nutritional or dietary changes that you were able to implement this term and the effects of these changes on your body composition and personal wellness.

_____

_____

_____

_____

_____

_____

_____

_____

_____

_____

III. List other lifestyle changes that you were able to make this term that may decrease your risk for disease. In a few sentences, explain how you feel about these changes and their impact on your overall well-being.

_____

_____

_____

_____

_____

_____

_____

_____

_____

_____

V. Indicate your total number of daily steps at the beginning of this course: ☐

Indicate your current total number of daily steps: ☐

VI. Briefly evaluate this course and its impact on your quality of life. Indicate what you feel will be needed for you to continue to adhere to an active and healthy lifestyle.

_____

_____

_____

_____

_____

_____

_____

_____

_____

_____

_____

_____

© Ken Redding/CORBIS

Appendixes

Exercise 1 *Step-Up*

Action: Step up and down using a box or chair approximately twelve to fifteen inches high. Conduct one set using the same leg each time you go up and then conduct a second set using the other leg. You could also alternate legs on each step-up cycle. You may increase the resistance by holding a child or some other object in your arms (hold the child or object close to the body to avoid increased strain in the lower back).

Muscles Developed: Gluteal muscles, quadriceps, gastrocnemius, and soleus

Photos © Fitness & Wellness, Inc.

Exercise 2 *Rowing Torso*

Action: Raise your arms laterally (abduction) to a horizontal position and bend your elbows to 90°. Have a partner apply enough pressure on your elbows to gradually force your arms forward (horizontal flexion) while you try to resist the pressure. Next, reverse the action, horizontally forcing the arms backward as your partner applies sufficient forward pressure to create resistance.

Muscles Developed: Posterior deltoid, rhomboids, and trapezius

© Fitness & Wellness, Inc.

Exercise 3 *Push-Up*

Action: Maintaining your body as straight as possible, flex the elbows, lowering the body until you almost touch the floor, then raise yourself back up to the starting position. If you are unable to perform the push-up as indicated, you can decrease the resistance by supporting the lower body with the knees rather than the feet (see illustration c) or using an incline plane and supporting your hands at a higher point than the floor (see illustration d). If you wish to increase the resistance, have someone else add resistance to your shoulders as you are coming back up (see illustrations e and f).

Muscles Developed: Triceps, deltoid, pectoralis major, erector spinae, and abdominals

Photos © Fitness & Wellness, Inc.

Exercise 4 *Abdominal Crunch and Bent-Leg Curl-Up*

Action: Start with your head and shoulders off the floor, arms crossed on your chest, and knees slightly bent (the greater the flexion of the knee, the more difficult the curl-up). Now curl up to about 30° (abdominal crunch—see illustration b) or curl all the way up (bent-leg curl-up), then return to the starting position without letting the head or shoulders touch the floor, or allowing the hips to come off the floor. If you allow the hips to raise off the floor and the head and shoulders to touch the floor, you will most likely "swing up" on the next sit-up, which minimizes the work of the abdominal muscles. If you cannot curl up with the arms on the chest, place the hands by the side of the hips or even help yourself up by holding on to your thighs (illustrations d and e). Do not perform the curl-up exercise with your legs completely extended, as this will cause strain on the lower back.

Muscles Developed: Abdominal muscles (crunch) and hip flexors (complete curl-up)

Photos © Fitness & Wellness, Inc.

NOTE: The bent-leg curl-up exercise should be used only by individuals of at least average fitness without a history of lower back problems. New participants and those with a history of lower back problems should use the abdominal crunch exercise in its place.

Exercise 5 **Leg Curl**

Action: Lie on the floor face down. Cross the right ankle over the left heel. Apply resistance with your right foot, while you bring the left foot up to 90° at the knee joint. (Apply enough resistance so that the left foot can only be brought up slowly.) Repeat the exercise, crossing the left ankle over the right heel.

Muscles Developed: Hamstrings (and quadriceps)

Photos © Fitness & Wellness, Inc.

Exercise 6 **Modified Dip**

Action: Place your hands and feet on opposite chairs with knees slightly bent (make sure that the chairs are well stabilized). Dip down at least to a 90° angle at the elbow joint, then return to the initial position. To increase the resistance, have someone else hold you down by the shoulders on the way up (see illustration c). You may also perform this exercise using a gymnasium bleacher or box and with the help of a partner, as illustrated in photo d.

Muscles Developed: Triceps, deltoid, and pectoralis major

Photos © Fitness & Wellness, Inc.

Exercise 7 *Pull-Up*

Action: Suspend yourself from a bar with a pronated grip (thumbs in). Pull your body up until your chin is above the bar, then lower the body slowly to the starting position. If you are unable to perform the pull-up as described, either have a partner hold your feet to push off and facilitate the movement upward—see illustrations c and d or use a lower bar and support your feet on the floor—see illustration e.

Muscles Developed: Biceps, brachioradialis, brachialis, trapezius, and latissimus dorsi

Photos © Fitness & Wellness, Inc.

Exercise 8 *Arm Curl*

Action: Using a palms-up grip, start with the arm completely extended (a), and with the aid of a sandbag or bucket filled (as needed) with sand or rocks, curl up as far as possible (b), then return to the initial position. Repeat the exercise with the other arm.

Muscles Developed: Biceps, brachioradialis, and brachialis

Photos © Fitness & Wellness, Inc.

Exercise 9 *Heel Raise*

Action: From a standing position with feet flat on the floor (a), raise and lower your body weight by moving at the ankle joint only (b). For added resistance, have someone else hold your shoulders down as you perform the exercise.

Muscles Developed: Gastrocnemius and soleus

Photos © Fitness & Wellness, Inc.

Exercise 10 *Leg Abduction and Adduction*

Action: Both participants sit on the floor. The person on the left places the feet on the inside of the other participant's feet. Simultaneously, the person on the left presses the legs laterally (to the outside—abduction), while the one on the right presses the legs medially (adduction). Hold the contraction for 5 to 10 seconds. Repeat the exercise at all three angles, and then reverse the pressing sequence. The person on the left places the feet on the outside and presses inward, while the one on the right presses outward.

Muscles Developed: Hip abductors (rectus femoris, sartori, gluteus medius and minimus), and adductors (pectineus, gracilis, adductor magnus, adductor longus, and adductor brevis)

Photos © Fitness & Wellness, Inc.

Exercise 11 *Reverse Crunch*

Action: Lie on your back with arms crossed on your chest and knees and hips flexed at 90° (a). Now attempt to raise the pelvis off the floor by lifting vertically from the knees and lower legs (b). This is a challenging exercise that may be difficult for beginners to perform.

Muscles Developed: Abdominals

Photos © Fitness & Wellness, Inc.

Exercise 12 *Pelvic Tilt*

Action: Lie flat on the floor with the knees bent at about a 90° angle (a). Tilt the pelvis by tightening the abdominal muscles, flattening your back against the floor, and raising the lower gluteal area ever so slightly off the floor (b). Hold the final position for several seconds. The exercise can also be performed against a wall (c).

Areas Stretched: Low-back muscles and ligaments.

Areas Strengthened: Abdominal and gluteal muscles

Photos © Fitness & Wellness, Inc.

Exercise 13 *Lateral Bridge*

Action: Lie on your side with legs bent (a: easier version) or straight (b: harder version) and support the upper body with your arm. Straighten your body by raising the hip off the floor, and hold the position for several seconds. Repeat the exercise with the other side of the body.

Muscles Developed: Abdominals (obliques and transversus abdominus) and quadratus lumborum (lower back)

Photos © Fitness & Wellness, Inc.

Exercise 14 *Prone Bridge*

Action: Starting in a prone position on a floor mat, balance yourself on the tips of your toes and elbows while attempting to maintain a straight body from heels to toes (do not arch the lower back). You can increase the difficulty of this exercise by placing your hands in front of you and straightening the arms (elbows off the floor).

Muscles Developed: Anterior and posterior muscle groups of the trunk and pelvis

© Fitness & Wellness, Inc.

Exercise 15 *Supine Bridge*

Action: Lie face up on the floor with the knees bent at about 120°. Do a pelvic tilt (Exercise 12, page 231) and maintain the pelvic tilt while you raise the hips off the floor until the upper body and upper legs are in a straight line. Hold this position for up to 5 seconds.

Areas Strengthened: Gluteal and abdominal flexor muscles

© Fitness & Wellness, Inc.

Strength-Training Exercises With Weights

Exercise 16 *Arm Curl*

Action: Use a supinated or palms-up grip, and start with the arms almost completely extended (a). Now curl up as far as possible (b), then return to the starting position.

Muscles Developed: Biceps, brachioradialis, and brachialis

Photos © Universal Gym Equipment, Inc.

Exercise 17 *Bench Press*

Action: Lie down on the bench with the head by the weight stack, the bench press bar above the chest, and place the feet on the bench (a). Grasp the bar handles and press upward until the arms are completely extended (b), then return to the original position. Do not arch the back during this exercise.

Muscles Developed: Pectoralis major, triceps, and deltoid

Photos © Nautilus Sports/Medical Industries, Inc.

Exercise 18 *Abdominal Crunch*

Action: Sit in an upright position and grasp the handles over your shoulders and crunch forward. Slowly return to the original position.

Muscles Developed: Abdominals

© Nautilus Sports/Medical Industries, Inc.

Exercise 19 *Leg Press*

Action: From a sitting position with the knees flexed at about 90° and both feet on the footrest (a), extend the legs fully (b), then return slowly to the starting position.

Muscles Developed: Quadriceps and gluteal muscles

Photos © Universal Gym Equipment, Inc.

Exercise 20 **Leg Curl**

Action: Lie with the face down on the bench, legs straight, and place the back of the feet under the padded bar (a). Curl up to at least 90° (b), and return to the original position.

Muscles Developed: Hamstrings

Photos © Universal Gym Equipment, Inc.

Exercise 21 **Lat Pull-Down**

Action: Starting from a sitting position, hold the exercise bar with a wide grip (a). Pull the bar down in front of you until it reaches the base of the neck (b), then return to the starting position.

Muscles Developed: Latissimus dorsi, pectoralis major, and biceps

Photos © Fitness & Wellness, Inc.

Exercise 22 **Heel Raise**

Action: Start with your feet either flat on the floor or the front of the feet on an elevated block (a), then raise and lower yourself by moving at the ankle joint only (b). If additional resistance is needed, you can use a squat strength-training machine.

Muscles Developed: Gastrocnemius and soleus

Photos © Universal Gym Equipment, Inc.

Exercise 23 **Triceps Extension**

Action: Using a palms-down grip, grasp the bar slightly closer than shoulder-width, and start with the elbows almost completely bent (a). Extend the arms fully (b), then return to starting position.

Muscles Developed: Triceps

Photos © Universal Gym Equipment, Inc.

Exercise 24   *Rotary Torso*

Action: Sit upright into the machine and place the elbows behind the padded bars. Rotate the torso as far as possible to one side and then return slowly to the starting position. Repeat the exercise to the opposite side.

Muscles Developed: Internal and external obliques (abdominal muscles)

© Nautilus Sports/Medical Industries, Inc.

Exercise 25   *Seated Back*

Action: Sit in the machine with your trunk flexed and the upper back against the shoulder pad. Place the feet under the padded bar and hold on with your hands to the bars on the sides (a). Start the exercise by pressing backward, simultaneously extending the trunk and hip joints (b). Slowly return to the original position.

Muscles Developed: Erector spinae and gluteus maximus

Photos © Universal Gym Equipment, Inc.

Exercise 26   *Rowing Torso*

Action: Sit in the machine with your arms in front of you, elbows bent and resting against the padded bars (a). Press back as far as possible, drawing the shoulder blades together (b). Return to the original position.

Muscles Developed: Posterior deltoid, rhomboids, and trapezius

Photos © Nautilus Sports/Medical Industries, Inc.

Exercise 27 **Back Extension**

Action: Place your feet under the ankle rollers and the hips over the padded seat. Start with the trunk in a flexed position and the arms crossed over the chest (a). Slowly extend the trunk to a horizontal position (b), hold the extension for 2 to 5 seconds, then slowly flex (lower) the trunk to the original position.

Muscles Developed: Erector spinae, gluteus maximus, and quadratus lumborum (lower back)

Photos © Fitness & Wellness, Inc.

Exercise 28 *Lateral Head Tilt*

Action: Slowly and gently tilt the head laterally. Repeat several times to each side.

Areas Stretched: Neck flexors and extensors and ligaments of the cervical spine

Exercise 29 *Arm Circles*

Action: Gently circle your arms all the way around. Conduct the exercise in both directions.

Areas Stretched: Shoulder muscles and ligaments

Exercise 30 *Side Stretch*

Action: Stand straight up, feet separated to shoulder width, and place your hands on your waist. Now move the upper body to one side and hold the final stretch for a few seconds. Repeat on the other side.

Areas Stretched: Muscles and ligaments in the pelvic region

Exercise 31 *Body Rotation*

Action: Place your arms slightly away from your body and rotate the trunk as far as possible, holding the final position for several seconds. Conduct the exercise for both the right and left sides of the body. You can also perform this exercise by standing about 2 feet away from the wall (back toward the wall), and then rotate the trunk, placing the hands against the wall.

Areas Stretched: Hip, abdominal, chest, back, neck, and shoulder muscles; hip and spinal ligaments

Exercise 32 *Chest Stretch*

Action: Place your hand on the shoulders of your partner, who will in turn push you down by your shoulders. Hold the final position for a few seconds.

Areas Stretched: Chest (pectoral) muscles and shoulder ligaments

Exercise 33 *Shoulder Hyperextension Stretch*

Action: Have a partner grasp your arms from behind by the wrists and slowly push them upward. Hold the final position for a few seconds.

Areas Stretched: Deltoid and pectoral muscles, and ligaments of the shoulder joint

© Fitness & Wellness, Inc.

Exercise 34 *Shoulder Rotation Stretch*

Action: With the aid of surgical tubing or an aluminum or wood stick, place the tubing or stick behind your back and grasp the two ends using a reverse (thumbs-out) grip. Slowly bring the tubing or stick over your head, keeping the elbows straight. Repeat several times (bring the hands closer together for additional stretch).

Areas Stretched: Deltoid, latissimus dorsi, and pectoral muscles; shoulder ligaments

Exercise 35 *Quad Stretch*

Action: Lie on your side and move one foot back by flexing the knee. Grasp the front of the ankle and pull the ankle toward the gluteal region. Hold for several seconds. Repeat with the other leg.

Areas Stretched: Quadriceps muscle, and knee and ankle ligaments

Exercise 36 *Heel Cord Stretch*

Action: Assume a push-up position, then bend one knee and stretch the opposite heel cord. Hold the stretched position for a few seconds. Alternate legs. You may also perform this exercise leaning against a wall or standing at the edge of a step, then stretch the heel downward.

Areas Stretched: Heel cord (Achilles tendon), gastrocnemius, and soleus muscles

Exercise 37 *Adductor Stretch*

Action: Stand with your feet about twice shoulder width and place your hands slightly above the knee. Flex one knee and slowly go down as far as possible, holding the final position for a few seconds. Repeat with the other leg.

Areas Stretched: Hip adductor muscles

Exercise 38 *Sitting Adductor Stretch*

Action: Sit on the floor and bring your feet in close to you, allowing the soles of the feet to touch each other. Now place your forearms (or elbows) on the inner part of the thigh and push the legs downward, holding the final stretch for several seconds.

Areas Stretched: Hip adductor muscles

Exercise 39 *Sit-and-Reach Stretch*

Action: Sit on the floor with legs together and gradually reach forward as far as possible. Hold the final position for a few seconds. This exercise may also be performed with the legs separated, reaching to each side as well as to the middle.

Areas Stretched: Hamstrings and lower back muscles, and lumbar spine ligaments

Exercise 40 *Triceps Stretch*

Action: Place the right hand behind your neck. Grasp the right arm above the elbow with the left hand. Gently pull the elbow backward. Repeat the exercise with the opposite arm.

Areas Stretched: Back of upper arm (triceps muscle) and shoulder joint

Exercise 41 *Single-Knee to Chest Stretch*

Action: Lie down flat on the floor. Bend one leg at approximately 100° and gradually pull the opposite leg toward your chest. Hold the final stretch for a few seconds. Switch legs and repeat the exercise.

Areas Stretched: Lower back and hamstring muscles, and lumbar spine ligaments

© Fitness & Wellness, Inc.

Exercise 44 *Sit-and-Reach Stretch*

See Exercise 39 in Appendix B.

Exercise 45 *Gluteal Stretch*

Action: Sit on the floor, bend the left leg and place your left ankle slightly above the right knee. Grasp the right thigh with both hands and gently pull the leg toward your chest. Repeat the exercise with the opposite leg.

Areas Stretched: Buttock area (gluteal muscles)

© Fitness & Wellness, Inc.

Exercise 42 *Double-Knee to Chest Stretch*

Action: Lie flat on the floor and then slowly curl up into a fetal position. Hold for a few seconds.

Areas Stretched: Upper and lower back and hamstring muscles; spinal ligaments

© Fitness & Wellness, Inc.

Exercise 43 *Upper and Lower Back Stretch*

Action: Sit on the floor and bring your feet in close to you, allowing the soles of the feet to touch each other. Hold on to your feet and gently bring your head and upper chest toward your feet.

Areas Stretched: Upper and lower back muscles and ligaments

© Fitness & Wellness, Inc.

Exercise 46 *Back Extension*

Action: Lie face down on the floor with the elbows by the chest, forearms on the floor, and the hands beneath the chin. Gently raise the trunk by extending the elbows until you reach an approximate 90° angle at the elbow joint. Be sure that the forearms remain in contact with the floor at all times. Hold the stretched position for a few seconds. DO NOT extend the back beyond this point. Hyperextension of the lower back may lead to or aggravate an already existing back problem.

Area Stretched: Abdominal region

Additional Benefit: Restore lower back curvature

© Fitness & Wellness, Inc.

Exercise 47　*Trunk Rotation and Lower Back Stretch*

Action: Sit on the floor and bend the right leg, placing the right foot on the outside of the left knee. Place the left elbow on the right knee and push against it. At the same time, try to rotate the trunk to the right (clockwise). Hold the final position for a few seconds. Repeat the exercise with the other side.

Areas Stretched: Lateral side of the hip and thigh; trunk, and lower back

© Fitness & Wellness, Inc.

Exercise 48　*Hip Flexors Stretch*

Action: Kneel down on an exercise mat, a soft surface, or place a towel under your knees. Raise the left knee off the floor and place the left foot about 3 feet in front of you. Place your left hand over your left knee and the right hand over the back of the right hip. Keeping the lower back flat, slowly move forward and downward as you apply gentle pressure over the right hip. Repeat the exercise with the opposite leg forward.

Areas Stretched: Flexor muscles in front of the hip joint

© Fitness & Wellness, Inc.

Exercise 49　*Cat Stretch*

Action: Kneel on the floor and place your hands in front of you (on the floor) about shoulder width apart. Relax your trunk and lower back (a). Now arch the spine and pull in your abdomen as far as you can and hold this position for a few seconds (b). Repeat the exercise 4–5 times.

Areas Stretched: Low back muscles and ligaments

Areas Strengthened: Abdominal and gluteal muscles

Photos © Fitness & Wellness, Inc.

Exercise 50　*Pelvic Clock*

Action: Lie face up on the floor with the knees bent at about 120°. Fully extend the hips as in the supine bridge (Exercise 15, page 232). Now progressively rotate the hips in a clockwise manner (2 o'clock, 4 o'clock, 6 o'clock, 8 o'clock, 10 o'clock, and 12 o'clock), holding each position in an isometric contraction for about 1 second. Repeat the exercise counterclockwise.

Areas Strengthened: Gluteal, abdominal, and hip flexor muscles

© Fitness & Wellness, Inc.

Exercise 51　*Pelvic Tilt*

See Exercise 12 in Appendix A, page 231).

Exercise 52　*Abdominal Crunch or Bent-Leg Curl-Up*

See Exercise 4 in Appendix A, page 228).

It is important that you do not stabilize your feet when performing either of these exercises, because doing so decreases the work of the abdominal muscles. Also, remember not to "swing up" but, rather, to curl up as you perform these exercises.

CONTRAINDICATED EXERCISES

Swan Stretch
Excessive strain on the spine; may harm intervertebral disks.

Alternative: Flexibility Exercise 46, page 239

Cradle
Excessive strain on the spine, knees, and shoulders.

Alternatives: Flexibility Exercises 46, 35, and 33, pages 239, 238, and 237

Windmill
Excessive strain on the spine and knees.

Alternatives: Flexibility Exercises 39 and 47, pages 238 and 240

Hurdler Stretch
Excessive strain on the bent knee.

Alternatives: Flexibility Exercises 35 and 39, page 238

The Hero
Excessive strain on the knees.

Alternatives: Flexibility Exercises 35 and 48, pages 238 and 240

Head Rolls
May injure neck disks.

Alternative: Flexibility Exercise 28, page 237

Straight-Leg Sit-Ups
These exercises strain the lower back.

Alternating Bent-Leg Sit-Ups

Alternatives: Strength Exercises 4 and 18, pages 228 and 233

Double-Leg Lift

Upright Double-Leg Lifts

V-Sits

All three of these exercises cause excessive strain on the spine and may harm disks.

Alternatives: Strength Exercises 4 and 18, pages 228 and 233

Sit-Ups with Hands Behind the Head

Excessive strain on the neck.

Alternatives: Strength Exercises 4 and 18, pages 228 and 233

Donkey Kicks

Excessive strain on the back, shoulders, and neck.

Alternatives: Flexibility Exercises 46, 48, and 28, pages 239, 240 and 237

Knee to Chest (with hands over the shin)

Excessive strain on the knee.

Alternatives: Flexibility Exercises 41 and 42, page 239

Standing Toe Touch

Excessive strain on the knee and lower back.

Alternative: Flexibility Exercise 39, page 238

Yoga Plow

Excessive strain on the spine, neck, and shoulders.

Alternatives: Flexibility Exercises 39, 41, 42, 43, and 45, pages 238 and 239

Full Squat

Excessive strain on the knees.

Alternatives: Flexibility Exercise 35, Strength Exercises 1, 19, pages 238, 227, and 233

CALORIC, PROTEIN, FAT, SATURATED FAT, CHOLESTEROL, AND CARBOHYDRATE CONTENT OF SELECTED FOODS

Food	Amount	Weight (g)	Calo-ries	Pro-tein (g)	Fat (g)	Sat. Fat (g)	Choles-terol (g)	Carbo-hydrate (g)
Apples, fresh, w/peel, lrg	1 ea	150	88	0.3	1	0.1	0	23
Applesauce, swtnd, w/o salt, cnd	1 cup	255	194	0.5	0	0.1	0	51
Apricots, pitted, fresh, whole	3 ea	114	55	1.6	0	0	0	13
Apricots, w/skin, in heavy syrup, cnd, whole	½ cup	120	100	0.6	0	0	0	26
Asparagus, spears, ckd w/o salt	4 ea	60	14	1.6	0	0	0	3
Avocado, Calif, fresh	½ ea	120	212	2.5	21	3.1	0	8
Bagel, plain, 3½" diameter	1 ea	68	187	7.1	1	0.1	0	36
Banana, fresh, med	1 ea	140	129	1.4	1	0.3	0	33
Bar, granola, hard	1 ea	24	113	2.4	5	0.6	0	15
Beans, black, mature, ckd w/o salt	1 cup	172	227	15.2	1	0.2	0	41
Beans, chickpea/garbanzo, mature, ckd	1 cup	164	269	14.5	4	0.4	0	45
Beans, frijoles/refried, cnd	½ cup	145	136	8	2	0.7	12	23
Beans, green, snap/string, ckd	½ cup	65	23	1.2	0	0	0	5
Beans, kidney, red, mature, cnd	1 cup	185	157	9.7	1	0.1	0	29
Beans, lima, fordhook, immature, ckd f/fzn w/o salt, drained	½ cup	85	85	5.2	0	0.1	0	16
Beans, mung, mature, sprouted, raw	½ cup	52	16	1.6	0	0	0	3
Beans, pinto, mature, ckd w/o salt	1 cup	171	234	14	1	0.2	0	44
Beef, chuck arm pot roast, brsd, choice, ¼" trim	3 oz	85	296	22.9	22	8.6	84	0
Beef, corned, cnd	3 oz	85	212	23	13	5.3	73	0
Beef, ground, hamburger patty, brld, well done, 16% fat	3 oz	85	225	24.3	13	5.3	84	0
Beef, ground, hamburger patty, brld, well done, 18% fat	3 oz	85	238	24	15	5.9	86	0
Beef, liver, fried	3 oz	85	184	22.7	7	2.3	410	7
Beef, T-bone steak, brld, choice, ¼" trim	3 oz	85	263	19.7	20	7.7	57	0
Beef, top sirloin steak, lean, brld, choice, ¼" trim	3 oz	85	172	25.8	7	2.6	76	0
Beer	12 fl-oz	360	148	1.1	0	0	0	13
Beer, light	12 fl-oz	354	99	0.7	0	0	0	5
Beets, cnd, drained, diced	½ cup	80	25	0.7	0	0	0	6
Biscuits, homemade	1 ea	35	124	2.5	6	1.5	1	16
Blueberries, fresh, bilberries	½ cup	73	41	0.5	0	0	0	10
Brandy, 86 proof	1 oz	28	70	0	0	0	0	0
Bread, banana, prep f/recipe w/veg shortening	1 pce	50	169	2.2	6	1.5	22	28
Bread, cracked wheat	1 pce	25	65	2.2	1	0.2	0	12
Bread, French	1 pce	35	96	3.1	1	0.2	0	18
Bread, mixed grain	1 pce	26	65	2.6	1	0.2	0	12
Bread, pita pocket, white	1 ea	60	165	5.5	1	0.1	0	33

Food	Amount	Weight (g)	Calories	Protein (g)	Fat (g)	Sat. Fat (g)	Cholesterol (g)	Carbohydrate (g)
Bread, pumpernickel	1 pce	32	80	2.8	1	0.1	0	15
Bread, rye	1 pce	25	65	2.1	1	0.2	0	12
Bread, white, f/recipe w/2% milk	1 pce	25	71	2	1	0.3	1	12
Bread, whole wheat	1 pce	25	62	2.4	1	0.2	0	12
Broccoli, med stalk, 8" long, ckd w/o add salt	1 ea	140	39	4.2	0	0.1	0	7
Broccoli, spear, raw, 5" long	1 ea	114	32	3.4	0	0.1	0	6
Brownie, chocolate, w/walnuts, prep f/rec	1 ea	20	93	1.2	6	1.5	15	10
Brussels Sprouts, ckd, drained	½ cup	78	30	2	0	0.1	0	7
Buns, hamburger	1 ea	40	114	3.4	2	0.5	0	20
Buns, hot dog/frankfurter	1 ea	40	114	3.4	2	0.5	0	20
Burger/Patty, vegetarian, Gardenburger, original	1 ea	71	130	8	3	1	11	18
Burger/Patty, vegetarian, soy	1 ea	71	142	14.9	6	1	0	6
Butter, salted	1 Tbs	5	36	0	4	2.5	11	0
Buttermilk, skim, cultured	1 cup	245	99	8.1	2	1.3	9	12
Cabbage, ckd w/o add salt, drained, shredded	½ cup	85	19	0.9	0	0	0	4
Cabbage, raw, shredded	½ cup	45	11	0.6	0	0	0	2
Cake, angel food, cmrcl prep	1 pce	60	155	3.5	0	0.1	0	35
Cake, carrot, w/cream cheese icing	1 pce	96	419	4.4	25	4.7	52	45
Cake, chocolate, w/chocolate icing, ⅛th	1 pce	69	253	2.8	11	3.3	29	38
Cake, devils food, marshmallow iced	1 pce	99	408	3.5	21	5.8	52	52
Cake, pound, w/butter	1 pce	30	116	1.7	6	3.5	66	15
Cake, white, w/chocolate icing	1 pce	71	259	1.8	8	3.7	13	46
Calamari/Squid, fried, mixed species	1 cup	150	262	26.9	11	2.8	390	12
Candy Bar, Almond Joy, fun size	1½ oz	42	196	1.8	11	7.3	2	24
Candy Bar, Mars almond	1 ea	50	234	4.1	12	3.6	8	31
Candy Bar, Milky Way, 2.1 oz bar	1 ea	60	254	2.7	10	4.7	8	43
Candy Bar, Special Dark sweet chocolate	1 ea	41	226	2	13	8.3	0	25
Candy, caramels, plain/chocolate	1 oz	28	107	1.3	2	1.8	2	22
Candy, hard, all flvrs	1 oz	28	110	0	0	0	0	27
Candy, Kisses, milk chocolate	1 oz	28	144	1.9	9	5.2	6	17
Candy, M & M's peanut chocolate	1 oz	28	144	2.7	7	2.9	3	17
Candy, M & M's plain chocolate	1 oz	28	138	1.2	6	3.7	4	20
Candy, milk chocolate, w/almonds	1 oz	28	147	2.5	10	4.8	5	15
Carrots, ckd w/o add salt, drained, slices	½ cup	73	33	0.8	0	0	0	8
Carrots, raw, whole, 7½" long	1 ea	81	35	0.8	0	0	0	8
Catsup/Ketchup	1 Tbs	15	16	0.2	0	0	0	4
Cauliflower, ckd, drained	½ cup	63	14	1.2	0	0	0	3
Celery, raw, med stalk, 8" long	1 ea	40	6	0.3	0	0	0	1
Cereal, 100% Bran, rte, dry	½ cup	33	89	4.1	2	0.3	0	24
Cereal, All-Bran, rte, dry	¼ cup	21	55	2.6	1	0.1	0	16
Cereal, Alpha-Bits, rte, dry	1 cup	28	110	2.2	1	0.1	0	24
Cereal, bran flakes, rte, dry	¾ cup	30	96	2.8	1	0.1	0	24
Cereal, Cheerios	1 cup	23	84	2.4	1	0.3	0	18

Food	Amount	Weight (g)	Calories	Protein (g)	Fat (g)	Sat. Fat (g)	Cholesterol (g)	Carbohydrate (g)
Cereal, Chex, corn, rte, dry	1 cup	28	105	2	0	0.1	0	24
Cereal, Chex, wheat, rte, dry	1 cup	46	159	4.8	1	0.2	0	37
Cereal, corn flakes, rte, dry	1 cup	25	91	1.6	0	0.1	0	22
Cereal, Corn Pops, rte, dry	1 cup	28	107	1	0	0.1	0	26
Cereal, Cream of Wheat, quick, ckd w/water	1 cup	244	132	3.7	0	0.1	0	27
Cereal, Crispy Rice, rte, dry	¾ cup	22	87	1.4	0	0	0	19
Cereal, Frosted Flakes, rte, dry	1 cup	35	135	1.4	0	0.1	0	32
Cereal, Frosted Mini Wheats, rte, dry	1 cup	55	186	5.2	1	0.2	0	45
Cereal, granola, rte, dry	½ cup	57	257	6	10	1.3	0	38
Cereal, Grape Nuts, rte, dry	½ cup	57	205	6.2	1	0.2	0	46
Cereal, Honey Bran, rte, dry	½ cup	30	102	2.6	1	0.2	0	25
Cereal, Life, plain, rte, dry	1 cup	44	167	4.3	2	0.3	0	35
Cereal, Mueslix, five grain muesli, rte, dry	1 cup	82	289	6.2	5	0.7	0	63
Cereal, Nutri-Grain, wheat, rte, dry	1 oz	28	101	2.4	0	0.1	0	24
Cereal, oatmeal, unsalted, ckd w/water	½ cup	120	74	3.1	1	0.2	0	13
Cereal, raisin bran, rte, dry	1 cup	49	155	3.9	1	0.1	0	38
Cereal, Shredded Wheat, sml biscuits, rte, dry	1 cup	19	68	2.1	0	0.1	0	15
Cereal, Smacks, rte, dry	1 cup	37	141	2.4	1	0.4	0	32
Cereal, Special K, rte, dry	1 cup	21	78	4.3	0	0	0	15
Cereal, Total, wheat, rte, dry	1 cup	33	116	3.3	1	0.2	0	26
Cereal, Wheaties, rte, dry	1 cup	29	106	3.1	1	0.2	0	23
Cheese Puffs/Cheetos	1 oz	28	155	2.1	10	1.8	1	15
Cheese Spread, low fat, low sod	1 pce	34	61	8.4	2	1.5	12	1
Cheese, American, proc, shredded	1 oz	28	105	6.2	9	5.5	26	0
Cheese, blue	1 oz	28	99	6	8	5.2	21	1
Cheese, cheddar, diced	1 oz	28	113	7	9	5.9	29	0
Cheese, feta	1 oz	28	74	4	6	4.2	25	1
Cheese, monterey jack, shredded	1 oz	28	105	6.9	8	5.3	25	0
Cheese, mozzarella, part skm mlk, low moist, shredded	1 oz	28	78	7.7	5	3	15	1
Cheese, parmesan, grated	1 Tbs	5	23	2.1	2	1	4	0
Cheese, ricotta, part skm	1 oz	28	39	3.2	2	1.4	9	1
Cheese, Swiss, shredded	1 oz	28	105	8	8	5	26	1
Cheesecake	1 pce	85	273	4.7	19	8.4	47	22
Cherries, sweet, fresh	10 ea	75	54	0.9	1	0.2	0	12
Chicken, broiler/fryer, breast, rstd	1 ea	98	193	29.2	8	2.1	82	0
Chicken, broiler/fryer, dark meat, w/o skin, rstd	3 oz	85	174	23.3	8	2.3	79	0
Chicken, broiler/fryer, drumstick, rstd	1 ea	52	112	14.1	6	1.6	47	0
Chicken, broiler/fryer, meat only, w/o skin, rstd	3 oz	85	162	24.6	6	1.7	76	0
Chips, corn	1 oz	28	151	1.8	9	1.3	0	16
Chips, tortilla, chili & lime	18 pce	28	110	2	2	0	0	22
Chips, tortilla, plain	1 oz	28	140	2	7	1.4	0	18
Cod, batter fried	3½ oz	100	173	17.4	8	1.6	50	7
Cod, stmd/poached	3½ oz	100	102	22.4	1	0.1	46	0

Food	Amount	Weight (g)	Calories	Protein (g)	Fat (g)	Sat. Fat (g)	Cholesterol (g)	Carbohydrate (g)
Coffee, brewed	¾ cup	180	4	0.2	0	0	0	1
Collards, ckd w/o add salt	½ cup	95	25	2	0	0	0	5
Cone, ice cream, wafer/cake type	1 ea	115	480	9.3	8	1.4	0	91
Cookie, chocolate chip, prep w/marg f/rec	2 ea	20	98	1.1	6	1.6	6	12
Cookie, chocolate sandwich, creme filled	4 ea	40	189	1.9	8	1.5	0	28
Cookie, fig bar	4 ea	56	195	2.1	4	0.6	0	40
Cookie, oatmeal raisin, prep f/rec	2 ea	26	113	1.7	4	0.8	9	18
Cookie, peanut butter, prep f/rec	2 ea	24	114	2.2	6	1.1	7	14
Cookie, shortbread, cmrcl, plain	4 ea	32	161	2	8	2	6	21
Cookie, vanilla, wafer type, 12–17% fat	10 ea	40	176	2	6	1.5	20	29
Coriander, raw	¼ cup	4	1	0.1	0	0	0	0
Corn, yellow, vac pack, cnd	½ cup	83	66	2	0	0.1	0	16
Cornbread, prep f/dry mix	1 ea	60	188	4.3	6	1.6	37	29
Cornmeal, yellow, degermed, enrich, dry	½ cup	120	439	10.2	2	0.3	0	93
Cottage Cheese, 2% fat	½ cup	113	101	15.5	2	1.4	9	4
Cottage Cheese, creamed, sml curd	½ cup	105	109	13.1	5	3	16	3
Crab, blue, cnd, drained	1 cup	135	134	27.7	2	0.3	120	0
Crackers, cheese	1 ea	10	50	1	3	0.9	1	6
Crackers, graham, plain/honey, 2½ square	2 ea	14	59	1	1	0.2	0	11
Crackers, matzoh, plain, svg	1 ea	28	111	2.8	0	0.1	0	23
Crackers, rye, wafers	2 ea	14	47	1.3	0	0	0	11
Crackers, saltine	1 ea	11	48	1	1	0.3	0	8
Crackers, standard, reg, snack type, round	1 ea	3	15	0.2	1	0.1	0	2
Crackers, Triscuit	1 ea	5	24	0.5	1	0.2	0	3
Crackers, wheat	1 ea	2	9	0.2	0	0.1	0	1
Cream Cheese	1 oz	28	98	2.1	10	6.2	31	1
Cream, light	1 Tbs	15	29	0.4	3	1.8	10	1
Cream, whipping, heavy	1 Tbs	15	52	0.3	6	3.5	21	0
Croissant, butter	1 ea	57	231	4.7	12	6.6	38	26
Cucumber, w/o skin, raw, sliced	½ cup	60	7	0.3	0	0	0	2
Dates, fresh, whole	10 ea	83	228	1.6	0	0.2	0	61
Dinner, chicken, cacciatore, w/noodles, low cal, fzn	1 ea	308	311	22.5	10	2.4	59	33
Doughnut, cake	1 ea	47	198	2.3	11	1.7	17	23
Doughnut, raised, glazed	1 ea	60	242	3.8	14	3.5	4	27
Egg Substitute, Egg Beaters, new	¼ cup	61	30	6	0	0	0	1
Egg Whites, raw	1 ea	33	16	3.5	0	0	0	0
Egg Yolks, raw, lrg	1 ea	17	61	2.8	5	1.6	218	0
Eggs, hard ckd/bld, lrg	1 ea	50	78	6.3	5	1.6	212	1
Eggs, scrambled, plain, lrg	1 ea	64	106	7.1	8	2.4	225	1
Eggs, whole, fried	1 ea	46	92	6.2	7	1.9	211	1
Entree, lasagna, w/meat, prep f/rec	1 pce	220	352	20.7	14	7.2	52	36
Entree, macaroni & cheese, prep f/rec w/margarine	½ cup	100	215	8.4	11	4.4	21	20

Food	Amount	Weight (g)	Calories	Protein (g)	Fat (g)	Sat. Fat (g)	Cholesterol (g)	Carbohydrate (g)
Entree, meatloaf, beef	1 pce	111	232	20.2	14	5.6	107	5
Entree, quiche, lorraine	1 pce	242	724	20.5	56	25.9	304	34
Entree, spaghetti, w/meatballs, prep f/rec	1 cup	248	332	18.6	12	3.3	74	39
Entree, spaghetti, w/tomato sauce & cheese, prep f/rec	1 cup	250	260	8.8	9	2	8	37
Figs, dried, unckd	1 ea	21	54	0.6	0	0	0	14
Fish Sticks/Portions, heated f/fzn, 4x1x.5	2 ea	56	152	8.8	7	1.8	63	13
Flour, all purpose, white, bleached, enrich	1 cup	125	455	12.9	1	0.2	0	95
Flour, whole wheat	1 cup	120	407	16.4	2	0.4	0	87
Frankfurter/Hot Dog, beef & pork, 10 pack	1 ea	57	182	6.4	17	6.1	28	1
Frankfurter/Hot Dog, beef, 8 pack	1 ea	57	180	6.8	16	6.9	35	1
Frankfurter/Hot Dog, turkey	1 ea	45	102	6.4	8	2.7	48	1
Frozen Yogurt, vanilla/strawberry, nonfat, sml scoop	4 oz	113	112	5.6	0	0.1	2	22
Fruit Cocktail, in heavy syrup, cnd	1 cup	245	179	1	0	0	0	46
Fruit Cocktail, in juice	1 cup	248	114	1.1	0	0	0	29
Fruit Punch, prep f/pwd	1 cup	240	89	0	0	0	0	23
Fudge, chocolate, prep f/rec	1 oz	28	107	0.5	2	1.4	4	22
Grapefruit, pink, fresh, 3¾" diameter	½ ea	123	37	0.7	0	0	0	9
Grapes, tokay/empress/red flame, fresh	10 ea	50	36	0.3	0	0.1	0	9
Haddock, fillet, brd, fried	3 oz	85	184	17.1	9	1.9	65	7
Halibut, Greenland, fillet, bkd/brld	3 oz	85	203	15.7	15	2.6	50	0
Honey, strained, extracted	1 Tbs	21	64	0.1	0	0	0	17
Hot Cocoa/Choc, prep f/rec w/whole milk	1 cup	250	192	9.8	6	3.6	20	29
Hummus/Hummos, raw	1 cup	246	421	12.1	21	3.1	0	50
Instant Breakfast, prep f/dry mix w/nonfat milk	1 cup	282	216	15.7	1	0.7	9	36
Instant Breakfast, prep f/dry mix w/whole milk	1 cup	281	280	15.4	9	5.4	38	36
Jam/Preserves, pkt	1 ea	14	39	0.1	0	0	0	10
Jelly	1 Tbs	18	51	0	0	0	0	13
Juice, apple, unswtnd, cnd/btld	½ cup	124	58	0.1	0	0	0	14
Juice, cranberry cocktail	1 cup	253	144	0	0	0	0	36
Juice, grape, unswtnd, btld/cnd	½ cup	127	77	0.7	0	0	0	19
Juice, grapefruit, unswtnd, cnd	½ cup	124	47	0.6	0	0	0	11
Juice, grapefruit, unswtnd, prep f/fzn conc	1 cup	247	101	1.4	0	0	0	24
Juice, lemon, fresh	1 Tbs	15	4	0.1	0	0	0	1
Juice, orange, prep f/fzn	½ cup	125	56	0.9	0	0	0	13
Juice, prune, w/o pulp	½ cup	88	60	0.7	0	0	0	14
Juice, tomato, w/salt, cnd	1 cup	244	41	1.9	0	0	0	10
Kale, ckd w/o add salt, drained	½ cup	55	15	1	0	0	0	3
Kiwi fruit/Chinese Gooseberries, fresh, med	1 ea	76	46	0.8	0	0	0	11

Food	Amount	Weight (g)	Calo-ries	Pro-tein (g)	Fat (g)	Sat. Fat (g)	Choles-terol (g)	Carbo-hydrate (g)
Lamb, leg, whole, lean, rstd, choice, ¼" trim	3 oz	85	162	24.1	7	2.3	76	0
Lamb, loin chop, lean, brld, choice, ¼" trim	3 oz	84	181	25.2	8	2.9	80	0
Lemonade, white, fzn conc	12 oz	340	615	1	1	0.1	0	160
Lentils, sprouts, stir fried	1 cup	124	125	10.9	1	0.1	0	26
Lentils, unsalted, ckd	1 cup	200	232	18	1	0.1	0	40
Lettuce, butterhead, Boston/bibb, leaf, raw	2 pce	15	2	0.2	0	0	0	0
Lettuce, romaine, raw, chpd	1 cup	55	8	0.9	0	0	0	1
Lobster, northern, stmd	1 cup	145	142	29.7	1	0.2	104	2
Lunchmeat Spread, liverwurst, cnd	1 oz	28	87	3.6	7	2.5	33	2
Lunchmeat, bologna, beef & pork	1 pce	28	88	3.3	8	3	15	1
Lunchmeat, bologna, turkey	2 pce	57	113	7.8	9	2.9	56	1
Lunchmeat, roast beef, deli style, pouch	3 oz	85	96	17.2	3	1.1	41	1
Lunchmeat, turkey breast, rstd, fat free	1 pce	28	24	4.2	0	0.1	9	1
Mayonnaise, imit, low cal	1 Tbs	15	35	0	3	0.5	4	2
Mayonnaise, soybean oil, w/salt	1 tsp	5	36	0.1	4	0.6	3	0
Melon, cantaloupe/musk, med 5" diameter	¼ ea	239	84	2.1	1	0.2	0	20
Melon, honeydew, fresh, wedge, ⅛ melon	1 pce	129	45	0.6	0	0	0	12
Milk Shake, chocolate, fast food	10 fl-oz	340	432	11.6	13	7.9	44	70
Milk, evaporated, whole, w/add vit A, cnd	½ cup	126	169	8.6	10	5.8	37	13
Milk, low fat, 1%, w/add vit A	1 cup	244	102	8	3	1.6	10	12
Milk, low fat, 2%, chocolate	1 cup	250	179	8	5	3.1	17	26
Milk, low fat, 2%, w/add vit A	1 cup	244	121	8.1	5	2.9	18	12
Milk, nonfat/skim, w/add vit A	1 cup	245	86	8.4	0	0.3	4	12
Milk, whole, 3.3%	1 cup	244	150	8	8	5.1	33	11
Milkshake, strawberry, fast food	10 fl-oz	340	384	11.6	10	5.9	37	64
Mixed Vegetables, cnd, drained	1 cup	182	86	4.7	0	0.1	0	17
Muffin, English, plain	1 ea	57	134	4.4	1	0.1	0	26
Muffin, English, plain, tstd	1 ea	52	133	4.4	1	0.1	0	26
Muffin, wheat bran, prep f/rec w/whole milk	1 ea	45	130	3.2	6	1.2	16	19
Mushrooms, raw, pces/slices	1 cup	35	9	1	0	0	0	1
Mustard Greens, ckd w/o add salt, drained	½ cup	70	10	1.6	0	0	0	1
Nuts, almonds, dried, unblanched, whole	¼ cup	36	208	7.7	18	1.4	0	7
Nuts, Brazil, dried, shelled, 32 kernels	1 oz	28	184	4	19	4.5	0	4
Nuts, cashews, dry rstd, salted	1 cup	137	786	21	63	12.5	0	45
Nuts, coconut, unswtnd, dried	½ cup	65	429	4.5	42	37.2	0	16
Nuts, peanuts, oil rstd, unsalted, chpd	1 oz	28	163	7.4	14	1.9	0	5
Nuts, pecans, dried, halves	1 oz	28	193	2.6	20	1.7	0	4
Nuts, walnuts, black, dried, chpd	1 oz	28	170	6.8	16	1	0	3

Food	Amount	Weight (g)	Calo-ries	Pro-tein (g)	Fat (g)	Sat. Fat (g)	Choles-terol (g)	Carbo-hydrate (g)
Oil, canola	1 cup	218	1927	0	218	15.5	0	0
Oil, corn	1 Tbs	15	133	0	15	1.9	0	0
Oil, olive	1 Tbs	15	133	0	15	2	0	0
Oil, peanut	1 cup	216	1909	0	216	36.5	0	0
Oil, safflower, greater than 70% linoleic	1 Tbs	15	133	0	15	0.9	0	0
Oil, soybean	1 tsp	5	44	0	5	0.7	0	0
Okra, bindi, ckd w/o add salt f/raw, drained, pods	8 ea	85	27	1.6	0	0	0	6
Olives, w/o pits, ripe, lrg, cnd	10 ea	44	51	0.4	5	0.6	0	3
Olives, w/o pits, ripe, sml, cnd	10 ea	32	37	0.3	3	0.5	0	2
Onions, yellow, ckd w/o add salt, drained, chpd	½ cup	105	46	1.4	0	0	0	11
Oranges, fresh, med	1 ea	180	85	1.7	0	0	0	21
Oysters, eastern, brd, fried, med	1 ea	45	89	3.9	6	1.4	36	5
Oysters, eastern, raw, wild	½ cup	120	82	8.5	3	0.9	64	5
Pancake, buckwheat, prep f/incomplete dry mix, 4"	1 ea	27	56	2.1	2	0.5	18	8
Pancake, plain, homemade, 4"	1 ea	73	166	4.7	7	1.5	43	21
Papaya, fresh, med	½ ea	227	89	1.4	0	0.1	0	22
Pasta, egg noodles, enrich, ckd	½ cup	80	106	3.8	1	0.2	26	20
Pasta, macaroni noodles, enrich, ckd	½ cup	70	99	3.3	0	0.1	0	20
Pasta, spaghetti noodles, enrich, salted, ckd	1 cup	140	197	6.7	1	0.1	0	40
Pasta, spaghetti noodles, whole wheat, ckd	1 cup	125	155	6.7	1	0.1	0	33
Pastry, cinnamon danish	1 ea	110	443	7.7	25	6.2	23	49
Peaches, fresh, sliced	½ cup	85	37	0.6	0	0	0	9
Peaches, in heavy syrup, cnd	½ tsp	96	71	0.4	0	0	0	19
Peaches, in juice, cnd, whole	½ tsp	77	34	0.5	0	0	0	9
Peanut Butter, smooth, salted	1 Tbs	32	190	8.1	16	3.3	0	6
Pears, bartlett, fresh, med	1 ea	180	106	0.7	1	0	0	27
Pears, in heavy syrup, cnd, halves	½ ea	103	76	0.2	0	0	0	20
Pears, in juice, cnd, halves	½ ea	77	38	0.3	0	0	0	10
Peas, cnd, drained	½ cup	85	59	3.8	0	0.1	0	11
Peas, green, ckd f/fzn w/o add salt, drained	½ cup	80	62	4.1	0	0	0	11
Peppers, bell, green, sweet, raw, med	1 ea	200	54	1.8	0	0.1	0	13
Peppers, bell, red, sweet, raw, sml	1 ea	74	20	0.7	0	0	0	5
Peppers, bell, yellow, sweet, raw, lrg	1 ea	186	50	1.9	0	0.1	0	12
Pickles, dill	1 ea	135	24	0.8	0	0.1	0	6
Pickles, sweet, med	1 ea	35	41	0.1	0	0	0	11
Pie, apple, bkd f/fzn, ⅛th of 8"	1 pce	118	280	2.2	13	4.5	0	40
Pie, blueberry, prep f/rec, ⅛th of 9"	1 pce	158	387	4.3	19	4.6	0	53
Pie, cherry, prep f/rec, ⅛th of 9"	1 pce	118	319	3.3	14	3.5	0	45
Pie, chocolate cream, rts, ⅛th of 8"	1 pce	175	532	4.5	34	8.7	9	59
Pie, lemon meringue, rts, ⅛th of 8"	1 pce	140	375	2.1	12	2.5	63	66
Pie, pecan, rts, ⅛th of 8"	1 pce	138	552	5.5	26	4.9	44	79
Pie, pumpkin, rts, ⅛th of 8"	1 pce	114	239	4.4	11	2	23	31
Pineapple, chunks, fresh	½ cup	78	38	0.3	0	0	0	10

Food	Amount	Weight (g)	Calories	Protein (g)	Fat (g)	Sat. Fat (g)	Cholesterol (g)	Carbohydrate (g)
Pineapple, in heavy syrup, cnd, tidbits	½ cup	128	100	0.4	0	0	0	26
Pineapple, in juice, cnd	½ cup	125	75	0.5	0	0	0	20
Popcorn, air popped, plain	1 cup	6	23	0.7	0	0	0	5
Popcorn, ckd in oil, salted	1 cup	11	55	1	3	0.5	0	6
Pork, bacon/cracklings, brld/pan fried/rstd	2 pce	15	86	4.6	7	2.6	13	0
Pork, cured, ham, reg, 11% fat, rstd	3 oz	85	151	19.2	8	2.7	50	0
Pork, ham, whole, rstd	3 oz	85	232	22.8	15	5.5	80	0
Pork, ribs, spareribs, brsd	3 oz	85	337	24.7	26	9.5	103	0
Potato Chips, plain, salted	10 pce	20	107	1.4	7	2.2	0	11
Potatoes, au gratin, prep w/milk & butter f/dry mix	1 cup	245	228	5.6	10	6.3	37	31
Potatoes, baked, w/flesh & skin, long	1 ea	202	220	4.6	0	0.1	0	51
Potatoes, hash browns, prep f/fzn	½ cup	78	170	2.5	9	3.5	0	22
Potatoes, mashed, w/whole milk	½ cup	105	81	2	1	0.3	2	18
Potatoes, sweet, flesh, bkd in skin, med, peeled	1 ea	146	150	2.5	0	0	0	35
Pretzels, hard, salted, twisted	1 oz	28	107	2.5	1	0.2	0	22
Prunes, dried	5 ea	61	146	1.6	0	0	0	38
Pudding, choc, rte, 5oz can	5 oz	142	189	3.8	6	1	4	32
Pudding, tapioca, 5oz can	5 oz	142	169	2.8	5	0.9	1	28
Pudding, vanilla, 5oz can	5 oz	142	185	3.3	5	0.8	10	31
Raisins, seedless, unpacked	1 oz	28	84	0.9	0	0	0	22
Raspberries, fresh	1 cup	123	60	1.1	1	0	0	14
Raspberries, swtnd, fzn	1 cup	250	400	10	15	9.1	12	62
Rice, brown, ckd	½ cup	96	107	2.5	1	0.2	0	22
Rice, white, reg, ckd	½ cup	103	134	2.8	0	0.1	0	29
Rice, wild, ckd	½ cup	100	101	4	0	0	0	21
Rolls, hard, white	1 ea	50	146	4.9	2	0.3	0	26
Salad Dressing, blue cheese/roquefort	1 Tbs	15	76	0.7	8	1.5	3	1
Salad Dressing, french	1 Tbs	16	69	0.1	7	1.5	0	3
Salad Dressing, French, low cal	1 Tbs	15	20	0	1	0.1	0	3
Salad Dressing, Italian	1 Tbs	15	70	0.1	7	1.1	0	2
Salad Dressing, Italian, diet, 2cal/tsp, cmrcl	1 Tbs	15	16	0	1	0.2	1	1
Salad Dressing, ranch	1 Tbs	15	80	0	8	1.2	5	0
Salad Dressing, thousand island	1 Tbs	15	57	0.1	5	0.9	4	2
Salad Dressing, thousand island, low cal	1 Tbs	15	24	0.1	2	0.2	2	2
Salad, chicken, w/celery	½ cup	78	268	10.6	25	3.1	48	1
Salad, pasta, garden primavera, prep f/dry	¾ cup	142	280	8	12	2.5	2	34
Salad, potato	½ cup	125	179	3.4	10	1.8	85	14
Salad, tuna	1 cup	205	383	32.9	19	3.2	27	19
Salami, beef & pork, dry	1 oz	28	117	6.4	10	3.4	22	1
Salmon, pink, w/bone, cnd, not drained	3 oz	85	118	16.8	5	1.3	47	0
Salmon, sockeye, fillet, bkd/brld	3 oz	85	184	23.2	9	1.6	74	0
Salsa, homemade, Mexican sauce	1 Tbs	15	3	0.1	0	0	0	1

Food	Amount	Weight (g)	Calories	Protein (g)	Fat (g)	Sat. Fat (g)	Cholesterol (g)	Carbohydrate (g)
Sandwich, bacon, lettuce & tomato, on soft white	1 ea	130	323	10.8	18	4.7	22	30
Sandwich, egg salad, on soft white	1 ea	111	361	9.1	24	4.2	149	29
Sandwich, peanut butter & jam, on soft white, unsalted	1 ea	100	348	11.5	15	3.1	2	46
Sandwich, reuben, grilled	1 ea	237	458	27.6	29	9.8	80	25
Sardines, Atlantic, w/bones, cnd in oil, drained	1 oz	28	58	6.9	3	0.4	40	0
Sauce, soy, made f/soy & wheat	1 Tbs	16	9	1.3	0	0	0	1
Sauce, teriyaki, rts	1 Tbs	18	15	1.1	0	0	0	3
Sauerkraut, w/liquid, cnd	½ cup	118	22	1.1	0	0	0	5
Sausage, pork, smkd, link	1 ea	68	265	15.1	22	7.7	46	1
Scallops, brd, fried, mixed species, lrg	2 ea	31	67	5.6	3	0.8	19	3
Seaweed, spirulina, dried	1 cup	119	345	68.4	9	3.2	0	28
Shrimp/Prawns, brd, fried, lrg	7 ea	85	206	18.2	10	1.8	150	10
Shrimp/Prawns, ckd, lrg	3 oz	85	84	17.8	1	0.2	166	0
Soda, cola	12 fl-oz	369	151	0	0	0	0	38
Soda, cola/Coke, diet, w/sacc, low sod	12 fl-oz	340	0	0	0	0	0	0
Soda, ginger ale	12 fl-oz	366	124	0	0	0	0	32
Soda, lemon lime	12 fl-oz	340	136	0	0	0	0	35
Soda, root beer	12 fl-oz	340	139	0	0	0	0	36
Sole/Flounder, fillet, bkd/brld	3 oz	85	99	20.5	1	0.3	58	0
Soup, beef bouillon/broth, cnd, prep w/water	1 cup	240	17	2.7	1	0.3	0	0
Soup, chicken noodle, prep w/water	1 cup	241	75	4	2	0.7	7	9
Soup, clam chowder, Manhattan, prep f/cnd	1 cup	244	112	12.3	2	0	10	11
Soup, clam chowder, New England, prep w/milk	1 cup	248	164	9.5	7	3	22	17
Soup, cream of chicken, prep w/milk	1 cup	248	191	7.5	11	4.6	27	15
Soup, cream of mushroom, prep w/milk	1 cup	245	201	6	13	5.1	20	15
Soup, minestrone, prep w/water	1 cup	241	82	4.3	3	0.6	2	11
Soup, pea, split, w/ham, prep w/water	1 cup	245	184	10	4	1.7	7	27
Soup, tomato, prep w/milk	1 cup	248	161	6.1	6	2.9	17	22
Soup, tomato, prep w/water	1 cup	245	86	2.1	2	0.4	0	17
Soup, vegetable beef, prep w/water	1 cup	245	78	5.6	2	0.9	5	10
Soup, vegetable, vegetarian, prep w/water	1 cup	250	75	2.2	2	0.3	0	12
Sour Cream, cultured	1 Tbs	14	30	0.4	3	1.8	6	1
Spinach, ckd w/o add salt, drained	½ cup	103	24	3.1	0	0	0	4
Spinach, raw, chpd	1 cup	55	12	1.6	0	0	0	2
Spinach, w/o add salt, cnd, drained	½ cup	103	24	2.9	1	0.1	0	4
Squash, acorn, ckd	1 cup	245	83	1.6	0	0	0	22
Squash, summer, ckd w/o add salt, drained	½ cup	90	18	0.8	0	0.1	0	4
Squash, winter, avg, bkd, mashed	½ cup	103	40	0.9	1	0.1	0	9
Strawberries, fresh, whole	1 cup	149	45	0.9	1	0	0	10
Strawberries, slices, swtnd, fzn	1 cup	250	240	1.3	0	0	0	65

Food	Amount	Weight (g)	Calo-ries	Pro-tein (g)	Fat (g)	Sat. Fat (g)	Choles-terol (g)	Carbo-hydrate (g)
Stuffing, bread, prep f/dry mix	½ cup	70	125	2.2	6	1.2	0	15
Sugar, beet/cane, brown, packed	1 tsp	5	19	0	0	0	0	5
Sugar, white, granulated	1 tsp	4	15	0	0	0	0	4
Syrup, maple	1 Tbs	20	52	0	0	0	0	13
Taco Shells	1 ea	10	47	0.7	2	0.3	0	7
Tangerines/Mandarin oranges, fresh, med	1 ea	116	51	0.7	0	0	0	13
Tea, brewed	¼ cup	180	2	0	0	0	0	1
Tempeh	1 cup	166	320	30.8	18	3.7	0	16
Tofu, firm, silken	½ cup	126	78	8.7	3	0.5	0	3
Tomatoes, red, ripe, raw, med, whole	1 ea	100	21	0.9	0	0	0	5
Tomatoes, red, ripe, w/o add salt, cnd, in liquid	½ cup	121	23	1.1	0	0	0	5
Tortilla/Taco/Tostada Shell, corn	1 ea	148	693	10.7	33	5	0	92
Trout, rainbow, fillet, bkd/brld, wild	3 oz	85	128	19.5	5	1.4	59	0
Tuna, light, cnd in oil, drained	3 oz	85	168	24.8	7	1.3	15	0
Tuna, light, cnd in water, drained	3½ oz	99	115	25.3	1	0.2	30	0
Turkey, average, w/o skin, rstd	3 oz	85	144	24.9	4	1.4	65	0
Turnip Greens, ckd f/fzn, drained	½ cup	73	22	2.4	0	0.1	0	4
Turnips, ckd w/add salt, raw, cubes	½ cup	78	16	0.6	0	0	0	4
Veal, loin, brsd	3 oz	85	241	25.7	15	5.7	100	0
Veal, loin, lean, brsd	3 oz	85	192	28.5	8	2.2	106	0
Vinegar, balsamic, 60 grain	1 Tbs	15	21	0	0	0		5
Watermelon, fresh, diced	1 cup	160	51	1	1	0.1	0	11
Wheat, bulgur, ckd	1 cup	135	112	4.2	0	0.1	0	25
Wheat, flakes, rolled, dry	1 cup	30	97	3.5	0	0	0	21
Wheat, germ, tstd	1 Tbs	6	23	1.7	1	0.1	0	3
Whiskey, 90 proof	2 fl-oz	42	110	0	0	0	0	0
Wine, cooler	4 oz	113	56	0.1	0	0	0	7
Wine, red	⅛ cup	30	22	0.1	0	0	0	1
Wine, Rose	2 fl-oz	59	42	0.1	0	0	0	1
Wine, white, med	2 fl-oz	59	40	0.1	0	0	0	0
Yogurt, fruit, low fat, 10g prot/8 oz	1 cup	227	231	9.9	2	1.6	10	43
Yogurt, plain, low fat, 12g prot/8 oz	8 oz	226	143	11.9	4	2.3	14	16

FAST FOOD RESTAURANTS

Food	Amount	Weight (g)	Calo-ries	Pro-tein (g)	Fat (g)	Sat. Fat (g)	Choles-terol (g)	Carbo-hydrate (g)
General								
Burrito, bean	1 ea	166	342	10.8	10	5.3	3	55
Chili, con carne	1 cup	255	258	24.8	8	3.5	135	22
Cole Slaw, fast food	1 cup	120	178	1.8	13	1.9	6	15
English Muffin, w/butter	1 ea	63	189	4.9	6	2.4	13	30
Entree, enchilada, cheese	1 ea	230	451	13.6	27	14.9	62	40
Hot Dog, plain	1 ea	98	242	10.4	15	5.1	44	18
Pancake, w/butter & syrup	2 ea	232	520	8.3	14	5.9	58	91
Sandwich, chicken, fillet, plain	1 ea	157	444	20.8	25	7.4	52	33
Sundae, hot fudge, fast food	1 ea	164	295	5.9	9	5.2	21	49
Arby's								
Salad, chef	1 ea	273	136	12.3	6	2.6	84	9
Sandwich, beef, Arby Q	1 ea	190	389	17.6	15	5.4	29	48

Food	Amount	Weight (g)	Calories	Protein (g)	Fat (g)	Sat. Fat (g)	Cholesterol (g)	Carbohydrate (g)
Sandwich, beef, French dip & swiss cheese	1 ea	154	369	24.7	16	7.5	58	31
Sandwich, beef 'n cheddar	1 ea	194	508	24.6	26	7.7	52	43
Sandwich, chicken, grilled, deluxe	1 ea	195	365	20	17	3	37	35
Sandwich, roast beef, regular	1 ea	155	383	22	18	6.9	43	35
Sauce, Arby's	½ oz	14	15	0.1	0	0	0	3
Sauce, horsey	½ oz	14	110	0.1	5	1.2	0	3
Burger King Corporation								
Cheeseburger, Whopper	1 ea	294	730	33	46	16	115	46
Croissant, w/egg, sausage & cheese	1 ea	110	375	13.8	29	10	162	16
Hamburger, Whopper	1 ea	270	640	27	39	11	90	45
Onion Rings, reg svg	3 ea	30	75	1	3	0.5	0	10
Potatoes, french fries, salted, med svg	1 ea	116	370	5	20	5	0	43
Sandwich, chicken, broiler	1 ea	168	373	20.3	20	4.1	54	28
Sandwich, fish, big	1 ea	255	700	26	41	6	90	56
Dunkin Donuts, Inc.								
Croissant, plain	1 ea	18	81	1.2	5	1.2	2	8
Hidden Valley								
Salad Dressing, ranch, reduced fat & cal	2 Tbs	28	58	0.5	5	0.9	10	2
International Dairy Queen Inc.								
Frozen Yogurt Cone, med	4 oz	113	148	5.1	1	0.3	3	32
Frozen Yogurt, nonfat	4 oz	113	133	4	0	0		28
Hamburger, homestyle	1 ea	138	290	17	12	5	45	29
Ice Cream Cone, vanilla, med	1 ea	142	237	5.7	6	4.3	22	38
Milk Shake, vanilla, med	1 ea	397	520	12	14	8	45	88
Onion Rings, svg	3 oz	85	241	3.8	12	3	0	29
Sandwich, fish, fillet	1 ea	182	396	17.1	17	3.7	48	42
Sundae, chocolate, med	1 ea	184	315	6.3	8	4.7	24	56
Jack In the Box								
Bowl, chicken, teriyaki	1 ea	502	670	26	4	1	15	128
Cheeseburger, Jumbo Jack	1 ea	296	640	31	38	15	105	44
Hamburger	1 ea	104	250	12	9	3.5	30	30
Hamburger, sourdough, jack	1 ea	233	690	34	45	15	105	37
Sandwich, chicken, supreme	1 ea	305	830	33	49	7	65	66
Kentucky Fried Chicken Corporation								
Chicken, leg, original recipe	1 ea	54	124	11.5	8	1.8	66	4
Chicken, wing, hot & spicy	1 ea	55	210	10	15	4	55	9
Chicken, wing, original recipe	1 ea	45	134	8.6	10	2.4	53	5
Long John Silver's								
Dinner, fish & fries, batter fried, 2pce	1 ea	261	610	27	37	7.9	60	52
McDonald's Nutrition Information Center								
Biscuit, sausage & egg	1 ea	175	541	17.7	36	9.8	241	34
Cheeseburger	1 ea	115	304	14.3	12	5.7	38	33
Cheeseburger, Quarter Pounder	1 ea	186	493	26	28	12.1	88	35
Chicken, nuggets, McNuggets, 4 pce, svg	1 ea	71	190	12	11	2.5	40	10

Food	Amount	Weight (g)	Calories	Protein (g)	Fat (g)	Sat. Fat (g)	Cholesterol (g)	Carbohydrate (g)
Danish, apple	1 ea	115	394	5.5	18	5.5	44	56
Frozen Yogurt Cone, vanilla, low fat	3 oz	85	142	3.8	4	2.8	19	22
Hamburger, Big Mac	1 ea	204	529	24.6	29	9.4	80	42
Hamburger, Quarter Pounder	1 ea	160	391	21.4	20	7.4	65	34
McMuffin, egg	1 ea	138	294	17.2	12	4.6	238	27
McMuffin, sausage	1 ea	135	434	15.7	28	9.6	54	31
Milk Shake, vanilla, sml	1 ea	289	355	10.8	9	5.9	39	58
Muffin, apple bran, fat free	1 ea	75	197	3.9	2	0.3	0	40
Pie, apple	1 ea	307	1037	12	52	14	0	136
Potatoes, french fries, sml svg	1 ea	68	210	3	10	1.5	0	26
Potatoes, hash browns	1 ea	55	135	1	8	1.6	0	15
Salad, garden, shaker	1 ea	149	100	7	6	3	75	4
Sandwich, Filet O Fish	1 ea	131	378	13.4	21	3.8	42	35
Sauce, sweet & sour, pkt 1	1⅛ oz	32	57	0	0	0	0	13
Pizza Hut, Inc.								
Pizza, cheese, pan, med, 12"	2 pce	205	495	22.8	21	9.5	47	53
Pizza, cheese, thin n' crispy, med, 12"	2 pce	148	350	18.8	14	6.8	43	36
Pizza, pepperoni, pan, med, 12"	2 pce	211	539	22.4	24	8.1	49	57
Pizza, pepperoni, personal pan	1 ea	255	637	27	28	10	55	69
Pizza, supreme, pan, med, 12"	2 pce	255	581	28	28	11.2	56	52
Subway International								
Sandwich, chicken breast, rstd, on white, 6"	1 ea	246	332	26	6	1	48	41
Sandwich, Italian bmt, on white, 6"	1 ea	246	445	21	21	8	56	39
Sandwich, meatball, on white, 6"	1 ea	260	404	18	16	6	33	44
Sandwich, roast beef, deli style	1 ea	180	245	13	4	1	13	38
Sandwich, tuna, w/lt mayonnaise, on wheat, 6"	1 ea	253	391	19	15	2	32	46
Sandwich, turkey, on white, 6"	1 ea	232	273	17	4	1	19	40
Taco Bell Inc.								
Burrito, beef, big supreme	1 ea	298	520	24	23	10	55	54
Burrito, seven layer	1 ea	234	438	13.2	19	5.8	21	55
Burrito, supreme	1 ea	255	440	17	19	8	35	51
Taco	1 ea	83	192	9.6	11	4.3	27	13
Taco, soft	1 ea	92	225	9.2	10	4.1	26	12
Wendy's Foods International								
Cheeseburger, w/bacon, jr	1 ea	170	393	20.5	19	7.5	58	35
Chicken, nuggets	6 pce	94	292	13.9	20	3.6	37	14
Frosty, dairy dessert, med	1 ea	298	440	11	11	7	50	73
Hamburger, bacon classic, big	1 ea	251	517	30.1	26	10.7	88	41
Salad, caesar, w/o dressing, side	1 ea	130	151	12.4	8	3.4	25	9
Salad, chicken, grilled, w/o dressing	1 ea	338	195	22.1	8	1.7	46	10
Salad, garden, deluxe, w/o dressing	1 ea	271	110	6.7	6	1	1	10
Salad, taco, w/o chips	1 ea	510	411	28.7	20	10.5	69	31
Sandwich, chicken, brd	1 ea	208	433	27.4	16	3.1	54	47
Sandwich, chicken, club	1 ea	220	483	30.6	20	4.4	64	48
Sandwich, chicken, grilled	1 ea	177	283	22.6	7	1.5	61	34

Food	Amount	Weight (g)	Calo-ries	Pro-tein (g)	Fat (g)	Sat. Fat (g)	Choles-terol (g)	Carbo-hydrate (g)
CONVENIENCE FOODS & MEALS								
El Charrito								
Entree, enchilada, beef, family size, 6 pack	1 ea	200	353	11.8	17	6.5	33	39
Healthy Choice								
Dinner, fish, herb baked, fzn	1 ea	273	300	14.1	6	1.3	31	48
Dinner, meatloaf, traditional, fzn	1 ea	340	316	15.3	5	2.5	37	52
Entree, burrito, chicken, con queso, fzn	1 ea	216	253	10.1	4	1.8	25	43
Entree, lasagna, roma, fzn	1 ea	284	311	19.3	7	2.2	26	44
Entree, spaghetti, bolognese, fzn	1 ea	284	280	14	6	2	30	43
Lean Cuisine								
Entree, chow mein, chicken, w/rice	1 ea	241	198	12.3	5	0.9	33	26
Entree, lasagna, w/meat sauce	1 ea	291	270	19	6	2.5	25	34
Entree, ravioli, cheese	1 ea	241	250	12	8	3	55	32
Entree, spaghetti, w/meatballs, fzn	1 ea	290	322	19.4	8	2.2	6	43
The Budget Gourmet								
Dinner, chicken, teriyaki, 3 dish	1 ea	340	360	20	12		55	44
Dinner, veal, parmigiana, 3 dish	1 ea	340	440	26	20		165	39
Entree, beef, sirloin tips, w/country gravy	1 ea	334	365	18.8	21		47	25
Entree, linguini, w/shrimp	1 ea	284	330	15	15		75	33
The Budget Gourmet-Slim Select								
Entree, stroganoff, beef	1 ea	238	269	17.3	10		58	28
Weight Watchers								
Entree, chow mein, chicken	1 ea	255	200	12	2	0.5	25	34

CHAPTER 1

1. W. M. Bortz II, "Disuse and Aging," *Journal of the American Medical Association*, 248 (1982): 1203–1208.
2. U. S. Department of Health and Human Services, Centers for Disease Control and Prevention, National Center for Health Statistics, *Deaths: Preliminary Data for 2003*, 53:15 (February 28, 2005).
3. T. A. Murphy and D. Murphy, *The Wellness for Life Workbook* (San Diego: Fitness Publications, 1987).
4. U. S. Department of Health and Human Services, *Physical Activity and Health: A Report of the Surgeon General* (Atlanta: U. S. Department of Health and Human Services, Centers for Disease Control and Prevention, National Center for Chronic Disease Prevention and Health Promotion, 1996).
5. National Academy of Sciences, Institute of Medicine, *Dietary Reference Intakes for Energy, Carbohydrates, Fiber, Fat, Protein and Amino Acids (Macronutrients)* (Washington, DC: National Academy Press, 2002).
6. U. S. Department of Health and Human Services, Department of Agriculture, *Dietary Guidelines for Americans 2005.* (Washington, DC: DHHS, 2005).
7. R. S. Paffenbarger, Jr., R. T. Hyde, A. L. Wing, and C. H. Steinmetz, "A Natural History of Athleticism and Cardiovascular Health," *Journal of the American Medical Association*, 252 (1984): 491–495.
8. S. N. Blair, H. W. Kohl III, R. S. Paffenbarger, Jr., D. G. Clark, K. H. Cooper, and L. W. Gibbons, "Physical Fitness and All-Cause Mortality: A Prospective Study of Healthy Men and Women," *Journal of the American Medical Association*, 262 (1989): 2395–2401.
9. S. N. Blair, H. W. Kohl III, C. E. Barlow, R. S. Paffenbarger, Jr., L. W. Gibbons, and C. A. Macera, "Changes in Physical Fitness and All-Cause Mortality: A Prospective Study of Healthy and Unhealthy Men," *Journal of the American Medical Association*, 273 (1995): 1193–1198.
10. I. Lee, C. Hsieh, and R. S. Paffenbarger, Jr., "Exercise Intensity and Longevity in Men: The Harvard Alumni Health Study," *Journal of the American Medical Association*, 273 (1995): 1179–1184.
11. U. S. Department of Health and Human Services, *Healthy People 2010 Objectives: Draft for Public Comment* (Washington DC, Public Health Service, 1998).
12. J. O. Prochaska, J. C. Norcross, and C. C. DiClemente, *Changing for Good* (New York: William Morrow and Co., 1994).
13. American College of Sports Medicine, *Guidelines for Exercise Testing and Prescription* (Philadelphia: Lippincott Williams & Wilkins, 2006).

CHAPTER 2

1. R. B. O'Hara et al., "Increased Volume Resistance Training: Effects upon Predicted Aerobic Fitness in a Select Group of Air Force Men," *ACSM's Health and Fitness Journal* 8, no. 4 (2004): 16–25.
2. American College of Sports Medicine, *Guidelines for Exercise Testing and Prescription* (Philadelphia: Lippincott Williams & Wilkins, 2006).
3. W. J. Evans, "Exercise, Nutrition and Aging," *Journal of Nutrition*, 122 (1992): 786–801.
4. R. A. Faulkner, E. J. Sprigings, A. McQuarrie, and R. D. Bell," A Partial Curl-Up Protocol for Adults Based on Analysis of Two Procedures," *Canadian Journal of Sports Science*, 14 (1989): 135–141; P. A. Macfarlane, "Out with the Sit-Up, in with the Curl-Up!," *JOPERD*, 64 (1993): 62–66; D. Knudson and D. Johnston, "Validity and Reliability of a Bench Trunk-Curl Up Test of Abdominal Endurance," *Journal of Strength and Conditioning Research*, 9 (1995): 165–169; R. Kjorstad. *Validity of Two Field Tests of Abdominal Strength and Muscular Endurance*, Unpublished master's thesis, Boise State University, 1997.
5. T. McNeill, D. Warwick, G. Anderson, and A. Schultz, "Trunk Strengths in Attempted Flexion, Extension, and Lateral Bending in Healthy Subjects and Patients with Low-Back Pain Disorders," *Spine*, 5 (1980): 529–536.
6. L. D. Robertson and H. Magnusdottir, "Evaluation of Criteria Associated with Abdominal Fitness Testing," *Research Quarterly for Exercise and Sport*, 58 (1987): 355–359; See note 5.
7. See note 7; G. L. Hall, R. K. Hetzler, D. Perrin, and A. Weltman, "Relationship of Timed Sit-Up Tests to Isokinetic Abdominal Strength," *Research Quarterly for Exercise and Sport*, 63 (1992): 80–84.
8. American College of Obstetricians and Gynecologists, *Guidelines for Exercise During Pregnancy*, 1994.
9. "Stretch Yourself Younger," *Consumer Reports on Health*, 11 (August 1999): 6–7.
10. J. H. Wilmore. *Exercise and Weight Control: Myths, Misconceptions, Gadgets, Gimmicks, and Quackery*, lecture given at annual meeting of American College of Sports Medicine, Indianapolis, June 1994.

CHAPTER 3

1. H. Atkinson, "Exercise for Longer Life: The Physician's Perspective," *Health News*, 3:7 (1997): 3.
2. American College of Sports Medicine, *Guidelines for Exercise Testing and Prescription* (Philadelphia: Lippincott Williams & Wilkins, 2006).
3. See note 2.
4. S. N. Blair, "Surgeon General's Report on Physical Fitness: The Inside Story," *ACSM's Health & Fitness Journal*, 1 (1997): 14–18.
5. R. F. DeBusk, U. Stenestrand, M. Sheehan, and W. L. Haskell, "Training Effects of Long Versus Short Bouts of Exercise in Healthy Subjects," *American Journal of Cardiology*, 65 (1990): 1010–1013.
6. National Academy of Sciences, Institute of Medicine, *Dietary Reference Intakes for Energy, Carbohydrates, Fiber, Fat,*

Protein and Amino Acids (Macronutrients) (Washington, DC: National Academy Press, 2002).

7. U. S. Department of Health and Human Services, Department of Agriculture, *Dietary Guidelines for Americans 2005* (Washington, DC: DHHS, 2005).

8. W. W. K. Hoeger, D. R. Hopkins, S. L. Barette, and D. F. Hale, "Relationship Between Repetitions and Selected Percentages of One Repetition Maximum: A Comparison Between Untrained and Trained Males and Females," *Journal of Applied Sport Science Research* 4, no. 2 (1990): 47–51.

9. See note 2.

10. See note 2.

11. Gatorade Sports Science Institute, "Core Strength Training," *Sports Science Exchange Roundtable* 13, no. 1 (2002): 1–4.

12. S. B. Thacker, J. Gilchrist, D. F. Stroup, and C. D. Kimsey., Jr., "The Impact of Stretching on Sports Injury Risk: A Systematic Review of the Literature," *Medicine and Science in Sports and Exercise*, 36 (2004): 371–378.

13. "Minimizing Back Pain," *Tufts University Health and Nutrition Letter* (New York: The Editors, May 1998).

14. R. Deyo, "Chiropractic Care for Back Pain: The Physician's Perspective," *HealthNews*, 4 (September 10, 1998).

15. A. Brownstein, "Chronic Back Pain Can Be Beaten," *Bottom Line Health*, 13 (October 1999): 3–4.

CHAPTER 4

1. J. L. Christi, L. M. Sheldahl, F. E. Tristani, L. S. Wann, K. B. Sagar, S. G. Levandoski, M. J. Ptacin, K. A. Sobocinski, and R. D. Morris, "Cardiovascular Regulation During Head-out Water Immersion Exercise," *Journal of Applied Physiology*, 69 (1990): 657–664; L. M. Sheldahl, F. E. Tristani, P. S. Clifford, C. V. Hughes, K. A. Sobocinski, and R. D. Morris, "Effect of Head-out Water Immersion on Cardiorespiratory Response to Dynamic Exercise," *Journal of American College of Cardiology*, 10 (1987): 1254–1258; J. Svedenhag and J. Seger, "Running on Land and in Water: Comparative Exercise Physiology," *Medicine and Science in Sports and Exercise*, 24 (1992): 1155–1160.

2. W. W. K. Hoeger, D. Hopkins, and D. Barber, "Physiologic Responses to Maximal Treadmill Running and Water Aerobic Exercise," *National Aquatics Journal*, 11 (1995): 4–7.

3. W. W. K. Hoeger, T. A. Spitzer-Gibson, N. Kaluhiokalani, R. K. M. Cardejon, and J. Kokkonen, "A Comparison of Physiological Responses to Self-Paced Water Aerobics and Self-Paced Treadmill Running," *International Council for Health, Physical Education, Recreation, Sport, and Dance Journal* 30, no. 4 (2004): 27–30.

4. W. W. K. Hoeger, T. S. Gibson, J. Moore, and D. R. Hopkins, "A Comparison of Selected Training Responses to Low Impact Aerobics and Water Aerobics," *National Aquatics Journal*, 9 (1993): 13–16.

5. E. J. Marcinick, J. Potts, G. Schlabach, S. Will, P. Dawson, and B. F. Hurley, "Effects of Strength Training on Lactate Threshold and Endurance Performance," *Medicine and Science in Sports and Exercise*, 23 (1991): 739–743.

CHAPTER 5

1. E. B. Rimm, A. Ascherio, E. Giovannucci, D. Spiegelman, M. J. Stampfer, and W. C. Willett, "Vegetable, Fruit, and Cereal Fiber Intake and Risk of Coronary Heart Disease Among Men," *Journal of the American Medical Association*, 275 (1996): 447–451.

2. National Academy of Sciences, Institute of Medicine. *Dietary Reference Intakes for Energy, Carbohydrates, Fiber, Fat, Protein and Amino Acids (Macronutrients)* (Washington, DC: National Academy Press, 2002).

3. "To E or Not to E?" *University of California at Berkeley Wellness Letter* (February 2005).

4. L. C. Clark et al., "Effects of Selenium Supplementation for Cancer Prevention in Patients with Carcinoma of the Skin: A Randomized Controlled Trial," *Journal of the American Medical Association*, 276 (1996): 1957–1963.

5. "Does This Mineral Prevent Cancer?" *University of California at Berkeley Wellness Letter*, 16:9 (2000): 1–2.

6. "The Merits of Multivitamins: EN's Guide to Choosing a Supplement," *Environmental Nutrition* 24, no. 6 (2001): 1.

7. American Psychiatric Association, *Diagnostic and Statistical Manual of Mental Disorders* (Washington, DC: APA, 1994).

8. See note 7.

9. U. S. Department of Health and Human Services, Department of Agriculture, *Dietary Guidelines for Americans 2005* (Washington, DC: DHHS, 2005).

CHAPTER 6

1. A. Must et al., "The Disease Burden Associated with Overweight and Obesity," *Journal of the American Medical Association*, 282 (1999): 1523–1529.

2. A. H. Mokdad, J. S. Marks, D. F. Stroup, and J. L. Gerberding, "Actual Causes of Death in the United States, 2000," *Journal of the American Medical Association* 291 (2004): 1238–1241.

3. R. Sturm and K. B. Wells, "Does Obesity Contribute as Much to Morbidity as Poverty or Smoking?" *Public Health* 115 (2001): 229–235.

4. E. E. Calle et. al., "Overweight, Obesity, and Mortality from Cancer in a Prospectively Studied Cohort of U. S. Adults," *New England Journal of Medicine*, 348 (2003): 1625–1638.

5. S. Thomsen, "A Steady Diet of Images," *BYU Magazine* 57, no. 3 (2003): 20–21.

6. G. D. Foster et al., "A Randomized Trial of a Low-Carbohydrate Diet for Obesity," *The New England Journal of Medicine* 348 (2003): 2082–2090; F. F. Samaha et al., "A Low-Carbohydrate as Compared with Low-Fat Diet in Severe Obesity," *The New England Journal of Medicine* 348 (2003): 2074–2081.

7. R. L. Leibel, M. Rosenbaum, and J. Hirsh, "Changes in Energy Expenditure Resulting from Altered Body Weight," *New England Journal of Medicine*, 332 (1995): 621–628.

8. American College of Sports Medicine, "Position Stand: Appropriate Intervention Strategies for Weight Loss and Prevention for Weight Regain for Adults," *Medicine and Science in Sports and Exercise* 33 (2001): 2145–2156.

9. J. H. Wilmore, "Exercise, Obesity, and Weight Control," *Physical Activity and Fitness Research Digest* (Washington DC: President's Council on Physical Fitness & Sports, 1994).

10. National Academy of Sciences, Institute of Medicine, *Dietary Reference Intakes for Energy, Carbohydrates, Fiber, Fat, Protein and Amino Acids (Macronutrients)* (Washington, DC: National Academy Press, 2002).

11. M. K. Serdula et al., "Prevalence of Attempting Weight Loss and Strategies for Controlling Weight," *Journal of the American Medical Association* 282 (1999): 1353–1358.

12. E. T. Poehlman et al., "Effects of Endurance and Resistance Training on Total Daily Energy Expenditure in Young Women: A Controlled Randomized Trial," *Journal of Clinical Endocrinology and Metabolism*, 87 (2002): 1004–1009; L. M. Van Etten et al., "Effect of an 18-wk Weight-training Program on Energy Expenditure and Physical Activity," *Journal of Applied Physiology*, 82 (1997): 298–304;. W. W. Campbell, M. C. Crim, V. R. Young, and W. J. Evans, "Increased Energy Requirements and Changes in Body Composition with Resistance Training in Older Adults," *American Journal of Clinical Nutrition*, 60 (1994): 167–175;

Z. Wang et al., "Resting Energy Expenditure: Systematic Organization and Critique of Prediction Methods," *Obesity Research*, 9 (2001): 331–336.

13. A. Tremblay, J. A. Simoneau, and C. Bouchard, "Impact of Exercise Intensity on Body Fatness and Skeletal Muscle Metabolism," *Metabolism* 43 (1994): 814–818.

14. W. W. K. Hoeger, C. Harris, E. M. Long, and D. R. Hopkins, "Four-Week Supplementation with a Natural Dietary Compound Produces Favorable Changes in Body Composition," *Advances in Therapy* 15, no. 5 (1998): 305–313; W. W. K. Hoeger, C. Harris, E. M. Long, R. L. Kjorstad, M. Welch, T. L. Hafner, D. R. Hopkins, "Dietary Supplementation with Chromium Picolinate/L-Carnitine Complex in Combination with Diet and Exercise Enhances Body Composition," *Journal of the American Nutraceutical Association* 2, no. 2 (1999): 40–45.

CHAPTER 7

1. H. E. Selye, *Stress Without Distress* (New York: Signet, 1974).

2. See Ray Rosenman, "Do You Have Type 'A' Behavior?" *Health and Fitness* (supplement): 1987; Redford Williams, *The Trusting Heart: Great News About Type A Behavior* (New York: Times Books, 1989): 120; Howard Friedman, *The Self-Healing Personality* (New York: Henry Holt & Co., 1991).

3. R. Williams, *The Trusting Heart: Great News About Type A Behavior* (New York: Times Book, Division of Random House, 1989).

4. D. Girdano and G. Everly, *Controlling Stress and Tension: A Holistic Approach* (Englewood Cliffs, NJ: Prentice Hall, 1992); W. Schafer, *Stress Management for Wellness* (Ft. Worth: HBJ College Publishers, 1995).

5. S. Bodian, "Meditate Your Way to Much Better Health," *Bottom Line Health* 18 (June 2004): 11–13.

6. D. Mueller, "Yoga Therapy," *ACSM's Health & Fitness Journal* 6, no. 1 (2002): 18–24.

7. S. C. Manchanda et al., "Retardation of Coronary Atherosclerosis With Yoga Lifestyle Intervention," *Journal of the Association of Physicians of India* 48 (2000): 687–694.

CHAPTER 8

1. E. R. Growald and A. Lusks, "Beyond Self," *American Health* (March 1988): 51–53.

2. U. S. Department of Health and Human Services, Centers for Disease Control and Prevention, National Center for Health Statistics, National Vital Statistics Reports, *Deaths: Preliminary Data for 2003*, 53:15 (February 28, 2005).

3. J. M. McGinnis and W. H. Foege, "Actual Causes of Death in the United States," *Journal of the American Medical Association*, 270 (1993): 2207–2212.

4. See note 2.

5. American Heart Association, *Heart Disease and Stroke Statistics—2005 Update* (Dallas: AHA, 2005).

6. S. N. Blair, H. W. Kohl III, R. S. Paffenbarger, Jr., D. G. Clark, K. H. Cooper, and L. W. Gibbons, "Physical Fitness and All-Cause Mortality: A Prospective Study of Healthy Men and Women," *Journal of the American Medical Association*, 262 (1989): 2395–2401.

7. "Water, Sodium, Potassium: The Verdict Is In," *University of California at Berkeley Wellness Letter* (Palm Coast, FL: The Editors, May 2004).

8. G. A. Kelley and Z. Tran, "Aerobic Exercise and Normotensive Adults: A Meta-analysis," *Medicine and Science in Sports and Exercise*, 27 (1995): 1371–1377.

9. R. Collins et al., "Blood Pressure, Stroke, and Coronary Heart Disease: Part 2, Short-term Reductions in Blood Pressure: Overview of Randomized Drug Trials in Their Epidemiological Context," *Lancet*, 335 (1990): 827–838.

10. S. N. Blair et al., "Influences of Cardiorespiratory Fitness and Other Precursors on Cardiovascular Disease and All-cause Mortality in Men and Women," *Journal of the American Medical Association*, 276 (1996): 205–210.

11. G. A. Kelley and K. S. Kelley, "Progressive Resistance Exercise and Resting Blood Pressure: A Meta-Analysis of Randomized Controlled Trials," *Hypertension*, 35 (2000): 838–843.

12. "Lipid Research Clinics Program: The Lipid Research Clinic Coronary Primary Prevention Trial Results," *Journal of the American Medical Association*, 251 (1984): 351–364.

13. American Heart Association, *Know the Facts, Get the Stats* (Dallas: AHA, 2003).

14. American Heart Association, *Heart and Stroke Facts* (Dallas: AHA, 1999).

15. "From Starring Role to Bit Part: Has the Curtain Come Down on Vitamin E?" *Environmental Nutrition* 25 no. 5 (May 2002): 1, 4.

16. E. B. Rimm, A. Ascherio, E. Giovannucci, D. Spiegelman, M. J. Stampfer, and W. C. Willett, "Vegetable, Fruit, and Cereal Fiber Intake and Risk of Coronary Heart Disease Among Men," *Journal of the American Medical Association*, 275 (1996): 447–451.

17. "The Homocysteine–CVD Connection," *HealthNews* (October 25, 1999).

18. "Inflammation May Be Key Cause of Heart Disease and More: Diet's Role," *Environmental Nutrition*, 27 no. 7 (July 2004): 1, 4.

19. S. Liu et al., "A Prospective Study of Dietary Glycemic Load, Carbohydrate Intake, and Risk of Coronary Heart Disease in the U. S.," *American Journal of Clinical Nutrition*, 71 (2000): 1455–1461.

20. G. M. Reaven, T. K. Strom, and B. Fox, *Syndrome X: Overcoming the Silent Killer that Can Give You a Heart Attack* (New York: Simon & Schuster, 2000).

21. See note 5.

22. American Cancer Society, *2005 Cancer Facts and Figures* (New York: ACS, 2005).

23. "Colorful Diet Helps Keep Cancer at Bay: Fruits and Vegetables Are Key," *Environmental Nutrition*, 24, no. 6 (2001): 1, 6.

24. L. Mitscher and V. Dolby, *The Green Tea Book–China's Fountain of Youth* (New York: Avery Press, 1997); L. Mitscher, "Strongest Known Disease-fighting Antioxidant," *Bottom Line Personal Health*, 18:4 (1997): 3.

25. N. Ahmad et al., "Green Tea Constituent Epigallocatechin-3-Gallate and Induction of Apoptosis and Cell Cycle Arrest in Human Carcinoma Cells," *Journal of the National Cancer Institute*, 89 (1997): 1881–1886.

26. I-Min Lee, "Exercise and Physical Health: Cancer and Immune Function," *Research Quarterly for Exercise and Sport*, 66 (1995): 286–291.

27. H. Weinstock, S. Berman, and W. Cates, "Sexually Transmitted Diseases Among American Youth: Incidence and Prevalence Estimates, 2000," *Perspectives on Sexual and Reproductive Health*, 36 (2004): 6–10.

CHAPTER 9

1. R. S. Paffenbarger, Jr., R. T. Hyde, A. L. Wing, and C. H. Steinmetz., "A Natural History of Athleticism and Cardiovascular Health," *Journal of the American Medical Association*, 252 (1984): 491–495.

2. S. N. Blair, H. W. Kohl III, R. S. Paffenbarger, Jr., D. G. Clark, K. H. Cooper, and L. W. Gibbons, "Physical Fitness and All-Cause Mortality: A Prospective Study of Healthy Men and Women," *Journal of the American Medical Association*, 262 (1989): 2395– 2401.

3. R. Hambrecht et al., "Various Intensities of Leisure Time Physical Activity in Patients with Coronary Artery Disease: Effects on Cardiorespiratory Fitness and Progression of Coronary Atherosclerotic Lesions," *Journal of the American College of Cardiology*, 22 (1993): 468–477.

4. C. L. Otis, B. Drinkwater, M. Johnson, A. Loucks, and J. Wilmore, "The Female Athlete Triad," *Medicine and Science in Sports and Exercise*, 29 (1997): i–ix.

5. American College of Obstetricians and Gynecologists. "Exercise During Pregnancy and the Postpartum Period." ACOG Committee Opinion No. 267, *International Journal of Gynecology and Obstetrics* 77 (2002): 79–81.

6. "New Advice About Bone Density Tests," *University of California at Berkeley Wellness Letter* 18, no. 10 (2002): 1–2.

7. M. T. Goodman et al., "Association of Dairy Products, Lactose, and Calcium with the Risk of Ovarian Cancer," *American Journal of Epidemiology* 156 (2002): 148–157.

8. Writing Group for the Women's Health Initiative, "Risks and Benefits of Combined Estrogen and Progestin in Healthy Postmenopausal Women: Principal Results from the Women's Health Initiative Randomized Controlled Trial," *Journal of the American Medical Association* 288 (2002): 321–333.

9. "Are Fruits and Vegetables Less Nutritious Today.?" *University of California Berkeley Wellness Letter*, 14:8 (1998): 1.

10. American College of Sports Medicine, "Position Stand: Exercise and Physical Activity for Older Adults," *Medicine and Science in Sports and Exercise*, 30 (1998): 992–1008.

11. F. W. Kash, J. L. Boyer, S. P. Van Camp, L. S. Verity, and J. P. Wallace. "The Effect of Physical Activity on Aerobic Power in Older Men (A Longitudinal Study): *The Physician and Sports Medicine*, 18:4 (1990): 73–83.

12. See note 10.

Chapter 1

1. a   2. e   3. d   4. c   5. c   6. b   7. b   8. d   9. a   10. e

Chapter 2

1. e   2. a   3. e   4. e   5. c   6. b   7. b   8. a   9. d   10. c

Chapter 3

1. d   2. c   3. c   4. d   5. a   6. c   7. b   8. c   9. e   10. e

Chapter 4

1. d   2. a   3. c   4. d   5. c   6. a   7. e   8. d   9. a   10. b

Chapter 5

1. b   2. e   3. c   4. d   5. d   6. a   7. a   8. c   9. a   10. e

Chapter 6

1. c   2. d   3. e   4. a   5. b   6. c   7. a   8. c   9. d   10. e

Chapter 7

1. a   2. c   3. c   4. e   5. b   6. e   7. e   8. a   9. e   10. c

Chapter 8

1. e   2. a   3. b   4. e   5. b   6. e   7. e   8. b   9. d   10. c

Chapter 9

1. b   2. e   3. e   4. d   5. d   6. e   7. b   8. a   9. e   10. c

Cover © Alan Becker/Getty Images

p. iii © Alan Becker/Getty Images; **p. v** © Ariel Skelley/CORBIS; **p. vi** © Steve Lupton/CORBIS; **p. vii** © Gulliver/zefa/CORBIS; **p. viii** © Ariel Skelley/CORBIS

Chapter 1

p. 1 © Ariel Skelley/CORBIS; **p. 2** © Fitness & Wellness, Inc.; **p. 4** © Fitness & Wellness, Inc.; **p. 8** © Fitness & Wellness, Inc.; **p. 14** © Fitness & Wellness, Inc.; **p. 17** © Fitness & Wellness, Inc.

Chapter 2

p. 25 © Paul Barton/CORBIS; **p. 26** © Fitness & Wellness, Inc.; **p. 28** © Fitness & Wellness, Inc.; **p. 29** © Fitness & Wellness, Inc.; **p. 31** © Fitness & Wellness, Inc.; **p. 32** © Fitness & Wellness, Inc.; **p. 33** © Fitness & Wellness, Inc.; **p. 34** © Fitness & Wellness, Inc.; **p. 36** © Fitness & Wellness, Inc.; **p. 37** © Fitness & Wellness, Inc.; **p. 38** © Fitness & Wellness, Inc.; **p. 39** © Fitness & Wellness, Inc.; **p. 41** (bottom left) © Life Measurement, Inc.; (all others) © Fitness & Wellness, Inc.

Chapter 3

p. 53 © Randy M. Ury/CORBIS; **p. 55** © Fitness & Wellness, Inc.; **p. 56** © Fitness & Wellness, Inc.; **p. 57** © Fitness & Wellness, Inc.; **p. 61** (bottom left) Eric Risberg; (all others) Fitness & Wellness, Inc.; **p. 66** © Fitness & Wellness, Inc.; **p. 67** © Fitness & Wellness, Inc.; **p. 72** © Fitness & Wellness, Inc.

Chapter 4

p. 87 © Don Mason/CORBIS; **p. 88** © Fitness & Wellness, Inc.; **p. 89** © Fitness & Wellness, Inc.; **p. 90** © (left) Fitness & Wellness, Inc.; (right) © Aero-belt Aerobics; **p. 91** © Fitness & Wellness, Inc.; **p. 92** Chuck Scheer, Boise State University; **p. 93** © Fitness & Wellness, Inc.; **p. 95** © Fitness & Wellness, Inc.; **p. 96** © Fitness & Wellness, Inc.; **p. 97** (left) © Fitness & Wellness, Inc.; (right) Eric Risberg

Chapter 5

p. 105 © Steve Lupton/CORBIS; **p. 106** © Fitness & Wellness, Inc.

Chapter 6

p. 127 © Michael Keller/CORBIS; **p. 123** (bottom) Eric Risberg; (all others) © Fitness & Wellness, Inc.; **p. 132** © 2001 PhotoDisc, Inc.; **p. 135** (top) © Fitness & Wellness, Inc.; (bottom) © Nautilus Sports/Medical Industries, Inc.; **p. 140** © Fitness & Wellness, Inc.

Chapter 7

p. 151 © Gulliver/zefa/CORBIS; **p. 153** © Fitness & Wellness, Inc.; **p. 154** © Fitness & Wellness, Inc.; **p. 158** © Fitness & Wellness, Inc.; **p. 160** © Fitness & Wellness, Inc.; **p. 161** © Fitness & Wellness, Inc.; **p. 163** © Fitness & Wellness, Inc.; **p. 166** © Fitness & Wellness, Inc.; **p. 167** © Fitness & Wellness, Inc.

Chapter 8

p. 171 © Lester Lefkowitz/CORBIS; **p. 179** © CORBIS; **p. 184** © Fitness & Wellness, Inc.; **p. 187** © 2001 PhotoDisc, Inc.; **p. 188** © Fitness & Wellness, Inc.

Chapter 9

p. 199 © Ariel Skelley/CORBIS; **p. 201** © Fitness & Wellness, Inc.; **p. 203** © Fitness & Wellness, Inc.; **p. 206** © Fitness & Wellness, Inc.; **p. 208** © Nautilus Sports/Medical Industries, Inc.; **p. 216** © Fitness & Wellness, Inc.

Appendixes

p. 225 © Ken Redding/CORBIS; **p. 227** © Fitness & Wellness, Inc.; **p. 228** © Fitness & Wellness, Inc.; **p. 229** © Fitness & Wellness, Inc.; **p. 230** © Fitness & Wellness, Inc.; **p. 231** © Fitness & Wellness, Inc.; **p. 232** © Fitness & Wellness, Inc.; **p. 233** (top two left, bottom two right) © Universal Gym Equipment, Inc.; (top two right, bottom left) © Nautilus Sports/ Medical Industries, Inc.; **p. 234** (top two right) © Fitness & Wellness, Inc.; (all others) © Universal Gym Equipment, Inc.; **p. 235** (middle two) © Universal Gym Equipment, Inc.; (all others) © Nautilus Sports/ Medical Industries, Inc.; **p. 236** © Fitness & Wellness, Inc.; **p. 237** © Fitness & Wellness, Inc.; **p. 238** © Fitness & Wellness, Inc.; **p. 239** © Fitness & Wellness, Inc.; **p. 240** © Fitness & Wellness, Inc.; **p. 241** © Fitness & Wellness, Inc.; **p. 242** © Fitness & Wellness, Inc.

A

Acquired immunodeficiency syndrome (AIDS) End stage of HIV infection, manifested by any of a number of diseases that arise when the body's immune system is compromised by HIV.

Action stage Stage of change in which people are actively changing a negative behavior or adopting a new, healthy behavior.

Activities of daily living Everyday behaviors that people normally do to function in life (cross the street, carry groceries, lift objects, do laundry, sweep floors).

Adequate Intakes (AI) The recommended amount of a nutrient intake when sufficient evidence is not available to calculate the EAR and subsequent RDA.

Aerobic dance A series of exercise routines performed to music; more commonly termed aerobics now.

Aerobic exercise Activity that requires oxygen to produce the necessary energy to carry out the activity.

Alcoholism Disease in which an individual loses control over drinking alcoholic beverages.

Altruism True concern for and action on behalf of others (opposite of egoism); a sincere desire to serve others above one's personal needs.

Amenorrhea Absence (primary amenorrhea) or cessation (secondary amenorrhea) of normal menstrual function.

Amino acids The basic building blocks of protein.

Anabolic steroids A synthetic version of the male sex hormone testosterone, which promotes muscle development and hypertrophy.

Android obesity Obesity pattern wherein individuals store fat primarily in the trunk or abdominal area.

Angiogenesis Capillary (blood vessel) formation into a tumor.

Anorexia nervosa An eating disorder characterized by self-imposed starvation to lose and then maintain very low body weight.

Antioxidants Compounds that prevent oxygen from combining with other substances it might damage.

Arrhythmias Irregular heart rhythms.

Atherosclerosis Fatty/cholesterol deposits in the walls of the arteries leading to formation of plaque.

B

Ballistic (or dynamic) stretching Exercises performed using jerky, rapid, and bouncy movements.

Basal metabolic rate (BMR) Lowest level of caloric intake necessary to sustain life.

Behavior modification The process used to permanently change negative behaviors in favor of positive behaviors that will lead to better health and well-being.

Benign Noncancerous.

Binge-eating disorder An eating disorder characterized by uncontrollable episodes of eating excessive amounts of food within a relatively short time.

Blood lipids (fat) Cholesterol and triglycerides.

Blood pressure A measure of the force exerted against the walls of the vessels by the blood flowing through them.

Body composition The fat and nonfat components of the human body.

Body Mass Index (BMI) An index that incorporates height and weight to estimate critical fat values at which risk for disease increases.

Bulimia nervosa An eating disorder characterized by a pattern of binge eating and purging.

C

C-reactive protein (CPR) A protein whose level in the blood increases with inflammation (which may be hidden deep in the body); elevation of this protein is an indicator of potential cardiovascular events.

Calorie The amount of heat necessary to raise the temperature of 1 gram of water 1° Centigrade; used to measure the energy value of food and the cost of physical activity.

Cancer Group of diseases characterized by uncontrolled growth and spread of abnormal cells into malignant tumors.

Carbohydrates Compounds composed of carbon, hydrogen, and oxygen that the body uses as its major source of energy.

Carcinogens Substances that contribute to the formation of cancers.

Carcinoma in situ Encapsulated malignant tumor that is found at an early stage and has not spread.

Cardiomyopathy A disease affecting the heart muscle.

Cardiorespiratory endurance Ability of the lungs, heart, and blood vessels to deliver adequate amounts of oxygen to the cells to meet the demands of prolonged physical activity.

Cardiorespiratory training zone The range of intensity at which a person should exercise to develop the cardiorespiratory system.

Cardiovascular diseases The array of conditions that affect the heart and blood vessels.

Carotenoids Pigment substances (more than 600) in plants, about 50 of which are precursors to vitamin A; the most potent carotenoid is beta-carotene.

Cholesterol A waxy substance, technically a steroid alcohol, found only in animal fats and oil; used in making cell membranes, as a building block for some hormones, in the fatty sheath around nerve fibers, and in other necessary substances.

Chronic diseases Illnesses that develop and last over a long time.

Chronic lower respiratory disease (CLRD) A group of diseases that limit air flow, such as chronic obstructive pulmonary disease, emphysema, and chronic bronchitis (all diseases of the respiratory system).

Chronological age Calendar age.

Chronotropic incompetence A condition in which the heart rate increases slowly during exercise and never reaches maximum.

Chylomicrons Molecules that transport triglycerides in the blood.

Cirrhosis A disease characterized by scarring of the liver.

Concentric muscle contraction A dynamic contraction in which the muscle shortens as it develops tension.

Contemplation stage Stage of change in which people are considering changing behavior in the next 6 months.

Contraindicated exercises Exercises that are not recommended because they pose potentially high risk for injury.

Cool-down A period at the end of an exercise session when exercise is tapered off.

Coronary heart disease (CHD) Condition in which the arteries that supply the heart muscle with oxygen and nutrients are narrowed by fatty deposits such as cholesterol and triglycerides.

Cross-training Using a combination of different aerobic activities to develop or maintain cardiorespiratory endurance.

Cruciferous vegetables Plants that produce cross-shaped leaves (cauliflower, broccoli, cabbage, Brussels sprouts, kohlrabi); these seem to have a protective effect against cancer.

D

Daily Values (DVs) Reference values for nutrients and food components used in food labels.

Deoxyribonucleic acid (DNA) Genetic substance of which genes are made; molecule that bears cell's genetic code.

Diabetes mellitus A condition in which blood glucose is unable to enter the cells because the pancreas either totally stops producing insulin or does not produce enough to meet the body's needs.

Diastolic blood pressure Pressure exerted by the blood against the walls of the arteries during the relaxation phase (diastole) of the heart.

Dietary Reference Intakes (DRIs) Four types of nutrient standards that are used to establish adequate amounts and maximum safe nutrient intakes in the diet: Estimated Average Requirements (EAR), Recommended Dietary Allowances (RDA), Adequate Intakes (AI), and Tolerable Upper Intake Levels (UL).

Distress Negative or harmful stress under which health and performance begin to deteriorate.

Duration of exercise Time exercising per session.

Dynamic exercise Strength training with muscle contraction that produces movement.

Dysmenorrhea Painful menstruation.

E

Eccentric muscle contraction A dynamic contraction in which the muscle lengthen as it develops tension.

Electrocardiogram (ECG or EKG) A recording of the electrical activity of the heart.

Energy-balancing equation A body weight formula stating that when caloric intake equals caloric output, weight remains unchanged.

Epidemiological The study of epidemic diseases.

Essential fat Body fat needed for normal physiological functions.

Essential nutrients Carbohydrates, fats, protein, vitamins, minerals, and water—the nutrients the human body requires for survival.

Estimated Average Requirements (EAR) The amount of a nutrient that meets the dietary needs in half the people.

Estimated energy requirement (EER) The average dietary energy (caloric) intake that is predicted to maintain energy balance in a healthy adult of defined age, gender, weight, height, and level of physical activity, consistent with good health.

Estrogen Female sex hormone; essential for bone formation and conservation of bone density.

Eustress Positive stress.

Exercise A type of physical activity that requires planned, structured, and repetitive bodily movement done to improve or maintain one or more components of physical fitness.

F

Fats (lipids) A class of nutrients that the body uses as a source of energy.

Female athlete triad Three interrelated disorders—disordered eating, amenorrhea, and bone mineral disorders—seen in some highly trained female athletes.

Ferritin Iron stored in the body.

Fiber Plant material that human digestive enzymes cannot digest.

Fight or flight Physiological response of the body to stress that prepares the individual to take action by stimulating the vital defense systems.

Fixed-resistance training Exercise with strength-training equipment that provides a constant amount of resistance through the range of motion.

Flexibility The achievable range of motion at a joint or group of joints without causing injury.

Free radicals Oxygen compounds produced in normal metabolism.

Free weights Barbells and dumbbells.

Frequency of exercise How often a person engages in an exercise session.

Functional fitness The physical capacity of the individual to meet ordinary and unexpected demands of daily life safely and effectively.

Functional independence Ability to carry out activities of daily living without assistance from other individuals.

G

General adaptation syndrome (GAS) A theoretical model that explains the body's adaptation to sustained stress, which includes three stages: alarm reaction, resistance, and exhaustion/recovery.

Goal The ultimate aim toward which effort is directed.

Gynoid obesity Obesity pattern wherein individuals store fat primarily around the hips and thighs.

H

Hatha yoga A yoga style that incorporates a series of static-stretching postures performed in specific sequences.

Health fitness standard The lowest fitness requirements for maintaining good health, decreasing the risk for chronic diseases, and lowering the incidence of muscular-skeletal injuries.

Health-related fitness A physical state encompassing cardiorespiratory endurance, muscular strength and endurance, muscular flexibility, and body composition.

Healthy life expectancy (HLE) Number of years a person is expected to live in good health; this number is obtained by subtracting ill-health years from overall life expectancy.

Heart rate reserve The difference between the maximal heart rate (MHR) and resting heart rate (RHR).

Hemoglobin Protein-iron compound in red blood cells that transports oxygen in the blood.

High-density lipoprotein (HDL) Cholesterol-transporting molecules in the blood (good cholesterol).

High-impact aerobics (HIA) Exercises incorporating movements in which both feet are off the ground at the same time momentarily.

Homeostasis A natural state of equilibrium. The body attempts to maintain this equilibrium by constantly reacting to external forces that attempt to disrupt this delicate balance.

Homocysteine Intermediate amino acid in the interconversion of two other amino acids: methionine and cysteine.

Human immunodeficiency virus (HIV) Virus that leads to acquired immunodeficiency syndrome (AIDS).

Hypertension Chronically elevated blood pressure.

Hypokinetic diseases Diseases related to a lack of physical activity.

Hypothermia A breakdown in the body's ability to generate heat, resulting in body temperature below 95°F.

I

Insulin-dependent diabetes mellitus (IDDM or Type 1) A form of diabetes in which the pancreas produces little or no insulin.

Intensity of exercise How hard a person has to exercise to improve cardiorespiratory endurance.

Intensity (in flexibility exercise) Degree of stretch.

Interval training A repeated series of exercise work bouts (intervals) interspersed with low-intensity or rest intervals.

Isokinetic exercise Strength training in which the equipment accommodates resistance to match the user's force through the full range of motion.

Isometric exercise Strength training with muscle contraction that produces little or no movement.

Isotonic exercise *See* Dynamic exercise.

L

Lean body mass Nonfat component of the human body.

Life expectancy Number of years a person is expected to live based on the person's birth year.

Lipoproteins Complex molecules that transport cholesterol in the bloodstream.

Locus of control The extent to which a person believes he or she can influence the external environment.

Low-density lipoprotein (LDL) Cholesterol-transporting molecules in the blood (bad cholesterol).

Low-impact aerobics (LIA) Exercises in which at least one foot is in contact with the ground or floor at all times.

M

Macronutrients The nutrients the body needs in proportionately large amounts; carbohydrates, fats, proteins, and water are examples.

Maintenance stage Stage of change in which people maintain behavioral change for up to 5 years.

Malignant Cancerous.

Maximal oxygen uptake (VO$_{2max}$) Maximum amount of oxygen the human body is able to utilize per minute of physical activity.

Meditation A mental exercise in which the objective is to gain control over one's attention, clearing the mind and blocking out stressors.

Megadoses For most vitamins, 10 times the RDA or more; for vitamins A and D, five and two times the RDA, respectively.

Melanoma The most virulent, rapidly spreading form of skin cancer.

MET Short for metabolic equivalent, the rate of energy expenditure at rest, or the equivalent of a VO$_2$ of 3.5 ml/kg/min.

Metabolic fitness Improvements in the metabolic profile through a moderate-intensity exercise program in spite of little or no improvement in health-related fitness components.

Metabolic profile Result of the assessment of diabetes and cardiovascular disease risk through plasma insulin, glucose, lipid, and lipoprotein levels.

Metabolic syndrome An array of metabolic abnormalities that contribute to the development of atherosclerosis triggered by resistance to insulin; these conditions include low HDL-cholesterol, high triglycerides, high blood pressure, and an increased blood clotting mechanism.

Metastasis Movement of bacteria or body cells from one part of the body to another.

Micronutrients The nutrients the body needs in small quantities—vitamins and minerals—that serve specific roles in transformation of energy and body tissue synthesis.

Minerals Inorganic elements needed by the body.

Mode of exercise Form of exercise (e.g., aerobic).

Moderate-impact aerobics (MIA) Aerobics that include plyometric training.

Motivation The desire and will to do something.

Muscular endurance Ability of a muscle to exert submaximal force repeatedly over a period of time.

Muscular hypertrophy An increase in muscle mass or size.

Muscular strength Ability to exert maximum force against resistance.

Myocardial infarction Heart attack; damage or death of an area of the heart muscle as a result of an obstructed artery to that area.

N

Negative resistance The lowering or eccentric phase of a repetition during the performance of a strength-training exercise.

Nitrosamines Potentially cancer-causing compounds formed when nitrites and nitrates—which are used to prevent the growth of harmful bacteria in processed meats—combine with other chemicals in the stomach.

Non-insulin-dependent diabetes mellitus (NIDDM or Type 2) A form of diabetes in which the pancreas either does not produce sufficient insulin or it produces adequate amounts but the cells become insulin-resistant, keeping glucose from entering the cell.

Nonresponders Individuals who exhibit small or no improvements in fitness compared with others who undergo the same training program.

Nutrients Substances found in food that provide energy, regulate metabolism, and help with growth and repair of body tissues.

Nutrition The science that studies the relationship of foods to optimal health and performance.

O

Obesity A chronic disease characterized by an excessively high amount of body fat (about 20 percent above recommended weight or a BMI at 30 or above).

Objectives Steps required to reach a goal.

Oligomenorrhea Irregular menstrual cycles.

One repetition maximum (1 RM) The maximal amount of resistance a person is able to lift in a single effort.

Opportunistic infections Diseases that arise in the absence of a healthy immune system that would fight them off in healthy people.

Osteoporosis Softening, deterioration, or loss of bone mass.

Overload principle Training concept holding that the demands placed on a body system must be increased systematically and progressively over time to cause physiologic adaptation.

Overweight Excess body weight when compared to a given standard such as height or recommended percent body fat.

P

Pedometer An electronic device that senses body motion and counts footsteps. Some pedometers also record distance, calories burned, speeds, and time spent being physically active.

Percent body fat (fat mass) Fat component of the body.

Personal trainer An exercise specialist who works one-on-one with an individual and is typically paid by the hour or exercise session.

Physical activity Bodily movement produced by skeletal muscles that requires energy expenditure and produces progressive health benefits.

Physical fitness The general capacity to adapt and respond favorably to physical effort.

Physical fitness standard Required criteria to achieve a high level of physical fitness; ability to do moderate to vigorous physical activity without undue fatigue.

Physiologic fitness Biological systems that are affected by physical activity; also the role of activity in disease prevention.

Physiological age Age based on the individual's functional and physical capacity.

Phytochemicals Compounds found in fruits and vegetables that block formation of cancerous tumors and disrupt the process of cancer.

Pilates Exercises that help strengthen the body's core by developing pelvic stability and abdominal control coupled with focused breathing patterns.

Plyometric training A form of exercise that requires forceful jumps or springing off the ground immediately after landing from a previous jump.

Positive resistance The lifting, pushing, or concentric phase of a repetition during the performance of a strength-training exercise.

Precontemplation stage Stage of change in which people are unwilling to change their behavior.

Preparation stage Stage of change in which people are getting ready to make a change within the coming month.

Principle of individuality Training concept that genetics plays a major role in individual responses to exercise training and these differences should be considered when designing exercise programs for different people.

Progressive muscle relaxation A relaxation technique that involves contracting, then relaxing muscle groups in the body in succession.

Progressive resistance training A gradual increase of resistance over a period of time.

Proprioceptive neuromuscular facilitation (PNF) A stretching technique in which muscles are stretched out progressively with intermittent isometric contractions.

Proteins A class of nutrients that the body uses to build and repair body tissues.

Q

Quackery/fraud The conscious promotion of unproven claims for profit.

R

Recommended body weight The weight at which there appears to be no harm to human health.

Recommended Dietary Allowances (RDA) The daily amount of a nutrient (statistically determined from the EARs) considered adequate to meet the known nutrient needs of almost 98 percent of all healthy people in the United States.

Registered dietitian (RD) A person with a college degree in dietetics who meets all certification and continuing education requirements of the American Dietetic Association or Dietitians of Canada.

Relapse Slipping or falling back into unhealthy behavior(s) or failing to maintain healthy behaviors.

Repetitions The number of times a movement is performed.

Resistance Amount of weight lifted.

Responders Individuals who exhibit improvements in fitness as a result of exercise training.

Resting metabolism The energy required to maintain the body's vital processes in the resting state.

Ribonucleic acid (RNA) Genetic material involved in the formation of cell proteins.

Risk factors Lifestyle and genetic variables that may lead to disease.

S

Sedentary Death Syndrome (SeDS) Deaths that are attributed to a lack of regular physical activity.

Set The number of repetitions performed for a given exercise.

Setpoint Body weight and body fat percentage unique to each person that is regulated by genetic and environmental factors.

Sexually transmitted infections (STIs) Communicable infections spread through sexual contact.

Shin splint Injury to the lower leg characterized by pain and irritation at the front of the leg.

Skill-related fitness Components of fitness important for successful motor performance in athletic events and in lifetime sports and activities.

Slow-sustained stretching Technique whereby the muscles are lengthened gradually through a joint's complete range of motion and the final position is held for several seconds.

SMART An acronym for Specific, Measurable, Attainable, Realistic, and Time-specific goals.

Specificity of training A principle holding that, for a muscle to increase in strength or endurance, the training program must be specific to obtain the desired effects.

Spirituality A sense of meaning and direction in life, a relationship to a higher being; encompasses freedom, prayer, faith, love, closeness to others, peace, joy, fulfillment, and altruism.

Step aerobics (SA) A form of exercise that combines stepping up and down from a bench with arm movements.

Storage fat Body fat stored in adipose tissue.

Stress The mental, emotional, and physiological response of the body to any situation that is new, threatening, frightening, or exciting.

Stress electrocardiogram (stress ECG) An exercise test during which the workload is gradually increased (until the subject reaches maximal fatigue), with blood pressure and 12-lead electrocardiographic monitoring throughout the test.

Stressor Stress-causing event.

Stretching Moving the joints beyond the accustomed range of motion.

Substrates Foods that are used as energy sources (carbohydrates, fat, protein).

Sun protection factor (SPF) Degree of protection offered by ingredients in sunscreen lotion; at least SPF 15 is recommended.

Supplements Tablets, pills, capsules, liquids, or powders that contain vitamins, minerals, amino acids, herbs, or fiber that are taken to increase the intake of these substances.

Synergistic action The effect of mixing two or more drugs, the effects of which can be much greater than the sum of two or more drugs acting by themselves.

Synergy A reaction in which the result is greater than the sum of its two parts.

Systolic blood pressure Pressure exerted by the blood against the walls of the arteries during the forceful contraction (systole) of the heart.

T

Termination/adoption stage Stage of change in which people have eliminated an undesirable behavior or maintained a positive behavior for more than 5 years.

Tolerable Upper Intake Levels (UL) The highest level of nutrient intake that appears to be safe for most healthy people without an increased risk of adverse effects.

Tolerable weight A realistic body weight that is close to the health fitness percent body fat standard.

Trans fatty acid Solidified fat formed by adding hydrogen to monounsaturated and polyunsaturated fats to increase shelf life.

Triglycerides Fats formed by glycerol and three fatty acids.

Type A Behavior pattern characteristic of a hard-driving, overambitious, aggressive, at times hostile and overly competitive person.

Type B Behavior pattern characteristic of a calm, casual, relaxed, and easy-going individual.

V

Variable-resistance training Exercise that utilizes special equipment with mechanical devices that provide differing amounts of resistance through the range of motion.

Vegetarians Individuals whose diet is of vegetable or plant origin.

Vigorous exercise An exercise intensity that is either above 6 METs, 60% of maximal oxygen uptake, or one that provides a "substantial" challenge to the individual.

Vitamins Organic substances essential for normal bodily metabolism, growth, and development.

W

Waist circumference (WC) A measurement to assess potential risk for disease based on intrabdominal fat content.

Warm-up A period preceding exercise when exercise begins slowly.

Wellness The constant and deliberate effort to stay healthy and achieve the highest potential for well-being.

Y

Yoga A school of thought in the Hindu religion that seeks to help the individual attain a higher level of spirituality and peace of mind.